SYSTEMATIC REVIEWS IN HEALTH CARE

Stata™ datasets and other additional information can be found on the book's web site:

www.systematicreviews.com

SYSTEMATIC REVIEWS IN HEALTH CARE:
META-ANALYSIS IN CONTEXT

Second edition

Edited by
Matthias Egger
Senior Lecturer in Epidemiology and Public Health Medicine, Division of Health Services Research and MRC Health Services Research Collaboration, Department of Social Medicine University of Bristol, UK

George Davey Smith
Professor of Clinical Epidemiology, Division of Epidemiology and MRC Health Services Research Collaboration, Department of Social Medicine, University of Bristol, UK

and

Douglas G Altman
Professor of Statistics in Medicine, ICRF Medical Statistics Group, Centre for Statistics in Medicine, Institute of Health Sciences, University of Oxford, UK

© BMJ Publishing Group 2001
Chapter 4 © Crown copyright 2000
Chapter 24 © Crown copyright 1995, 2000
Chapters 25 and 26 © The Cochrane Collaboration 2000

First published in 1995
by the BMJ Publishing Group, BMA House, Tavistock Square,
London WC1H 9JR

www.bmjbooks.com

First edition 1995
Second impression 1997
Second edition 2001
Second impression 2001
Third impression 2003
Fourth impression 2003
Fifth impression 2005

British Library Cataloguing in Publication Data

A catalogue record for this book is available from the British Library

ISBN 0-7279-1488-X

Typeset by Phoenix Photosetting, Chatham, Kent
Printed and bound by TJ International Ltd, Padstow, Cornwall

Contents

Contributors

Douglas G Altman
Professor of Statistics in Medicine
ICRF Medical Statistics Group
Centre for Statistics in Medicine
Institute of Health Sciences
University of Oxford
Oxford, UK

Gerd Antes
Director
German Cochrane Centre
Institut für Medizinische Biometrie und Medizinische Informatik
University of Freiburg
Freiburg i.B., Germany

Michael J Bradburn
Medical Statistician
ICRF Medical Statistics Group
Centre for Statistics in Medicine
Institute of Health Sciences
University of Oxford, Oxford, UK

Iain Chalmers
Director
UK Cochrane Centre
NHS Research and Development Programme
Oxford, UK

Michael J Clarke
Associate Director (Research)
UK Cochrane Centre
NHS Research and Development Programme
and
Overviews' Co-ordinator
Clinical Trials Service Unit
Oxford, UK

George Davey Smith
Professor of Clinical Epidemiology
Division of Epidemiology and MRC Health Services Research
  Collaboration
Department of Social Medicine
University of Bristol
Bristol, UK

Jonathan J Deeks
Senior Medical Statistician
Systematic Review Development Programme
Centre for Statistics in Medicine
Institute of Health Sciences
University of Oxford
Oxford, UK

Kay Dickersin
Associate Professor
Department of Community Health
Brown University
Rhode Island, USA

Catherine Dubé
Department of Medicine
Division of Gastro-enterology
University of Ottawa
Ottawa, Canada

Shah Ebrahim
Professor in Epidemiology of Ageing
Division of Epidemiology and MRC Health Services Research
  Collaboration
Department of Social Medicine
University of Bristol
Bristol, UK

Martin Eccles
Professor of Clinical Effectiveness
Centre for Health Services Research
University of Newcastle upon Tyne
Newcastle upon Tyne, UK

Matthias Egger
Senior Lecturer in Epidemiology and Public Health Medicine
Division of Health Services Research and MRC Health Services
    Research Collaboration
Department of Social Medicine
University of Bristol
Bristol, UK

Nick Freemantle
Reader in Epidemiology and Biostatistics
Medicines Evaluation Group
Centre for Health Economics
University of York
York, UK

J A Muir Gray
Director
Institute of Health Sciences
University of Oxford
Oxford, UK

Peter Jüni
Research Fellow
MRC Health Services Research Collaboration
Department of Social Medicine
University of Bristol
Bristol, UK

Carol Lefebvre
Information Specialist
UK Cochrane Centre
NHS Research and Development Programme
Oxford, UK

James Mason
Senior Research Fellow
Medicines Evaluation Group
Centre for Health Economics
University of York
York, UK

Finlay A McAlister
Assistant Professor
Division of General Internal Medicine
University of Alberta Hospital
Edmonton, Canada

David Moher
Director
Thomas C Chalmers Centre for Systematic Reviews
Children's Hospital of Eastern Ontario Research Institute
University of Ottawa
Ottawa, Canada

Miranda Mugford
Professor of Health Economics
School of Health Policy and Practice
University of East Anglia
Norwich, UK

Keith O'Rourke
Statistician
Clinical Epidemiology Unit
Loeb Research Institute
Ottawa Hospital
Ottawa, Canada

Andrew D Oxman
Director
Health Services Research Unit
National Institute of Public Health
Oslo, Norway

Martin Schneider
Specialist Registrar in Internal Medicine
Department of Medicine
University Hospitals
Geneva, Switzerland

Stephen J Sharp
Medical Statistician
GlaxoWellcome Research and Development
London, UK

Beverley Shea
Loeb Health Research Institute
Clinical Epidemiology Unit
Ottawa Hospital
University of Ottawa
Ottawa, Canada

Jonathan A C Sterne
Senior Lecturer in Medical Statistics
Division of Epidemiology and MRC Health Services Research
    Collaboration
Department of Social Medicine
University of Bristol
Bristol, UK

Lesley A Stewart
Head
Meta-Analysis Group
MRC Clinical Trials Unit
London, UK

Alexander J Sutton
Lecturer in Medical Statistics
Department of Epidemiology and Public Health
University of Leicester
Leicester, UK

Simon G Thompson
Director
MRC Biostatistics Unit
Institute of Public Health
University of Cambridge
Cambridge, UK

Foreword

"If, as is sometimes supposed, science consisted in nothing but the laborious accumulation of facts, it would soon come to a standstill, crushed, as it were, under its own weight. The suggestion of a new idea, or the detection of a law, supersedes much that has previously been a burden on the memory, and by introducing order and coherence facilitates the retention of the remainder in an available form.... Two processes are thus at work side by side, the reception of new material and the digestion and assimilation of the old; and as both are essential we may spare ourselves the discussion of their relative importance. One remark, however, should be made. The work which deserves, but I am afraid does not always receive, the most credit is that in which discovery and explanation go hand in hand, in which not only are new facts presented, but their relation to old ones is pointed out."[1]

The above quotation is from the presidential address given by Lord Rayleigh, Professor of Physics at Cambridge University, at the meeting of the British Association for the Advancement of Science held in Montreal in 1884. More than a century later, research funding agencies, research ethics committees, researchers and journal editors in the field of health research have only just begun to take Lord Rayleigh's injunction seriously. Research synthesis has a long history and has been developed in many spheres of scientific activity.[2] Social scientists in the United States, in particular, have been actively discussing, developing and applying methods for this kind of research for more than quarter of a century,[3–5] and, when the quality of the original research has been adequate, research syntheses have had an important impact on policy and practice.[6,7]

It was not until the late 1980s that Cynthia Mulrow[8] and Andy Oxman[9] began to spell out, for a medical readership, the scientific issues that need to be addressed in research synthesis. During the 1990s, there was an encouraging growth of respect for scientific principles among those preparing "stand alone" reviews, particularly reviews of research on the effects of health care interventions. Unfortunately, there is still little evidence that the same scientific principles are recognised as relevant in preparing the "discussion" sections of reports of new research. An analysis of papers in five influential general medical journals showed that the results of new studies are only very rarely presented in the context of systematic reviews of relevant earlier studies.[10]

In an important step in the right direction, the *British Medical Journal*, acknowledging the cumulative nature of scientific evidence, now publishes with each report of new research a summary of what is already known on the topic addressed, and what the new study has added.

As a result of the slow progress in adopting scientifically defensible methods of research synthesis in health care, the limited resources made available for research continue to be squandered on ill-conceived studies,[11] and avoidable confusion continues to result from failure to review research systematically and set the results of new studies in the context of other relevant research. As a result, patients and others continue to suffer unnecessarily.[12]

Take, for example, the disastrous effects of giving class 1 anti-arrhythmic drugs to people having heart attacks, which has been estimated to have caused tens of thousands of premature deaths in the United States alone.[13] The fact that the theoretical potential of these drugs was not being realised in practice could have been recognised many years earlier than it was. The warning signs were there in one of the first systematic reviews of controlled trials in health care,[14] yet more than 50 trials of these drugs were conducted over nearly two decades[15] before official warnings about their lethal impact were issued. Had the new data generated by each one of these trials been presented within the context of systematic reviews of the results of all previous trials, the lethal potential of this class of drugs would have become clear earlier, and an iatrogenic disaster would have been contained, if not avoided.

Failure to improve the quality of reviews by taking steps to reduce biases and the effects of the play of chance – whether in "stand alone" reviews or in reports of new evidence – will continue to have adverse consequences for people using health services. The first edition of this book helped to raise awareness of this,[16] and its main messages were well received. However, the call to improve the scientific quality of reviews has not been accepted by everyone. In 1998, for example, editors at the *New England Journal of Medicine* rejected a commentary they had commissioned because they felt that their readers would not understand its main message – that meta-analysis (statistical synthesis of the results of separate but similar studies) could not be expected to reduce biases in reviews, but only to reduce imprecision.[17] The journal's rejection was particularly ironic in view of the fact that it had published one of the earliest and most important systematic reviews ever done.[18]

It was because of the widespread and incautious use of the term "meta-analysis" that the term "systematic reviews" was chosen as the title for the first edition of this book.[16] Although meta-analysis may reduce statistical imprecision and may sometimes hint at biases in reviews (for example through tests of homogeneity, or funnel plots), it can never prevent biases. As in many forms of research, even elegant statistical manipulations, when performed on biased rubble, are incapable of generating unbiased precious stones. As Matthias Egger has put it – the diamond used to represent a summary statistic cannot be assumed to be the jewel in the crown!

The term "meta-analysis" has become so attractive to some people that they have dubbed themselves "meta-analysts", and so repellent to others that they have lampooned it with dismissive "synonyms" such as "mega-silliness"[19] and "shmeta-analysis".[20] Current discussions about ways of reducing biases and imprecision in reviews of research must not be allowed to be held hostage by ambiguous use of the term 'meta-analysis'. Hopefully, both the title and the organisation of the contents of this second edition of the book will help to promote more informed and specific criticisms of reviews, and set meta-analysis in a proper context.

Interest in methods for research synthesis among health researchers and practitioners has burgeoned during the five years that have passed between the first and second editions of this book. Whereas the first edition[16] had eight chapters and was just over 100 pages long, the current edition has 26 chapters and is nearly 500 pages long. The first edition of the book contained a methodological bibliography of less than 400 citations. Because that bibliography has now grown to over 2500 citations, it is now published and updated regularly in *The Cochrane Methodology Register*.[21] These differences reflect the breathtaking pace of methodological developments in this sphere of research. Against this background it is easy to understand why I am so glad that Matthias Egger and George Davey Smith – who have contributed so importantly to these developments – agreed to co-edit the second edition of this book with Doug Altman.

After an introductory editorial chapter, the new edition begins with six chapters concerned principally with preventing and detecting biases in systematic reviews of controlled experiments. The important issue of investigating variability within and between studies is tackled in the four chapters that follow. The "methodological tiger country" of systematic reviews of observational studies is then explored in three chapters. Statistical methods and computer software are addressed in a section with four chapters. The book concludes with six chapters about using systematic reviews in practice, and two about the present and future of the Cochrane Collaboration.

Looking ahead, I hope that there will have been a number of further developments in this field before the third edition of the book is prepared. First and foremost, there needs to be wider acknowledgement of the essential truth of Lord Rayleigh's injunction, particularly within the research community and among funders. Not only is research synthesis an essential process for taking stock of the dividends resulting from the investment of effort and other resources in research, it is also intellectually and methodologically challenging, and this should be reflected in the criteria used to judge the worth of academic work. Hopefully we will have seen the back of the naïve notion that when the results of systematic reviews differ from those of large trials, the latter should be assumed to be "the truth".[22]

Second, I hope that people preparing systematic reviews, rather than having to detect and try to take account of biases retrospectively, will increasingly be able to draw on material that is less likely to be biased. Greater efforts are needed to reduce biases in the individual studies that will contribute to reviews.[23] Reporting biases need to be reduced by registration of studies prior to their results being known, and by researchers recognising that they have an ethical and scientific responsibility to report findings of well-designed studies, regardless of the results.[24] And I hope that there will be greater collaboration in designing and conducting systematic reviews prospectively, as a contribution to reducing biases in the review process, as pioneered in the International Multicentre Pooled Analysis of Colon Cancer Trials.[25]

Third, the quality of reviews of observational studies must be improved to address questions about aetiology, diagnostic accuracy, risk prediction and prognosis.[26] These questions cannot usually be tackled using controlled experiments, so this makes systematic reviews of the relevant research more complex. Consumers of research results are frequently confused by conflicting claims about the accuracy of a diagnostic test, or the importance of a postulated aetiological or prognostic factor. They need systematic reviews that explore whether these differences of opinion simply reflect differences in the extent to which biases and the play of chance have been controlled in studies with apparently conflicting results. A rejection of meta-analysis in these circumstances[20] should not be used as an excuse for jettisoning attempts to reduces biases in reviews of such observational data.

Fourth, by the time the next edition of this book is published it should be possible to build on assessments of individual empirical studies that have addressed methodological questions, such as those published in the *Cochrane Collaboration Methods Groups Newsletter*,[27] and instead, take account of up-to-date, systematic reviews of such studies. Several such methodological reviews are currently being prepared, and they should begin to appear in *The Cochrane Library* in 2001.

Finally, I hope that social scientists, health researchers and lay people will be cooperating more frequently in efforts to improve both the science of research synthesis and the design of new studies. Lay people can help to ensure that researchers address important questions, and investigate outcomes that really matter.[28,29] Social scientists have a rich experience of research synthesis, which remains largely untapped by health researchers, and they have an especially important role to play in designing reviews and new research to assess the effects of complex interventions and to detect psychologically mediated effects of interventions.[30,31] Health researchers, for their part, should help lay people to understand the benefits and limitations of systematic reviews, and encourage social scientists to learn from the methodological developments that have arisen from the recent, intense activity in reviews of health care interventions. Indeed, five years from now there may be a case for reverting to the original title of the book – *Systematic Reviews* – to reflect the fact that improving the quality of research synthesis presents similar challenges across the whole spectrum of scientific activity.

Iain Chalmers

Acknowledgements

I am grateful to Mike Clarke, Paul Glasziou, Dave Sackett, and the editors for help in preparing this foreword.

1 Rayleigh, The Right Hon Lord. *Presidential address at the 54th meeting of the British Association for the Advancement of Science, Montreal, August/September 1884.* London: John Murray. 1889:3–23.

2 Chalmers I, Hedges LV, Cooper H. A brief history of research synthesis. *Eval Health Prof* (in press).

3 Glass GV. Primary, secondary and meta-analysis of research. *Educat Res* 1976;**5**:3–8.

4 Lipsey MW, Wilson DB. The efficacy of psychological, educational, and behavioral treatment. *Am Psychol* 1993;**48**:1181–209.

5 Cooper H, Hedges LV. *The handbook of research synthesis.* New York: Russell Sage Foundation, 1994.

6 Chelimsky E. *Politics, Policy, and Research Synthesis.* Keynote address before the National Conference on Research Synthesis, sponsored by the Russell Sage Foundation, Washington DC, 21 June 1994.

7 Hunt M. *How science takes stock: the story of meta-analysis.* New York: Russell Sage Foundation, 1997.

8 Mulrow CD. The medical review article: state of the science. *Ann Int Med* 1987;**106**:485–8.

9 Oxman AD, Guyatt GH. Guidelines for reading literature reviews. *Can Med Assoc J* 1988;**138**:697–703.
10 Clarke M, Chalmers I. Discussion sections in reports of controlled trials published in general medical journals: islands in search of continents? *JAMA* 1998;**280**:280–2.
11 Soares K, McGrath J, Adams C. Evidence and tardive dyskinesia. *Lancet* 1996;**347**:1696–7.
12 Antman EM, Lau J, Kupelnick B, Mosteller F, Chalmers TC. A comparison of results of meta-analyses of randomized control trials and recommendations of clinical experts. *JAMA* 1992;**268**:240–8.
13 Moore T. *Deadly Medicine*. New York: Simon and Schuster, 1995.
14 Furberg CD. Effect of anti-arrhythmic drugs on mortality after myocardial infarction. *Am J Cardiol* 1983;**52**:32C–36C.
15 Teo KK, Yusuf S, Furberg CD. Effects of prophylactic anti-arrhythmic drug therapy in acute myocardial infarction. *JAMA* 1993;**270**:1589–95.
16 Chalmers I, Altman DG. *Systematic reviews*. London: BMJ, 1995.
17 Sackett DL, Glasziou P, Chalmers I. *Meta-analysis may reduce imprecision, but it can't reduce bias*. Unpublished commentary commissioned by the New England Journal of Medicine, 1997.
18 Stampfer MJ, Goldhaber SZ, Yusuf S, Peto R, Hennekens CH. Effect of intravenous streptokinase on acute myocardial infarction: pooled results from randomized trials. *N Engl J Med* 1982;**307**:1180–2.
19 Eysenck HJ. An exercise in mega-silliness. *Am Psychol* 1978;**33**:517.
20 Shapiro S. Meta-analysis/shmeta-analysis. *Am J Epidemiol* 1994;**140**:771–8.
21 *Cochrane Methodology Register*. In: *The Cochrane Library*, Issue 1. Oxford: Update Software, 2001.
22 Ioannidis JP, Cappelleri JC, Lau J. Issues in comparisons between meta-analyses and large trials. *JAMA* 1998;**279**:1089–93.
23 Chalmers I. Unbiased, relevant, and reliable assessments in health care. *BMJ* 1998;**317**:1167–8.
24 Chalmers I, Altman DG. How can medical journals help prevent poor medical research? Some opportunities presented by electronic publishing. *Lancet* 1999;**353**:490–3.
25 International Multicentre Pooled Analysis of Colon Cancer Trials (IMPACT). Efficacy of adjuvant fluorouracil and folinic acid in colon cancer. *Lancet* 1995;**345**:939–44.
26 Stroup DF, Berlin JA, Morton SC, Olkin I, Williamson GD, Rennie D, Moher D, Becker BJ, Sipe TA, Thacker SB. Meta-analysis of observational studies in epidemiology: a proposal for reporting. Meta-analysis Of Observational Studies in Epidemiology (MOOSE) group. *JAMA* 2000;**283**:2008–12.
27 Clarke M, Hopewell S (eds). *The Cochrane Collaboration Methods Groups Newsletter*. vol 4, 2000.
28 Chalmers I. What do I want from health research and researchers when I am a patient? *BMJ* 1995;**310**:1315–18.
29 Oliver S. Users of health services: following their agenda. In: Hood S, Mayall B, Oliver S (eds). *Critical issues in social research*. Buckingham: Open University Press, 1999:139–153.
30 Boruch RF. *Randomized experiments for planning and evaluation*. Thousand Oaks: Sage Publications,1997.
31 Oakley A. *Experiments in knowing*. Oxford: Polity Press, 2000.

Introduction

1 Rationale, potentials, and promise of systematic reviews

MATTHIAS EGGER, GEORGE DAVEY SMITH, KEITH O'ROURKE

Summary points

- Reviews are essential tools for health care workers, researchers, consumers and policy makers who want to keep up with the evidence that is accumulating in their field.
- Systematic reviews allow for a more objective appraisal of the evidence than traditional narrative reviews and may thus contribute to resolve uncertainty when original research, reviews, and editorials disagree.
- Meta-analysis, if appropriate, will enhance the precision of estimates of treatment effects, leading to reduced probability of false negative results, and potentially to a more timely introduction of effective treatments.
- Exploratory analyses, e.g. regarding subgroups of patients who are likely to respond particularly well to a treatment (or the reverse), may generate promising new research questions to be addressed in future studies.
- Systematic reviews may demonstrate the lack of adequate evidence and thus identify areas where further studies are needed.

The volume of data that need to be considered by practitioners and researchers is constantly expanding. In many areas it has become simply impossible for the individual to read, critically evaluate and synthesise the state of current knowledge, let alone keep updating this on a regular basis. Reviews have become essential tools for anybody who wants to keep up with the new evidence that is accumulating in his or her field of interest. Reviews are also required to identify areas where the

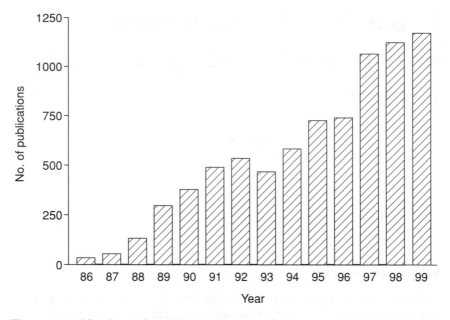

Figure 1.1 Number of publications concerning meta-analysis, 1986–1999. Results from MEDLINE search using text word and medical subject (MESH) heading "meta-analysis" and text word "systematic review".

available evidence is insufficient and further studies are required. However, since Mulrow[1] and Oxman and Guyatt[2] drew attention to the poor quality of narrative reviews it has become clear that conventional reviews are an unreliable source of information. In response to this situation there has, in recent years, been increasing focus on formal methods of systematically reviewing studies, to produce explicitly formulated, reproducible, and up-to-date summaries of the effects of health care interventions. This is illustrated by the sharp increase in the number of reviews that used formal methods to synthesise evidence (Figure 1.1).

In this chapter we will attempt to clarify terminology and scope, provide some historical background, and examine the potentials and promise of systematic reviews and meta-analysis.

Systematic review, overview or meta-analysis?

A number of terms are used concurrently to describe the process of systematically reviewing and integrating research evidence, including "systematic review", "meta-analysis", "research synthesis", "overview" and "pooling". In the foreword to the first edition of this book, Chalmers and Altman[2] defined systematic review as a review that has been prepared using a systematic approach to minimising biases and random errors which is documented in a materials and methods section. A systematic review may, or may not, include a meta-analysis: a statistical analysis of the results from independent studies, which generally aims to produce a single estimate of a treatment effect.[4] The distinction between systematic review and meta-analysis, which will be used throughout this book, is important because it is always appropriate and desirable to systematically review a body of data, but it may sometimes be inappropriate, or even misleading, to statistically pool results from separate studies.[5] Indeed, it is our impression that reviewers often find it hard to resist the temptation of combining studies even when such meta-analysis is questionable or clearly inappropriate.

The scope of meta-analysis

As discussed in detail in Chapter 12, a clear distinction should be made between meta-analysis of randomised controlled trials and meta-analysis of epidemiological studies. Consider a set of trials of high methodological quality that examined the same intervention in comparable patient populations: each trial will provide an unbiased estimate of the same underlying treatment effect. The variability that is observed between the trials can confidently be attributed to random variation and meta-analysis should provide an equally unbiased estimate of the treatment effect, with an increase in the precision of this estimate. A fundamentally different situation arises in the case of epidemiological studies, for example case-control studies, cross-sectional studies or cohort studies. Due to the effects of confounding and bias, such observational studies may produce estimates of associations that deviate from the underlying effect in ways that may systematically differ from chance. Combining a set of epidemiological studies will thus often provide spuriously precise, but biased, estimates of associations. The thorough consideration of heterogeneity between observational study results, in particular of possible sources of confounding and bias, will generally provide more insights than the mechanistic calculation of an overall measure of effect (see Chapters 9 and 12 for examples of observational meta-analyses).

The fundamental difference that exists between observational studies and randomised controlled trials does not mean that the latter are immune to bias. Publication bias and other reporting biases (see Chapter 3) may distort the evidence from both trials and observational studies. Bias may also be introduced if the methodological quality of

5

controlled trials is inadequate[6,7] (Chapter 5). It is crucial to understand the limitations of meta-analysis and the importance of exploring sources of heterogeneity and bias (Chapters 8–11), and much emphasis will be given to these issues in this book.

Historical notes

Efforts to compile summaries of research for medical practitioners who struggle with the amount of information that is relevant to medical practice are not new. Chalmers and Tröhler[8] drew attention to two journals published in the 18th century in Leipzig and Edinburgh, *Comentarii de rebus in scientia naturali et medicina gestis* and *Medical and Philosophical Commentaries*, which published critical appraisals of

---

Box 1.1 From Laplace and Gauss to the first textbook of meta-analysis

Astronomers long ago noticed that observations of the same objects differed even when made by the same observers under similar conditions. The calculation of the mean as a more precise value than a single measurement had appeared by the end of the 17th century.[9] By the late 1700s probability models were being used to represent the uncertainty of observations that was caused by measurement error. Laplace decided to write these models not as the probability that an observation equalled the true value plus some error but as the truth plus the "probability of some error". In doing this he recognised that as probabilities of independent errors multiply he could determine the most likely joint errors, the concept which is at the heart of maximum likelihood estimation.[10] Laplace's method of combining and quantifying uncertainty in the combination of observations required an explicit probability distribution for errors in the individual observations and no acceptable one existed. Gauss drew on empirical experience and argued that a probability distribution corresponding to what is today referred to as the Normal or Gaussian distribution would be best. This remained speculative until Laplace's formulation of the central limit theorem – that for large sample sizes the error distribution will always be close to Normally distributed. Hence, Gauss's method was more than just a good guess but justified by the central limit theorem. Most statistical techniques used today in meta-analysis follow from Gauss's and Laplace's work. Airy disseminated their work in his 1861 "textbook" on "meta-analysis" for astronomers (Figure 1.2) which included the first formulation of a random effects model to allow for heterogeneity in the results.[11] Airy offered practical advice and argued for the use of judgement to determine what type of statistical model should be used.

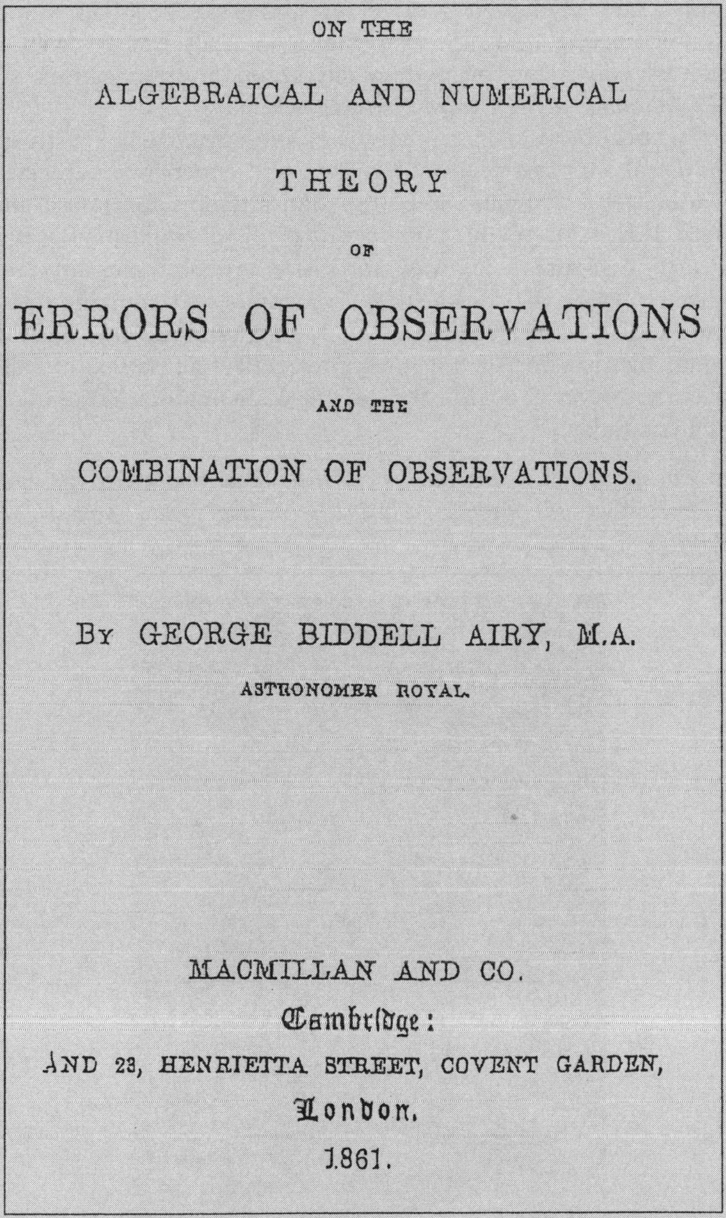

ON THE

ALGEBRAICAL AND NUMERICAL

THEORY

OF

ERRORS OF OBSERVATIONS

AND THE

COMBINATION OF OBSERVATIONS.

By GEORGE BIDDELL AIRY, M.A.

ASTRONOMER ROYAL.

MACMILLAN AND CO.

Cambridge:

AND 23, HENRIETTA STREET, COVENT GARDEN,

London.

1861.

Figure 1.2 The title page of what may be seen as the first "textbook" of meta-analysis, published in 1861.

important new books in medicine, including, for example, William Withering's now classic *Account of the foxglove* (1785) on the use of digitalis for treating heart disease. These journals can be seen as the 18th century equivalents of modern day secondary publications such as the *ACP Journal Club* or *Evidence based medicine*.

The statistical basis of meta-analysis reaches back to the 17th century when in astronomy and geodesy intuition and experience suggested that combinations of data might be better than attempts to choose amongst them (see Box 1.1). In the 20th century the distinguished statistician Karl Pearson (Figure 1.3), was, in 1904, probably the first medical researcher reporting the use of formal techniques to combine data from different studies. The rationale for pooling studies put forward by Pearson in his account on the preventive effect of serum inoculations against enteric fever,[12] is still one of the main reasons for undertaking meta-analysis today:

> *"Many of the groups ... are far too small to allow of any definite opinion being formed at all, having regard to the size of the probable error involved".*[12]

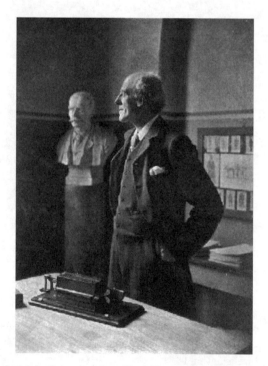

Figure 1.3 Distinguished statistician Karl Pearson is seen as the first medical researcher to use formal techniques to combine data from different studies.

However, such techniques were not widely used in medicine for many years to come. In contrast to medicine, the social sciences and in particular psychology and educational research, developed an early interest in the synthesis of research findings. In the 1930s, 80 experiments examining the "potency of moral instruction in modifying conduct" were systematically reviewed.[13] In 1976 the psychologist Glass coined the term "meta-analysis" in a paper entitled "Primary, secondary and meta-analysis of research".[14] Three years later the British physician and epidemiologist Archie Cochrane drew attention to the fact that people who want to make informed decisions about health care do not have ready access to reliable reviews of the available evidence.[15] In the 1980s meta-analysis became increasingly popular in medicine, particularly in the fields of cardiovascular disease,[16,17] oncology,[18] and perinatal care.[19] Meta-analysis of epidemiological studies[20,21] and "cross design synthesis",[22] the integration of observational data with the results from meta-analyses of randomised clinical trials was also advocated. In the 1990s the foundation of the Cochrane Collaboration (see Chapters 25 and 26) facilitated numerous developments, many of which are documented in this book.

Why do we need systematic reviews? A patient with myocardial infarction in 1981

A likely scenario in the early 1980s, when discussing the discharge of a patient who had suffered an uncomplicated myocardial infarction, is as follows: a keen junior doctor asks whether the patient should receive a beta-blocker for secondary prevention of a future cardiac event. After a moment of silence the consultant states that this was a question which should be discussed in detail at the Journal Club on Thursday. The junior doctor (who now regrets that she asked the question) is told to assemble and present the relevant literature. It is late in the evening when she makes her way to the library. The MEDLINE search identifies four clinical trials.[23–26] When reviewing the conclusions from these trials (Table 1.1) the doctor finds them to be rather confusing and contradictory. Her consultant points out that the sheer amount of research published makes it impossible to keep track of and critically appraise individual studies. He recommends a good review article. Back in the library the junior doctor finds an article which the *BMJ* published in 1981 in a "Regular Reviews" section.[27] This narrative review concluded:

> *Thus, despite claims that they reduce arrhythmias, cardiac work, and infarct size, we still have no clear evidence that beta-blockers improve long-term survival after infarction despite almost 20 years of clinical trials.*[27]

Table 1.1 Conclusions from four randomised controlled trials of beta-blockers in secondary prevention after myocardial infarction.

The mortality and hospital readmission rates were not significantly different in the two groups. This also applied to the incidence of cardiac failure, exertional dyspnoea, and frequency of ventricular ectopic beats.

Reynolds and Whitlock[23]

Until the results of further trials are reported long-term beta-adrenoceptor blockade (possibly up to two years) is recommended after uncomplicated anterior myocardial infarction.

Multicentre International Study[24]

The trial was designed to detect a 50% reduction in mortality and this was not shown. The non-fatal reinfarction rate was similar in both groups.

Baber *et al.*[25]

We conclude that long-term treatment with timolol in patients surviving acute myocardial infarction reduces mortality and the rate of reinfarction.

The Norwegian Multicentre Study Group[26]

The junior doctor is relieved. She presents the findings of the review article, the Journal Club is a full success and the patient is discharged without a beta-blocker.

Narrative reviews

Traditional narrative reviews have a number of disadvantages that systematic reviews may overcome. First, the classical review is subjective and therefore prone to bias and error.[28] Mulrow showed that among 50 reviews published in the mid 1980s in leading general medicine journals, 49 reviews did not specify the source of the information and failed to perform a standardised assessment of the methodological quality of studies.[1] Our junior doctor could have consulted another review of the same topic, published in the *European Heart Journal* in the same year. This review concluded that "it seems perfectly reasonable to treat patients who have survived an infarction with timolol".[29] Without guidance by formal rules, reviewers will inevitably disagree about issues as basic as what types of studies it is appropriate to include and how to balance the quantitative evidence they provide. Selective inclusion of studies that support the author's view is common. This is illustrated by the observation that the frequency of citation of clinical trials is related to their outcome, with studies in line with the prevailing opinion being quoted more frequently than unsupportive studies[30,31] Once a set of studies has been assembled a common way to review the results is to count the number of studies supporting various sides of an issue and to choose the view receiving the most votes. This procedure is clearly unsound, since it ignores sample size, effect size, and research design. It is thus hardly surprising that reviewers using traditional methods often reach opposite conclusions[1] and miss small, but potentially important, differences.[32] In controversial areas the conclusions drawn from a given body of evidence may be associated more with the speciality of the reviewer than with the available data.[33] By systematically identifying, scrutinising, tabulating, and perhaps integrating all relevant studies, systematic reviews allow a more objective appraisal, which can help to resolve uncertainties when the original research, classical reviews and editorial comments disagree.

Limitations of a single study

A single study often fails to detect, or exclude with certainty, a modest, albeit relevant, difference in the effects of two therapies. A trial may thus show no statistically significant treatment effect when in reality such an effect exists – it may produce a false negative result. An examination of clinical trials which reported no statistically significant differences between experimental and control therapy has shown that false negative results in health care research are common. For a clinically relevant difference in outcome the probability of missing this effect given the trial size was greater than 20% in 115 (85%) of the 136 trials examined.[34] Similarly, a recent examination of 1941 trials relevant to the treatment of schizophrenia showed that only 58 (3%) studies were large enough to detect an important improvement.[35] The number of patients included in trials is thus often inadequate, a situation which has changed little over recent years.[34] In some cases, however, the required sample size may be difficult to achieve. A drug which reduces the risk of death from myocardial infarction by 10% could, for example, delay many thousands of deaths each year in the UK alone. In order to detect such an effect with 90% certainty over ten thousand patients in each treatment group would be needed.[36]

The meta-analytic approach appears to be an attractive alternative to such a large, expensive and logistically problematic study. Data from patients in trials evaluating the same or a similar drug in a number of smaller, but comparable, studies are considered. Methods used for meta-analysis employ a weighted average of the results in which the larger trials have more influence than the smaller ones. Comparisons are made exclusively between patients enrolled in the same study. As discussed in detail in chapter 15, there are a variety of statistical techniques available for this purpose.[37,38] In this way the necessary number of patients may be reached, and relatively small effects can be detected or excluded with confidence. Systematic reviews can also contribute to considerations regarding the applicability of study results. The findings

11

of a particular study might be felt to be valid only for a population of patients with the same characteristics as those investigated in the trial. If many trials exist in different groups of patients, with similar results being seen in the various trials, then it can be concluded that the effect of the intervention under study has some generality. By putting together all available data meta-analyses are also better placed than individual trials to answer questions regarding whether or not an overall study result varies among subgroups, e.g. among men and women; older and younger patients or participants with different degrees of severity of disease.

A more transparent appraisal

An important advantage of systematic reviews is that they render the review process transparent. In traditional narrative reviews it is often not clear how the conclusions follow from the data examined. In an adequately presented systematic review it should be possible for readers to replicate the quantitative component of the argument. To facilitate this, it is valuable if the data included in meta-analyses are either presented in full or made available to interested readers by the authors. The increased openness required leads to the replacement of unhelpful descriptors such as "no clear evidence", "some evidence of a trend", "a weak relationship" and "a strong relationship".[39] Furthermore, performing a meta-analysis may lead to reviewers moving beyond the conclusions authors present in the abstract of papers, to a thorough examination of the actual data.

The epidemiology of results

The tabulation, exploration and evaluation of results are important components of systematic reviews. This can be taken further to explore sources of heterogeneity and test new hypotheses that were not posed in individual studies, for example using "meta-regression" techniques (see also Chapters 8–11). This has been termed the "epidemiology of results" where the findings of an original study replace the individual as the unit of analysis.[40] However, it must be born in mind that although the studies included may be controlled experiments, the meta-analysis itself is subject to many biases inherent in observational studies.[41] Aggregation or ecological bias[42] is also a problem unless individual patient data is available (see Chapter 6). Systematic reviews can, nevertheless, lead to the identification of the most promising or the most urgent research question, and may permit a more accurate calculation of the sample sizes needed in future studies (see Chapter 24). This is illustrated by an early meta-analysis of four trials that compared different methods of monitoring the fetus during labour.[43] The meta-analysis led to the hypothesis that, compared with intermittent auscultation, continuous fetal heart monitoring reduced the risk of neonatal seizures. This hypothesis was subsequently confirmed in a single randomised trial of almost seven times the size of the four previous studies combined.[44]

What was the evidence in 1981? Cumulative meta-analysis

What conclusions would our junior doctor have reached if she had had access to a meta-analysis? Numerous meta-analyses of trials examining the effect of beta-antagonists have been published since 1981.[17,45–48] Figure 1.4 shows the results from the most recent analysis that included 33 randomised comparisons of beta-blockers versus placebo or alternative treatment in patients who had had a myocardial infarction.[48] These trials were published between 1967 and 1997. The combined relative risk indicates that beta-blockade starting after the acute infarction reduces subsequent premature mortality by an estimated 20% (relative risk 0.80). A useful way to show the evidence that was available in 1981 and at other points in time is to perform a *cumulative* meta-analysis.[49]

Cumulative meta-analysis is defined as the repeated performance of meta-analysis whenever a new relevant trial becomes available for inclusion. This allows the retrospective identification of the point in time when a treatment effect first reached conventional levels of statistical significance. In the case of beta-blockade in secondary prevention of myocardial infarction, a statistically significant beneficial effect ($P < 0.05$) became evident by 1981 (Figure 1.5). Subsequent trials in a further 15 000 patients simply confirmed this result. This situation has been taken to suggest that further studies in large numbers of patients may be at best superfluous and costly, if not unethical,[50] once a statistically significant treatment effect is evident from meta-analysis of the existing smaller trials.

Similarly, Lau *et al.* showed that for the trials of intravenous streptokinase in acute myocardial infarction, a statistically significant ($P = 0.01$) combined difference in total mortality was achieved by 1973[49] (Figure 1.6). At that time, 2432 patients had been randomised in eight small trials. The results of the subsequent 25 studies which included the large GISSI-1 and ISIS-2 trials[51,52] and enrolled a total of 34 542 additional patients reduced the significance level to $P = 0.001$ in 1979, $P = 0.0001$ in 1986 and to $P < 0.00001$ when the first mega-trial appeared, narrowing the confidence intervals around an essentially unchanged

13

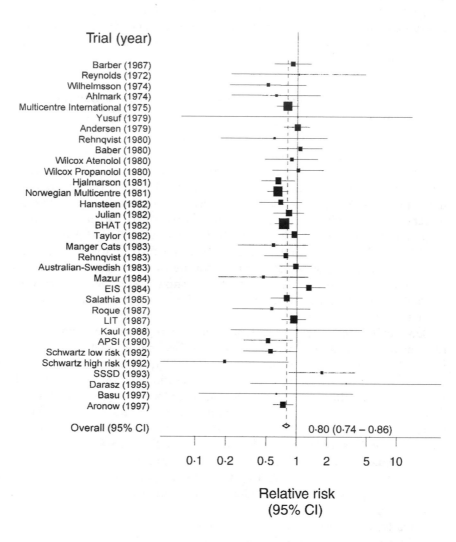

Figure 1.4 "Forest plot" showing mortality results from trials of beta-blockers in secondary prevention after myocardial infarction. Trials are ordered by year of publication. The black square and horizontal line correspond to the trials' risk ratio and 95% confidence intervals. The area of the black squares reflects the weight each trial contributes in the meta-analysis. The diamond represents the combined relative risk with its 95% confidence interval, indicating a 20% reduction in the odds of death. See Chapter 2 for a detailed description of forest plots. Adapted from Freemantle et al.[48]

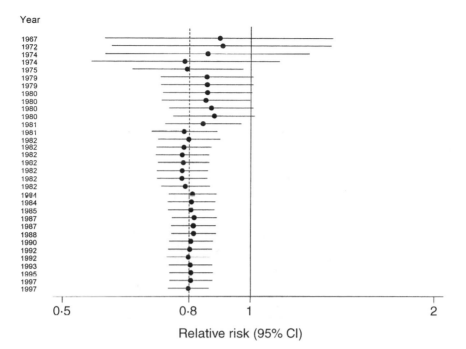

Figure 1.5 Cumulative meta-analysis of controlled trials of beta-blockers after myocardial infarction. The data correspond to Figure 1.4. A statistically significant (P < 0·05) beneficial effect on mortality became evident in 1981.

estimate of about 20% reduction in the risk of death. Interestingly, at least one country licensed streptokinase for use in myocardial infarction before GISSI-1[51] was published, whereas many national authorities waited for this trial to appear and some waited a further two years for the results of ISIS-2[52] (Figure 1.6).

Another application of cumulative meta-analysis has been to correlate the accruing evidence with the recommendations made by experts in review articles and text books. Antman *et al.* showed for thrombolytic drugs that recommendations for routine use first appeared in 1987, 14 years after a statistically significant (P = 0·01) beneficial effect became evident in cumulative meta-analysis.[53] Conversely, the prophylactic use of lidocaine continued to be recommended for routine use in myocardial infarction despite the lack of evidence for any beneficial effect, and the possibility of a harmful effect being evident in the meta-analysis.

15

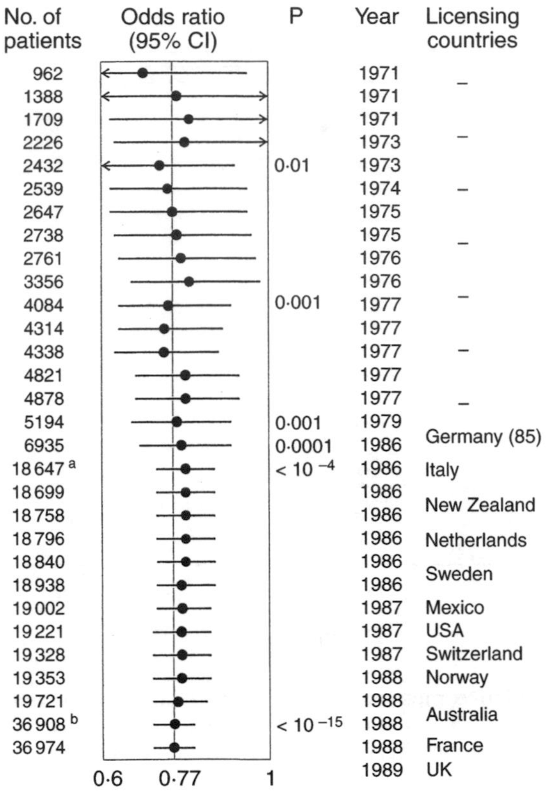

No. of patients	Odds ratio (95% CI)	P	Year	Licensing countries
962			1971	–
1388			1971	
1709			1971	
2226			1973	–
2432		0·01	1973	
2539			1974	–
2647			1975	
2738			1975	–
2761			1976	
3356			1976	
4084		0·001	1977	–
4314			1977	
4338			1977	–
4821			1977	
4878			1977	–
5194		0·001	1979	
6935		0·0001	1986	Germany (85)
18 647 [a]		< 10 [−4]	1986	Italy
18 699			1986	
18 758			1986	New Zealand
18 796			1986	Netherlands
18 840			1986	
18 938			1986	Sweden
19 002			1987	Mexico
19 221			1987	USA
19 328			1987	Switzerland
19 353			1988	Norway
19 721			1988	
36 908 [b]		< 10 [−15]	1988	Australia
36 974			1988	France
	0·6 0·77 1		1989	UK

Figure 1.6 Cumulative meta-analysis of randomised controlled trials of intravenous streptokinase in myocardial infarction. The number of patients randomised in a total of 33 trials, and national authorities licensing streptokinase for use in myocardial infarction are also shown. [a]Includes GISSI-1; [b]ISIS-2.

Conclusions

Systematic review including, if appropriate, a formal meta-analysis is clearly superior to the narrative approach to reviewing research. In addition to providing a precise estimate of the overall treatment effect in some instances, appropriate examination of heterogeneity across individual studies can produce useful information with which to guide rational and cost effective treatment decisions. Systematic reviews are also important to demonstrate areas where the available evidence is insufficient and where new, adequately sized trials are required.

Acknowledgements

We are grateful to Sir David Cox for providing key references to early statistical work and to Iain Chalmers for his comments on an earlier draft of this chapter. We thank Dr T Johansson and G Enocksson (Pharmacia AB, Stockholm) and Dr A Schirmer and Dr M Thimme (Behring AG, Marburg) for providing data on licensing of streptokinase in different countries. This chapter draws on material published earlier in the *BMJ*.[54]

1 Mulrow CD. The medical review article: state of the science. *Ann Intern Med* 1987;**106**:485–8.
2 Oxman AD, Guyatt GH. Guidelines for reading literature reviews. *Can Med Assoc J* 1988;**138**:697–703.
3 Chalmers I, Altman D (eds). *Systematic reviews*. London: BMJ Publishing Group, 1995.
4 Huque MF. Experiences with meta-analysis in NDA submissions. *Proc Biopharmac Sec Am Stat Assoc* 1988;**2**:28–33.
5 O'Rourke K, Detsky AS. Meta-analysis in medical research: strong encouragement for higher quality in individual research efforts. *J Clin Epidemiol* 1989;**42**:1021–4.
6 Schulz KF, Chalmers I, Hayes RJ, Altman D. Empirical evidence of bias. Dimensions of methodological quality associated with estimates of treatment effects in controlled trials. *JAMA* 1995;**273**:408–12.
7 Moher D, Pham B, Jones A, *et al.* Does quality of reports of randomised trials affect estimates of intervention efficacy reported in meta-analyses? *Lancet* 1998;**352**:609–13.
8 Chalmers I, Tröhler U. Helping physicians to keep abreast of the medical literature: Medical and philosophical commentaries, 1773–1795. *Ann Intern Med* 2000; **133**: 238–43.
9 Plackett RL. Studies in the history of probability and statistics: VII. The principle of the arithmetic mean. *Biometrika* 1958;**1958**:130–5.
10 Stigler SM. *The history of statistics. The measurement of uncertainty before 1900*. Cambridge, MA: The Belknap Press of Harvard University Press, 1990.
11 Airy GB. *On the algebraical and numerical theory of errors of observations and the combinations of observations*. London: Macmillan, 1861.
12 Pearson K. Report on certain enteric fever inoculation statistics. *BMJ* 1904;**3**:1243–6.
13 Peters CC. Summary of the Penn State experiments on the influence of instruction in character education. *J Educat Sociol* 1933;**7**:269–72.
14 Glass GV. Primary, secondary and meta-analysis of research. *Educat Res* 1976;**5**:3–8.
15 Cochrane AL. 1931–1971: a critical review, with particular reference to the medical profession. In: *Medicines for the year 2000*. London: Office of Health Economics, 1979:1–11.
16 Baber NS, Lewis JA. Confidence in results of beta-blocker postinfarction trials. *BMJ* 1982; **284**:1749–50.
17 Yusuf S, Peto R, Lewis J, Collins R, Sleight P. Beta blockade during and after myocardial infarction: an overview of the randomized trials. *Prog Cardiovasc Dis* 1985;**17**:335–71.
18 Early Breast Cancer Trialists' Collaborative Group. Effects of adjuvant tamoxifen and of cytotoxic therapy on mortality in early breast cancer. An overview of 61 randomized trials among 28 896 women. *N Engl J Med* 1988;**319**:1681–92.
19 Chalmers I, Enkin M, Keirse M. *Effective care during pregnancy and childbirth*. Oxford: Oxford University Press, 1989.
20 Greenland S. Quantitative methods in the review of epidemiologic literature. *Epidemiol Rev* 1987;**9**:1–30.
21 Friedenreich CM. Methods for pooled analyses of epidemiologic studies. *Epidemiology* 1993;**4**:295–302.

22 General Accounting Office. *Cross design synthesis: a new strategy for medical effectiveness research*. Washington, DC: GAO, 1992.
23 Reynolds JL, Whitlock RML. Effects of a beta-adrenergic receptor blocker in myocardial infarctation treated for one year from onset. *Br Heart J* 1972;**34**:252–9.
24 Multicentre International Study: supplementary report. Reduction in mortality after myocardial infarction with long-term beta-adrenoceptor blockade. *BMJ* 1977;**2**:419–21.
25 Baber NS, Wainwright Evans D, Howitt G, *et al.* Multicentre post-infarction trial of propranolol in 49 hospitals in the United Kingdom, Italy and Yugoslavia. *Br Heart J* 1980;**44**:96–100.
26 The Norwegian Multicenter Study Group. Timolol-induced reduction in mortality and reinfarction in patients surviving acute myocardial infarction. *N Engl J Med* 1981;**304**:801–7.
27 Mitchell JRA. Timolol after myocardial infarction: an answer or a new set of questions? *BMJ* 1981;**282**:1565–70.
28 Teagarden JR. Meta-analysis: whither narrative review? *Pharmacotherapy* 1989;**9**:274–84.
29 Hampton JR. The use of beta blockers for the reduction of mortality after myocardial infarction. *Eur Heart J* 1981;**2**:259–68.
30 Ravnskov U. Cholesterol lowering trials in coronary heart disease: frequency of citation and outcome. *BMJ* 1992;**305**:15–19.
31 Gøtzsche PC. Reference bias in reports of drug trials. *BMJ* 1987;**295**:654–6.
32 Cooper H, Rosenthal R. Statistical versus traditional procedures for summarising research findings. *Psychol Bull* 1980;**87**:442–9.
33 Chalmers TC, Frank CS, Reitman D. Minimizing the three stages of publication bias. *JAMA* 1990;**263**:1392–5.
34 Freiman JA, Chalmers TC, Smith H, Kuebler RR. The importance of beta, the type II error, and sample size in the design and interpretation of the randomized controlled trial. In: Bailar JC, Mosteller F, eds. *Medical uses of statistics*. Boston, MA: NEJM Books, 1992:357–73.
35 Thornley B, Adams C. Content and quality of 2000 controlled trials in schizophrenia over 50 years. *BMJ* 1998;**317**:1181–4.
36 Collins R, Keech A, Peto R, *et al.* Cholesterol and total mortality: need for larger trials. *BMJ* 1992;**304**:1689.
37 Berlin J, Laird NM, Sacks HS, Chalmers TC. A comparison of statistical methods for combining event rates from clinical trials. *Stat Med* 1989;**8**:141–51.
38 Fleiss JL. The statistical basis of meta-analysis. *Stat Meth Med Res* 1993;**2**:121–45.
39 Rosenthal R. An evaluation of procedures and results. In: Wachter KW, Straf ML, eds. *The future of meta-analysis*. New York: Russel Sage Foundation, 1990:123–33.
40 Jenicek M. Meta-analysis in medicine. Where we are and where we want to go. *J Clin Epidemiol* 1989;**42**:35–44.
41 Gelber RD, Goldhirsch A. Interpretation of results from subset analyses within overviews of randomized clinical trials. *Stat Med* 1987;**6**:371–8.
42 Piantadosi S, Byar DP, Green SB. The ecological fallacy. *Am J Epidemiol* 1988;**127**:893–904.
43 Chalmers I. Randomised controlled trials of fetal monitoring 1973–1977. In: Thalhammer O, Baumgarten K, Pollak A, eds. *Perinatal medicine*. Stuttgart: Thieme, 1979:260–5.
44 MacDonald D, Grant A, Sheridan-Pereira M, Boylan P, Chalmers I. The Dublin randomised controlled trial of intrapartum fetal heart rate monitoring. *Am J Obstet Gynecol* 1985;**152**:524–39.
45 Beta-Blocker Pooling Project Research Group. The beta-blocker pooling project (BBPP): subgroup findings from randomized trials in post-infarction trials. *Eur Heart J* 1988;**9**:8–16.
46 Goldstein S. Review of beta blocker myocardial infarction trials. *Clin Cardiol* 1989;**12**:54–7.
47 Soriano JB, Hoes AW, Meems L, Grobbee DE. Increased survival with beta-blockers: importance of ancillary properties. *Prog Cardiovasc Dis* 1997;**39**:445–56.
48 Freemantle N, Cleland J, Young P, Mason J, Harrison J. Beta blockade after

myocardial infarction: systematic review and meta regression analysis. *BMJ* 1999;**318**:1730-7.

49 Lau J, Antman EM, Jimenez-Silva J, Kupelnick B, Mosteller F, Chalmers TC. Cumulative meta-analysis of therapeutic trials for myocardial infarction. *N Engl J Med* 1992;**327**:248-54.

50 Murphy DJ, Povar GJ, Pawlson LG. Setting limits in clinical medicine. *Arch Intern Med* 1994;**154**:505-12.

51 Gruppo Italiano per lo Studio della Streptochinasi nell'Infarto Miocardico (GISSI). Effectiveness of intravenous thrombolytic treatment in acute myocardial infarction. *Lancet* 1986;**i**:397-402.

52 ISIS-2 Collaborative Group. Randomised trial of intravenous streptokinase, oral aspirin, both, or neither among 17187 cases of suspected acute myocardial infarction: ISIS-2. *Lancet* 1988;**ii**:349-60.

53 Antman EM, Lau J, Kupelnick B, Mosteller F, Chalmers TC. A comparison of results of meta-analyses of randomized control trials and recommendations of clinical experts. *JAMA* 1992;**268**:240-8.

54 Egger M, Davey Smith G. Meta-analysis: potentials and promise. *BMJ* 1997;**315**:1371-4.

Part I: Systematic reviews of controlled trials

2 Principles of and procedures for systematic reviews

MATTHIAS EGGER, GEORGE DAVEY SMITH

Summary points

- Reviews and meta-analyses should be as carefully planned as any other research project, with a detailed written protocol prepared in advance.
- The formulation of the review question, the a priori definition of eligibility criteria for trials to be included, a comprehensive search for such trials and an assessment of their methodological quality, are central to high quality reviews.
- The graphical display of results from individual studies on a common scale ("Forest plot") is an important step, which allows a visual examination of the degree of heterogeneity between studies.
- There are different statistical methods for combining the data in meta-analysis but there is no single "correct" method. A thorough sensitivity analysis should always be performed to assess the robustness of combined estimates to different assumptions, methods and inclusion criteria and to investigate the possible influence of bias.
- When interpreting results, reviewers should consider the importance of beneficial and harmful effects of interventions in absolute and relative terms and address economic implications and implications for future research.

Systematic reviews allow a more objective appraisal of the evidence than traditional narrative reviews and may thus contribute to resolve uncertainty when original research, reviews and editorials disagree. Systematic reviews are also important to identify questions to be addressed in future studies. As will be discussed in the subsequent chapter, ill conducted reviews and meta-analyses may, however, be biased due to exclusion of relevant studies, the inclusion of inadequate studies or the inappropriate statistical combination of studies. Such bias can be minimised if a few basic principles are observed. Here we will introduce these principles and give an overview of the practical steps involved in performing systematic reviews. We will focus on systematic reviews of controlled trials but the basic principles are applicable to reviews of any type of study (see Chapters 12–14 for a discussion of systematic reviews of observational studies). Also, we assume here that the review is based on summary information obtained from published papers, or from the authors. Systematic reviews and meta-analyses based on individual patient data are discussed in Chapter 6. We stress that the present chapter can only serve as an elementary introduction. Readers who want to perform systematic reviews should consult the ensuing chapters and consider joining forces with the Cochrane Collaboration (see Chapters 25 and 26).

Developing a review protocol

Systematic reviews should be viewed as observational studies of the evidence. The steps involved, summarised in Box 2.1, are similar to any other research undertaking: formulation of the problem to be addressed, collection and analysis of the data, and interpretation of the results. Likewise, a detailed study protocol which clearly states the question to be addressed, the subgroups of interest, and the methods and criteria to be employed for identifying and selecting relevant studies and extracting and analysing information should be written in advance. This is important to avoid bias being introduced by decisions that are influenced by the data. For example, studies which produced unexpected or undesired results may be excluded by *post hoc* changes to the inclusion criteria. Similarly, unplanned data-driven subgroup analyses are likely to produce spurious results.[1,2] The review protocol should ideally be conceived by a group of reviewers with expertise both in the content area and the science of research synthesis.

Objectives and eligibility criteria

The formulation of detailed objectives is at the heart of any research project. This should include the definition of study participants, interventions, outcomes and settings. As with patient inclusion and exclusion criteria in clinical studies, eligibility criteria can then be defined for the type of studies to be included. They relate to the quality of trials and to

24

Box 2.1 Steps in conducting a systematic review*

1 Formulate review question

2 Define inclusion and exclusion criteria
- participants
- interventions and comparisons
- outcomes
- study designs and methodological quality

3 Locate studies (see also Chapter 4)
Develop search strategy considering the following sources:
- *The Cochrane Controlled Trials Register* (CCTR)
- electronic databases and trials registers not covered by CCTR
- checking of reference lists
- handsearching of key journals
- personal communication with experts in the field

4 Select studies
- have eligibility checked by more than one observer
- develop strategy to resolve disagreements
- keep log of excluded studies, with reasons for exclusions

5 Assess study quality (see also Chapter 5)
- consider assessment by more than one observer
- use simple checklists rather than quality scales
- always assess concealment of treatment allocation, blinding and handling of patient attrition
- consider blinding of observers to authors, institutions and journals

6 Extract data
- design and pilot data extraction form
- consider data extraction by more than one observer
- consider blinding of observers to authors, institutions and journals

7 Analyse and present results (see also Chapters 8–11, 15, 16)
- tabulate results from individual studies
- examine forest plot
- explore possible sources of heterogeneity
- consider meta-analysis of all trials or subgroups of trials
- perform sensitivity analyses, examine funnel plots
- make list of excluded studies available to interested readers

8 Interpret results (see also Chapters 19–24)
- consider limitations, including publication and related biases
- consider strength of evidence
- consider applicability
- consider numbers-needed-to-treat to benefit / harm
- consider economic implications
- consider implications for future research

* Points 1–7 should be addressed in the review protocol.

the combinability of patients, treatments, outcomes and lengths of follow-up. As discussed in detail in Chapter 5, quality and design features of clinical trials can influence the results.[3-5] Ideally, only controlled trials with proper patient randomisation which report on all initially included patients according to the intention-to-treat principle and with an objective, preferably blinded, outcome assessment would be considered for inclusion.[6] Formulating assessments regarding study quality can be a subjective process, however, especially since the information reported is often inadequate for this purpose.[7-10] It is therefore generally preferable to define only basic inclusion criteria, to assess the methodological quality of component studies, and to perform a thorough sensitivity analysis, as illustrated below.

Literature search

The search strategy for the identification of the relevant studies should be clearly delineated. As discussed in Chapter 4, identifying controlled trials for systematic reviews has become more straightforward in recent years. Appropriate terms to index randomised trials and controlled trials were introduced in the widely used bibliographic databases MEDLINE and EMBASE by the mid 1990s. However, tens of thousands of trial reports had been included prior to the introduction of these terms. In a painstaking effort the Cochrane Collaboration checked the titles and abstracts of almost 300 000 MEDLINE and EMBASE records which were then re-tagged as clinical trials if appropriate. It was important to examine both MEDLINE and EMBASE because the overlap in journals covered by the two databases is only about 34%.[11] The majority of journals indexed in MEDLINE are published in the US whereas EMBASE has better coverage of European journals (see Box 4.1 in Chapter 4 for a detailed comparison of MEDLINE and EMBASE). Re-tagging continues in MEDLINE and EMBASE and projects to cover other databases are ongoing or planned. Finally, thousands of reports of controlled trials have been identified by manual searches ("handsearching") of journals, conference proceedings and other sources.

All trials identified in the re-tagging and handsearching projects have been included in the *The Cochrane Controlled Trials Register* which is available in the Cochrane Library on CD ROM or online (see Chapter 25). This register currently includes over 250 000 records and is clearly the best single source of published trials for inclusion in systematic reviews. Searches of MEDLINE and EMBASE are, however, still required to identify trials that were published recently (see the search strategy described in Chapter 4). Specialised databases, conference proceedings and the bibliographies of review articles, monographs and the located studies should be scrutinised as well. Finally, the searching by hand of key journals should be considered, keeping in mind that many journals are already being searched by the Cochrane Collaboration.

The search should be extended to include unpublished studies, as their results may systematically differ from published trials. As discussed in Chapter 3, a systematic review which is restricted to published evidence may produce distorted results due to publication bias. Registration of trials at the time they are established (and before their results become known) would eliminate the risk of publication bias.[12] A number of such registers have been set up in recent years and access to these has improved, for example through the Cochrane Collaboration's *Register of Registers* or the internet-based *meta*Register of Controlled Trials which has been established by the publisher Current Science (see Chapters 4 and 24). Colleagues, experts in the field, contacts in the pharmaceutical industry and other informal channels can also be important sources of information on unpublished and ongoing trials.

Selection of studies, assessment of methodological quality and data extraction

Decisions regarding the inclusion or exclusion of individual studies often involve some degree of subjectivity. It is therefore useful to have two observers checking eligibility of candidate studies, with disagreements being resolved by discussion or a third reviewer.

Randomised controlled trials provide the best evidence of the efficacy of medical interventions but they are not immune to bias. Studies relating methodological features of trials to their results have shown that trial quality influences effect sizes.[4,5,13] Inadequate concealment of treatment allocation, resulting, for example, from the use of open random number tables, is on average associated with larger treatment effects.[4,5,13] Larger effects were also found if trials were not double-blind.[4] In some instances effects may also be overestimated if some participants, for example, those not adhering to study medications, were excluded from the analysis.[14-16] Although widely recommended, the assessment of the methodological quality of clinical trials is a matter of ongoing debate.[7] This is reflected by the large number of different quality scales and checklists that are available.[10,17] Empirical evidence[10] and theoretical considerations[18] suggests that although summary quality scores may in some circumstances provide a useful overall assessment, scales should not generally be used to assess the quality of trials in systematic reviews. Rather, as discussed in Chapter 5, the relevant methodological aspects should be identified in the study protocol, and assessed individually.

27

Again, independent assessment by more than one observer is desirable. Blinding of observers to the names of the authors and their institutions, the names of the journals, sources of funding and acknowledgments should also be considered as this may lead to more consistent assessments.[19] Blinding involves photocopying of papers removing the title page and concealing journal identifications and other characteristics with a black marker, or scanning the text of papers into a computer and preparing standardised formats.[20,21] This is time consuming and potential benefits may not always justify the additional costs.[22]

It is important that two independent observers extract the data, so errors can be avoided. A standardised record form is needed for this purpose. Data extraction forms should be carefully designed, piloted and revised if necessary. Electronic data collection forms have a number of advantages, including the combination of data abstraction and data entry in one step, and the automatic detection of inconsistencies between data recorded by different observers. However, the complexities involved in programming and revising electronic forms should not be underestimated.[23]

Presenting, combining and interpreting results

Once studies have been selected, critically appraised and data extracted the characteristics of included studies should be presented in tabular form. Table 2.1 shows the characteristics of the long term trials that were included in a systematic review[24] of the effect of beta blockade in secondary prevention after myocardial infarction (we mentioned this example in Chapter 1 and will return to it later in this chapter). Freemantle et al.[24] included all parallel group randomised trials that examined the effectiveness of beta blockers versus placebo or alternative treatment in patients who had had a myocardial infarction. The authors searched 11 bibliographic databases, including dissertation abstracts and grey literature databases, examined existing reviews and checked the reference lists of each identified study. Freemantle et al. identified 31 trials of at least six months' duration which contributed 33 comparisons of beta blocker with control groups (Table 2.1).

Standardised outcome measure

Individual results have to be expressed in a standardised format to allow for comparison between studies. If the endpoint is binary (e.g. disease versus no disease, or dead versus alive) then relative risks or odds ratios are often calculated. The odds ratio has convenient mathematical properties, which allow for ease in the combination of data and

Table 2.1 Characteristics of long term trials comparing beta blockers with control. Adapted from Freemantle et al.[24]

Author	Year	Drug	Study duration (years)	Concealment of treatment allocation	Double-blind	Mortality (No./total no.) Beta blocker	Control
Barber	1967	Practolol	2	Unclear	Unclear	33/ 207	38/ 213
Reynolds	1972	Alprenolol	1	Yes	Yes	3/ 38	3/ 39
Ahlmark	1974	Alprenolol	2	Unclear	Unclear	5/ 69	11/ 93
Wilhelmsson	1974	Alprenolol	2	Unclear	Yes	7/ 114	14/ 116
Multicentre International	1975	Practolol	2	Unclear	Yes	102/ 1533	127/ 1520
Yusuf	1979	Atenolol	1	Unclear	Yes	1/ 11	1/ 11
Andersen	1979	Alprenolol	1	Unclear	Yes	61/238	62/242
Rehnqvist	1980	Metoprolol	1	Unclear	Unclear	4/59	6/52
Baber	1980	Propranolol	0·75	Unclear	Yes	28/355	27/365
Wilcox (Atenolol)	1980	Atenolol	1	Yes	Yes	17/132	19/129
Wilcox (Propanolol)	1980	Propranolol	1	Yes	Yes	19/ 127	19/ 129
Hjalmarson	1981	Metoprolol	2	Unclear	No	40/ 698	62/ 697
Norwegian Multicentre	1981	Timolol	1·4	Unclear	Yes	98/ 945	152/ 939
Hansteen	1982	Propranolol	1	Unclear	Yes	25/ 278	37/ 282
Julian	1982	Sotalol	1	Yes	Yes	64/ 873	52/ 583
BHAT	1982	Propranolol	2·1	Yes	Yes	138/ 1916	188/ 1921
Taylor	1982	Oxprenolol	4	Done	Yes	60/ 632	48/ 471
Manger Cats	1983	Metoprolol	1	Unclear	Yes	9/ 273	16/ 280
Rehnqvist	1983	Metoprolol	3	Unclear	Yes	25/ 154	31/ 147
Australian-Swedish	1983	Pindolol	2	Unclear	Yes	45/ 263	47/ 266
Mazur	1984	Propranolol	1·5	Unclear	No	5/ 101	11/ 103
EIS	1984	Oxprenolol	1	Unclear	Yes	57/ 853	45/ 883
Salathia	1985	Metoprolol	1	Unclear	Yes	49/ 416	52/ 348
Roqué	1987	Timolol	2	Unclear	Yes	7/ 102	12/ 98
LIT	1987	Metoprolol	1·5	Unclear	Yes	86/ 1195	93/ 1200
Kaul	1988	Propranolol	0·5	Unclear	Yes	3/ 25	3/ 25
ASPI	1990	Acebutolol	0·87	Yes	Yes	17/ 298	34/ 309
Schwartz (high risk)	1992	Oxprenolol	1·8	Unclear	No	2/ 48	12/ 56
Schwartz (low risk)	1992	Oxprenolol	1·8	Unclear	Yes	15/ 437	27/ 432
SSSD	1993	Metoprolol	3	Unclear	No	17/ 130	9/ 123
Darasz	1995	Xamoterol	0·5	Unclear	Yes	3/ 23	1/ 24
Basu	1997	Carvedilol	0·5	Unclear	Yes	2/ 75	3/ 71
Aronow	1997	Propranolol	1	Unclear	Unclear	44/ 79	60/ 79

the testing of the overall effect for statistical significance, but, as discussed in Box 2.2, the odds ratio will differ from the relative risk if the outcome is common. Relative risks should probably be prefered over odds ratios because they are more intuitively comprehensible to most people.[25,26] Absolute measures such as the absolute risk reduction or the number of patients needed to be treated for one person to benefit[27] are more helpful when applying results in clinical practice (see below). If the outcome is continuous and measurements are made on the same scale (e.g. blood pressure measured in mm Hg) the mean difference between the treatment and control groups is used. If trials measured outcomes in different ways, differences may be presented in standard deviation units, rather than as absolute differences. For example, the efficacy of non-steroidal antiinflammatory drugs for reducing pain in patients with rheumatoid arthritis was measured using different scales.[28] The choice and calculation of appropriate summary statistics is covered in detail in Chapters 15 and 16.

Graphical display

Results from each trial are usefully graphically displayed together with their confidence intervals in a "forest plot", a form of presentation developed in the 1980s by Richard Peto's group in Oxford. Figure 2.1 represents the forest plot for the trials of beta-blockers in secondary prevention after myocardial infarction which we mentioned in Chapter 1.[24] Each study is represented by a black square and a horizontal line which correspond to the point estimate and the 95% confidence intervals of the relative risk. The 95% confidence intervals would contain the true underlying effect in 95% of the occasions, if the study was repeated again and again. The solid vertical line corresponds to no effect of treatment (relative risk 1·0). If the confidence interval includes 1, then the difference in the effect of experimental and control therapy is not statistically significant at conventional levels (P > 0·05). The confidence interval of most studies cross this line. The area of the black squares reflects the weight of the study in the meta-analysis (see below).

A logarithmic scale was used for plotting the relative risk in Figure 2.2. There are a number of reasons why ratio measures are best plotted on logarithmic scales.[29] Most importantly, the value of a risk ratio and its reciprocal, for example 0·5 and 2, which represent risk ratios of the same magnitude but opposite directions, will be equidistant from 1·0. Studies with relative risks below and above 1·0 will take up equal space on the graph and thus visually appear to be equally important. Also, confidence intervals will be symmetrical around the point estimate.

30

Box 2.2 Odds ratio or relative risk?

Odds ratios are often used in order to bring the results of different trials into a standardised format. What is an odds ratio and how does it relate to the relative risk? The *odds* is defined as the number of patients who fulfill the criteria for a given endpoint divided by the number of patients who do not. For example, the odds of diarrhoea during treatment with an antibiotic in a group of 10 patients may be 4 to 6 (4 with diarrhoea divided by 6 without, 0·66), as compared to 1 to 9 (0·11) in a control group. A bookmaker (a person who takes bets, especially on horse-races, calculates odds, and pays out winnings) would, of course, refer to this as nine to one. The *odds ratio* of treatment to control group in this example is 6 (0·66 divided by 0·11). The risk, on the other hand, is calculated as the number of patients with diarrhoea divided by all patients. It would be 4 in 10 in the treatment group and 1 in 10 in the control group, for a risk ratio, or a *relative risk*, of 4 (0·4 divided by 0·1). As shown in Figure 2.1, the odds ratio will be close to the relative risk if the endpoint occurs relatively infrequently, say in less than 15%. If the outcome is more common, as in the diarrhoea example, then the odds ratio will differ increasingly from the relative risk. The choice of binary outcome measures is discussed in detail in Chapter 16.

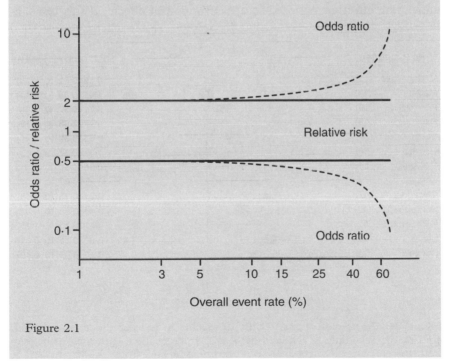

Figure 2.1

31

Heterogeneity between study results

The thoughtful consideration of heterogeneity between study results is an important aspect of systematic reviews.[30,31] As mentioned above, this should start when writing the review protocol, by defining potential sources of heterogeneity and planning appropriate subgroup analyses. Once the data have been assembled, simple inspection of the forest plot is informative. The results from the beta-blocker trials are fairly homogeneous, clustering between a relative risk of 0·5 and 1·0, with widely overlapping confidence intervals (Figure 2.2). In contrast, trials of BCG vaccination for prevention of tuberculosis[32] (Figure 2.3) are clearly heterogeneous. The findings of the UK trial, which indicate substantial benefit of BCG vaccination are not compatible with those from the Madras or Puerto Rico trials which suggest little effect or only a modest benefit. There is no overlap in the confidence intervals of the three trials. Other graphical representations, discussed elsewhere, are particularly useful to detect and investigate heterogeneity. These include Galbraith plots[29] (see Chapter 9), L'Abbé plots[33] (see Chapters 8, 10 and 16) and funnel plots[34] (see Chapter 11).

Statistical tests of homogeneity (also called tests for heterogeneity) assess whether the individual study results are likely to reflect a single underlying effect, as opposed to a distribution of effects. If this test fails

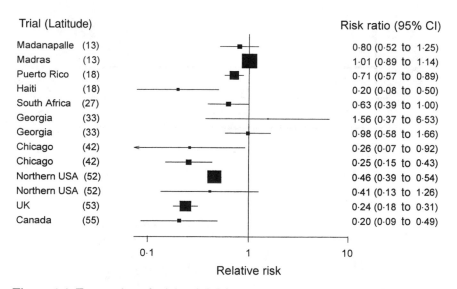

Figure 2.3 Forest plot of trials of BCG vaccine to prevent tuberculosis. Trials are ordered according to the latitude of the study location, expressed as degrees from the equator. No meta-analysis is shown. Adapted from Colditz et al.[32]

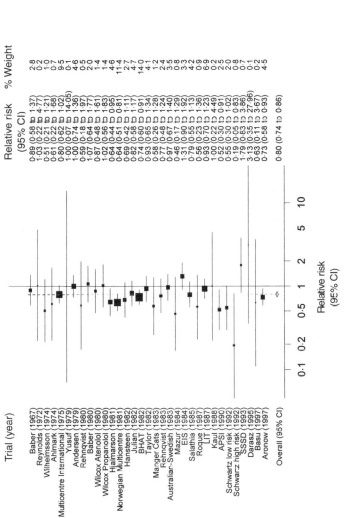

Figure 2.2 Forest plot showing total mortality from trials of beta-blockers in secondary prevention after myocardial infarction. The black square and horizontal line correspond to the relative risk and 95% confidence intervals. The area of the black squares reflects the weight each trial contributes to the meta-analysis. The diamond at the bottom of the graph represents the combined relative risk and its 95% confidence interval, indicating a 20% reduction in the risk of death. The solid vertical line corresponds to no effect of treatment (relative risk 1·0), the dotted vertical line to the combined relative risk (0·8). The relative risk, 95% confidence interval and weights are also given in tabular form. The graph was produced in STATA (see Chapter 18). Adapted from Freemantle et al.[24]

to detect heterogeneity among results, then it is assumed that the differences observed between individual studies are a consequence of sampling variation and simply due to chance. A chi-square test of homogeneity gives P = 0·25 for the beta-blocker trials but P < 0·001 for the BCG trials. The BCG trials are an extreme example, however, and a major limitation of statistical tests of homogeneity is their lack of power – they often fail to reject the null hypothesis of homogeneous results even if substantial inter-study differences exist. Reviewers should therefore not assume that a non-significant test of heterogeneity excludes important heterogeneity. Heterogeneity between study results should not be seen as purely a problem for systematic reviews, since it also provides an opportunity for examining why treatment effects differ in different circumstances, as discussed below and in Chapters 8 and 9.

Methods for estimating a combined effect estimate

If, after careful consideration, a meta-analysis is deemed appropriate, the last step consists in estimating an overall effect by combining the data. Two principles are important. Firstly, simply pooling the data from different studies and treating them as one large study would fail to preserve the randomisation and introduce bias and confounding. For example, a recent review and "meta-analysis" of the literature on the role of male circumcision in HIV transmission concluded that the risk of HIV infection was lower in uncircumcised men.[35] However, the analysis was performed by simply pooling the data from 33 diverse studies. A re-analysis stratifying the data by study found that an intact foreskin was in fact associated with an increased risk of HIV infection.[36] Confounding by study thus led to a change in the direction of the association (a case of "Simpson's paradox" in epidemiological parlance[37]). The unit of the trial must therefore always be maintained when combining data.

Secondly, simply calculating an arithmetic mean would be inappropriate. The results from small studies are more subject to the play of chance and should, therefore, be given less weight. Methods used for meta-analysis employ a weighted average of the results in which the larger trials generally have more influence than the smaller ones. There are a variety of statistical techniques available for this purpose (see Chapter 15), which can be broadly classified into two models.[38] The difference consists in the way the variability of the results *between* the studies is treated. The "*fixed effects*" model considers this variability as exclusively due to random variation and individual studies are simply weighted by their precision.[39] Therefore, if all the studies were infinitely large they would give identical results. The main alternative, the "*random effects*" model,[40] assumes a different underlying effect for each study and takes this into consideration as an additional source of variation. Effects are assumed to be randomly distributed and the central point of this distribution is the focus of the combined effect estimate. The random effects model leads to relatively more weight being given to smaller studies and to wider confidence intervals than the fixed effects model. The use of random effects models has been advocated if there is heterogeneity between study results. This is problematic, however. Rather than simply ignoring it after applying some statistical model, the approach to heterogeneity should be to scrutinise, and attempt to explain it.[30,31]

While neither of the two models can be said to be "correct", a substantial difference in the combined effect calculated by the fixed and random effects models will be seen only if studies are markedly heterogeneous, as in the case of the BCG trials (Table 2.2). Combining trials using a random effects model indicates that BCG vaccination halves the the risk of tuberculosis, whereas fixed effects analysis indicates that the risk is only reduced by 35%. This is essentially explained by the different weight given to the large Madras trial which showed no protective effect of vaccination (41% of the total weight with fixed effects model, 10% with random effects model, Table 2.2). Both analyses are probably misguided. As shown in Figure 2.2, BCG vaccination appears to be effective at higher latitudes but not in warmer regions, possibly because

Table 2.2 Meta-analysis of trials of BCG vaccination to prevent tuberculosis using a fixed effects and random effects model. Note the differences in the weight allocated to individual studies. The raw data (from Colditz et al.[32]) are given in Chapter 18.

Trial	Relative risk (95% CI)	Fixed effects weight (%)	Random effects weight (%)
Madanapalle	0·80 (0·52 to 1·25)	3·20	8·88
Madras	1·01 (0·89 to 1·14)	41·40	10·22
Puerto Rico	0·71 (0·57 to 0·89)	13·21	9·93
Haiti	0·20 (0·08 to 0·50)	0·73	6·00
South Africa	0·63 (0·39 to 1·00)	2·91	8·75
Georgia	0·98 (0·58 to 1·66)	0·31	3·80
Georgia	1·56 (0·37 to 6·53)	2·30	8·40
Chicago	0·26 (0·07 to 0·92)	0·40	4·40
Chicago	0·25 (0·15 to 0·43)	2·25	8·37
Northern USA	0·41 (0·13 to 1·26)	23·75	10·12
Northern USA	0·46 (0·39 to 0·54)	0·50	5·05
UK	0·24 (0·18 to 0·31)	8·20	9·71
Canada	0·20 (0·09 to 0·49)	0·84	6·34
Combined relative risks		0·65 (0·60 to 0·70)	0·49 (0·35 to 0·70)

exposure to certain environmental mycobacteria acts as a "natural" BCG inoculation in warmer regions.[41] In this situation it is more meaningful to quantify how the effect varies according to latitude than to calculate an overall estimate of effect which will be misleading, independent of the model used (see Chapter 18 for further analyses of the BCG trials).

Bayesian meta-analysis

There are other statistical approaches, which some feel are more appropriate than either of the above. One uses Bayes' theorem, named after the 18th century English clergyman Thomas Bayes.[42-44] Bayesian statisticians express their belief about the size of an effect by specifying some prior probability distribution before seeing the data – and then update that belief by deriving a posterior probability distribution, taking the data into account.[45] Bayesian models are available in both a fixed and random effects framework but published applications have usually been based on the random effects assumption. The confidence interval (or more correctly in bayesian terminology: the 95% credible interval which covers 95% of the posterior probability distribution) will be slightly wider than that derived from using the conventional models.[46,47] Bayesian methods allow probability statements to be made directly regarding, for example, the comparative effects of two treatments ("the probability that treatment A is better than B is 0·99").[48] Bayesian approaches to meta-analysis can integrate other sources of evidence, for example findings from observational studies or expert opinion and are particularly useful for analysing the relationship between treatment benefit and underlying risk (see Chapter 10).[44,49] Finally, they provide a natural framework for cumulative meta-analysis.[49,50]

Bayesian approaches are, however, controversial because the definition of prior probability will often involve subjective assessments and opinion which runs against the principles of systematic review. Furthermore, analyses are complex to implement and time consuming. More methodological research is required to define the appropriate place of bayesian methods in systematic reviews and meta-analysis.[44,49]

Sensitivity analysis

There will often be diverging opinions on the correct method for performing a particular meta-analysis. The robustness of the findings to different assumptions should therefore always be examined in a thorough sensitivity analysis. This is illustrated in Figure 2.4 for the beta-blocker after myocardial infarction meta-analysis.[24] First, the overall

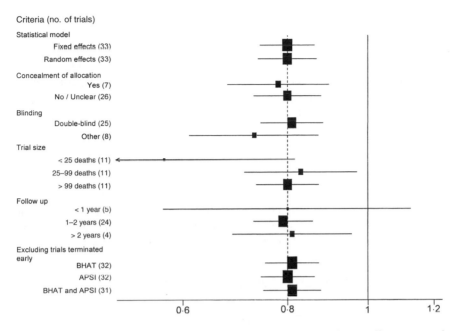

Figure 2.4 Sensitivity analyses examining the robustness of the effect on total mortality of beta-blockers in secondary prevention after myocardial infarction. The dotted vertical line corresponds to the combined relative risk from the fixed effects model (0·8).

effect was calculated by different statistical methods, both using a fixed and a random effects model. It is evident from the figure that the overall estimate is virtually identical and that confidence intervals are only slightly wider when using the random effects model. This is explained by the relatively small amount of between trial variation present in this meta-analysis.

Methodological quality was assessed in terms of concealment of allocation of study participants to beta-blocker or control groups and blinding of patients and investigators.[24] Figure 2.4 shows that the estimated treatment effect was similar for studies with and without concealment of treatment allocation. The eight studies that were not double-blind indicated more benefit than the 25 double-blind trials but confidence intervals overlap widely. Statistically significant results are more likely to get published than non-significant findings[51] and this can distort the findings of meta-analyses (see Chapter 3). Whether such publication bias is present can be examined by stratifying the analysis by study size. Smaller effects can be statistically significant in larger studies. If publication bias is present, it is expected that of published studies, the larger ones will report the smaller effects. The figure shows that in the present example this is indeed the case with the 11 smallest trials (25 deaths or less) showing the largest effect. However, exclusion of the smaller studies has little effect on the overall estimate. Studies varied in terms of length of follow up but this again had little effect on estimates. Finally, two trials[52,53] were terminated earlier than anticipated on the grounds of the results from interim analyses. Estimates of treatment effects from trials which were stopped early because of a significant treatment difference are liable to be biased away from the null value. Bias may thus be introduced in a meta-analysis which includes such trials.[54] Exclusion of these trials, however, again affects the overall estimate only marginally.

The sensitivity analysis thus shows that the results from this meta-analysis are robust to the choice of the statistical method and to the exclusion of trials of lesser quality or of studies terminated early. It also suggests that publication bias is unlikely to have distorted its findings.

Relative or absolute measures of effect?

The relative risk of death associated with the use of beta-blockers after myocardial infarction is 0·80 (95% confidence interval 0·74 to 0·86) (Figure 2.2). The *relative risk reduction*, obtained by substracting the relative risk from 1 and expressing the result as a percentage, is 20% (95% confidence interval 14 to 26%). The relative measures ignore the underlying absolute risk. The risk of death among patients who have survived the acute phase of myocardial infarction, however, varies widely.[55] For example, among patients with three or more cardiac risk factors, the probability of death at two years after discharge ranged from 24 to 60%.[55] Conversely, two-year mortality among patients with no risk factors was less than three percent. The *absolute risk reduction*, or risk difference, reflects both the underlying risk without therapy and the risk reduction associated with therapy. Taking the reciprocal of the risk difference gives the number of patients who need to be treated to prevent one event, which is abbreviated to NNT or NNT(benefit).[27] The number of patients that need to be treated to harm one patient, denoted as NNH or, more appropriately, NNT(harm)[56] can also be calculated.

For a baseline risk of one per cent per year, the absolute risk difference indicates that two deaths are prevented per 1000 treated patients (Table 2.3). This corresponds to 500 patients (1 divided by 0·002) treated for one year to prevent one death. Conversely, if the risk is above 10%, less than 50 patients have to be treated to prevent one fatal event. Many clinicians would probably decide not to treat patients at very low risk, considering the large number of patients who would

Table 2.3 Beta-blockade in secondary prevention after myocardial infarction. Absolute risk reductions and numbers-needed-to-treat for one year to prevent one death, NNT(benefit), for different levels of control group mortality.

One-year mortality risk among controls (%)	Absolute risk reduction	NNT(benefit)
1	0·002	500
3	0·006	167
5	0·01	100
10	0·02	50
20	0·04	25
30	0·06	17
40	0·08	13
50	0·1	10

Calculations assume a constant relative risk reduction of 20%.

have to be exposed to the adverse effects of beta-blockade to postpone one death. Appraising the NNT from a patient's estimated risk without treatment, and the relative risk reduction with treatment, is a helpful aid when making a decision in an individual patient. A nomogram to determine NNTs at the bedside is available[57] and confidence intervals can be calculated.[56]

Meta-analysis using absolute effect measures such as the risk difference may be useful to illustrate the range of absolute effects across studies. The *combined* risk difference (and the NNT calculated from it) will, however, be essentially determined by the number and size of trials in low, intermediate and high-risk patients. Combined results will thus be applicable only to patients at levels of risk corresponding to the average risk of the trial participants. It is therefore generally more meaningful to use relative effect measures when summarising the evidence while considering absolute measures when applying it to a specific clinical or public health situation. The use of numbers-needed-to-treat in meta-analysis is discussed in more detail in Chapter 20.

Conclusions

Systematic reviews involve structuring the processes through which a thorough review of previous research is carried out. The issues of the completeness of the evidence identified, the quality of component studies and the combinability of evidence are made explicit. How likely is it that publication and related biases have been avoided? Is it sensible to combine the individual trials in meta-analysis or is there heterogeneity between individual study results which renders the calculation of an overall estimate questionable? If meta-analysis was performed, how robust are the results to changes in assumptions? Finally, has the analysis contributed to the process of making rational health care decisions? These issues will be considered in more depth in the following chapters.

Acknowledgements

This chapter draws on material published earlier in the *BMJ*.[58]

We are grateful to Iain Chalmers for helpful comments on an earlier draft of this chapter.

1 Gelber RD, Goldhirsch A. From the overview to the patient: how to interpret meta-analysis data. *Recent Results Cancer Res* 1993;**127**:167–76.
2 Oxman AD, Guyatt GH. A consumer's guide to subgroup analyses. *Ann Intern Med* 1992;**116**:78–84.
3 Sacks H, Chalmers TC, Smith H Jr. Randomized versus historical controls for clinical trials. *Am J Med* 1982;**72**:233–40.
4 Schulz KF, Chalmers I, Hayes RJ, Altman D. Empirical evidence of bias. Dimensions of methodological quality associated with estimates of treatment effects in controlled trials. *JAMA* 1995;**273**:408–12.
5 Moher D, Pham B, Jones A, *et al.* Does quality of reports of randomised trials affect estimates of intervention efficacy reported in meta-analyses? *Lancet* 1998;**352**:609–13.
6 Prendiville W, Elbourne D, Chalmers I. The effects of routine oxytocic administration in the management of the third stage of labour: an overview of the evidence from controlled trials. *Br J Obstet Gynaecol* 1988;**95**:3–16.
7 Moher D, Jadad AR, Tugwell P. Assessing the quality of randomized controlled trials. Current issues and future directions. *Int J Technol Assess Hlth Care* 1996;**12**:195–208.
8 Begg C, Cho M, Eastwood S, *et al.* Improving the quality of reporting of randomized controlled trials. The CONSORT statement. *JAMA* 1996;**276**:637–9.
9 Schulz KF. Randomised trials, human nature, and reporting guidelines. *Lancet* 1996;**348**:596–8.
10 Jüni P, Witschi A, Bloch R, Egger M. The hazards of scoring the quality of clinical trial for meta-analysis. *JAMA* 1999;**282**:1054–60.
11 Smith BJ, Darzins PJ, Quinn M, Heller RF. Modern methods of searching the medical literature. *Med J Aust* 1992;**157**:603–11.
12 Dickersin K. Research registers. In: Cooper H, Hedges LV, eds. *The handbook of research synthesis.* New York: Russell Sage Foundation, 1994.
13 Chalmers TC, Celano P, Sacks HS, Smith H. Bias in treatment assignment in controlled clinical trials. *N Engl J Med* 1983;**309**:1358–61.
14 Sackett DL, Gent M. Controversy in counting and attributing events in clinical trials. *N Engl J Med* 1979;**301**:1410–12.
15 Peduzzi P, Wittes J, Detre K, Holford T. Analysis as-randomized and the problem of non-adherence: an example from the veterans affairs randomized trial of coronary artery bypass surgery. *Stat Med* 1993;**12**:1185–95.
16 May GS, Demets DL, Friedman LM, Furberg C, Passamani E. The randomized clinical trial: bias in analysis. *Circulation* 1981;**64**:669–73.
17 Moher D, Jadad AR, Nichol G, Penman M, Tugwell P, Walsh S. Assessing the quality of randomized controlled trials: an annotated bibliography of scales and checklists. *Controlled Clin Trials* 1995;**16**:62–73.
18 Greenland S. Quality scores are useless and potentially misleading. *Am J Epidemiol* 1994;**140**:300–2.
19 Jadad AR, Moore RA, Carrol D, *et al.* Assessing the quality of reports of randomized clinical trials: is blinding necessary? *Controlled Clin Trials* 1996;**17**:1–12.

20 Chalmers TC. Problems induced by meta-analyses. *Stat Med* 1991;**10**:971–80.
21 Moher D, Fortin P, Jadad AR, *et al.* Completeness of reporting of trials published in languages other than English: implications for conduct and reporting of systematic reviews. *Lancet* 1996;**347**:363–6.
22 Berlin JA, on behalf of University of Pennsylvania Meta-analysis Blinding Study Group. Does blinding of readers affect the results of meta-analyses? *Lancet* 1997;**350**:185–6.
23 *Cochrane Reviewer's Handbook* (updated July 1999). In: *The Cochrane Library* (database on disk and CD-ROM). *The Cochrane Collaboration*. Oxford: Update Software, 1999.
24 Freemantle N, Cleland J, Young P, Mason J, Harrison J. Beta blockade after myocardial infarction: systematic review and meta regression analysis. *BMJ* 1999;**318**:1730–7.
25 Sackett DL, Deeks JJ, Altman D. Down with odds ratios! *Evidence-Based Med* 1996;**1**:164–7.
26 Deeks J. When can odds ratios mislead? *BMJ* 1998;**317**:1155.
27 Laupacis A, Sackett DL, Roberts RS. An assessment of clinically useful measures of the consequences of treatment. *N Engl J Med* 1988;**318**:1728–33.
28 Gøtzsche PC. Sensitivity of effect variables in rheumatoid arthritis: a meta-analysis of 130 placebo controlled NSAID trials. *J Clin Epidemiol* 1990;**43**:1313–18.
29 Galbraith R. A note on graphical presentation of estimated odds ratios from several clinical trials. *Stat Med* 1988;**7**:889–94.
30 Bailey K. Inter-study differences: how should they influence the interpretation and analysis of results? *Stat Med* 1987;**6**:351–8.
31 Thompson SG. Why sources of heterogeneity in meta-analysis should be investigated. *BMJ* 1994;**309**:1351–5.
32 Colditz GA, Brewer TF, Berkley CS, *et al.* Efficacy of BCG vaccine in the prevention of tuberculosis. *JAMA* 1994;**271**:698–702.
33 L'Abbé KA, Detsky AS, O'Rourke K. Meta-analysis in clinical research. *Ann Intern Med* 1987;**107**:224–33.
34 Light RJ, Pillemer DB. *Summing up. The science of reviewing research.* Cambridge, MA: Harvard University Press, 1984.
35 Van Howe RS. Circumcision and HIV infection: review of the literature and meta-analysis. *Int J STD AIDS* 1999;**10**:8–16.
36 O'Farrell N, Egger M. Circumcision in men and the prevalence of HIV infection: a meta-analysis revisited. *Int J STD AIDS* 2000; **11**:137–42.
37 Last JM. *A dictionary of epidemiology.* New York: Oxford University Press, 1995.
38 Berlin J, Laird NM, Sacks HS, Chalmers TC. A comparison of statistical methods for combining event rates from clinical trials. *Stat Med* 1989;**8**:141–51.
39 Yusuf S, Peto R, Lewis J, Collins R, Sleight P. Beta blockade during and after myocardial infarction: an overview of the randomized trials. *Prog Cardiovasc Dis* 1985;**17**:335–71.
40 DerSimonian R, Laird N. Meta-analysis in clinical trials. *Controlled Clin Trials* 1986;**7**:177–88.
41 Fine PEM. Variation in protection by BCG: implications of and for heterologous immunity. *Lancet* 1995;**346**:1339–45.
42 Carlin JB. Meta-analysis for 2 × 2 tables: a Bayesian approach. *Stat Med* 1992;**11**:141–58.
43 Bland JM, Altman DG. Bayesians and frequentists. *BMJ* 1998;**317**:1151.
44 Spiegelhalter DJ, Myles JP, Jones DR, Abrams KR. An introduction to bayesian methods in health technology assessment. *BMJ* 1999;**319**:508–12.
45 Lilford RJ, Braunholtz D. The statistical basis of public policy: a paradigm shift is overdue. *BMJ* 1996;**313**:603–7.
46 Su XY, Li Wan Po A. Combining event rates from clinical trials: comparison of bayesian and classical methods. *Ann Pharmacother* 1996;**30**:460–5.
47 Thompson SG, Smith TC, Sharp SJ. Investigating underlying risk as a source of heterogeneity in meta-analysis. *Stat Med* 1997;**16**:2741–58.
48 Fredman L. Bayesian statistical methods. *BMJ* 1996;**313**:569–70.
49 Song F, Abrams KR, Jones DR, Sheldon TA. Systematic reviews of trials and other studies. *Health Technol Assess* 1998;**2(19)**.

41

50 Eddy DM, Hasselblad V, Shachter R. *Meta-analysis by the confidence profile method. The statistical synthesis of evidence.* Boston: Academic Press, 1992.
51 Easterbrook PJ, Berlin J, Gopalan R, Matthews DR. Publication bias in clinical research. *Lancet* 1991;**337**:867–72.
52 Anon. A randomized trial of propranolol in patients with acute myocardial infarction. I. Mortality results. *JAMA* 1982;**247**:1707–14.
53 Boissel JP, Leizorovicz A, Picolet H, Ducruet T. Efficacy of acebutolol after acute myocardial infarction (the APSI trial). The APSI Investigators. *Am J Cardiol* 1990;**66**:24C–31C.
54 Green S, Fleming TR, Emerson S. Effects on overviews of early stopping rules for clinical trials. *Stat Med* 1987;**6**:361–7.
55 The Multicenter Postinfarction Research Group. Risk stratification and survival after myocardial infarction. *N Engl J Med* 1983;**309**:331–6.
56 Altman DG. Confidence intervals for the number needed to treat. *BMJ* 1998;**317**:1309–12.
57 Chatellier G, Zapletal E, Lemaitre D, Menard J, Degoulet P. The number needed to treat: a clinically useful nomogram in its proper context. *BMJ* 1996;**312**:426–9.
58 Egger M, Davey Smith G, Phillips AN. Meta-analysis: principles and procedures. *BMJ* 1997;**315**:1533–7.

3 Problems and limitations in conducting systematic reviews

MATTHIAS EGGER, KAY DICKERSIN,
GEORGE DAVEY SMITH

Summary points

- There are numerous ways in which bias can be introduced in reviews and meta-analyses of controlled clinical trials.
- If the methodological quality of trials is inadequate then the findings of reviews of this material may also be compromised.
- Publication bias can distort findings because trials with statistically significant results are more likely to get published, and more likely to be published without delay, than trials without significant results.
- Among published trials, those with significant results are more likely to get published in English, more likely to be cited, and more likely to be published more than once which means that they will also be more likely to be identified and included in reviews.
- The choice of the outcome that is reported can be influenced by the results. The outcome with the most favourable findings will generally be reported, which may introduce bias.
- Criteria for inclusion of studies into a review may be influenced by knowledge of the results of the set of potential studies.
- The definition of eligibility criteria for trials to be included, a comprehensive search for such trials, and an assessment of their methodological quality are central to systematic reviews. Systematic reviews are thus more likely to avoid bias than traditional, narrative reviews.

Systematic reviews and meta-analyses have received a mixed reception since the outset. Those on the receiving end have rejected what they see as exercises in "mega-silliness"[1] and the authors of a highly distinguished series of systematic reviews of care during pregnancy and childhood[2] have been dubbed as terrorists ("an obstetrical Baader-Meinhof gang"[3]). Some statisticians think that meta-analysis "represents the unacceptable face of statisticism"[4] and to clinicians objecting to the findings of meta-analyses "a tool has become a weapon".[5] Others "still prefer the conventional narrative review article".[6] At the other end of the spectrum, the application of a technique which basically consists of calculating a weighted average has been described as "Newtonian"[7] and it has been suggested that with the advent of meta-analysis there is no place left for the narrative review article.[8] As may be imagined, the truth is likely to lie somewhere between these extreme views.

This mixed reception is not surprising considering that several examples exist of meta-analyses of small trials whose findings were later contradicted by a single large randomised trial (Figure 3.1).[9,10] Also, systematic reviews addressing the same issue have reached opposite conclusions.[11] For example, one group reviewing trials comparing low-molecular-weight (LMW) heparins and standard heparin in the prevention of thrombosis following surgery concluded that "LMW heparins seem to have a higher benefit to risk ratio than unfractionated heparin in preventing perioperative thrombosis",[12] while another group of reviewers considered that "there is at present no convincing evidence that in general surgery patients LMW heparins, compared with standard heparin, generate a clinically important improvement in the benefit to risk ratio".[21] The differences between these

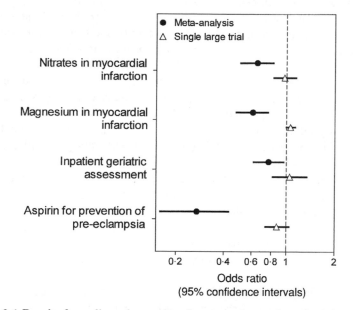

Figure 3.1 Results from discordant pairs of meta-analyses of small trials and single large trials: effect of nitrates[13,14] and magnesium[15,16] on mortality in acute myocardial infarction, effect of inpatient geriatric assessment on mortality in the elderly,[17,18] and effect of aspirin on the risk of pre-eclampsia.[19,20]

Table 3.1 Characteristics of two systematic reviews of clinical trials which addressed the same issue but reached opposite conclusions: low-molecular-weight (LMW) heparin compared with standard heparin in the prevention of perioperative thrombosis.

Characteristic	Leizorovicz et al.[12]	Nurmohamed et al.[21]
Literature search		
Years covered	1984–91	1984–91
Search for unpublished data	Yes	No
Language restrictions	None	English, German, French
Accepted methods to detect deep-vein thrombosis	Fibrinogen uptake test, thermographic DeVeTherm test, Doppler ultrasonography, phlebography	Fibrinogen uptake test in general surgery patients, phlebography for orthopaedic surgery patients
Assessment of trial quality	No	Eight-point scale
Analysis		
Number of studies included	39	23*
Number of patients included	12 375	8172
Statistical model	Fixed effects	Fixed effects
Stratified by trial quality	No	Yes
Conclusions	LMW heparins have higher benefit to risk ratio in preventing perioperative thrombosis	There is no convincing evidence that in general surgery patients LMW heparins have a higher benefit to risk ratio

* Thirteen studies were considered to be of high methodological quality.

reviews are summarised in Table 3.1. The literature search was free of language restrictions and attempts were made to identify unpublished studies in one review[12] but not the other.[21] One group of reviewers[21] based their conclusion on a subgroup of trials, which they considered to possess the highest methodological strength, while the other group[12] did not consider the quality of trials.

Contrary to one of the central objectives of systematic reviews, to reduce uncertainty, such contradictory reports may contribute to the confusion, a situation that has arisen in other fields, for example when assessing calcium antagonists or cholesterol-lowering interventions in hypertension and coronary heart disease, or mammography for breast cancer screening.[22–24] In this chapter we will review the problems and limitations of systematic reviews and meta-analyses.

Garbage in – garbage out?

The quality of component trials is of crucial importance: if the "raw material" is flawed, then the findings of reviews of this material may also be compromised. Clearly, the trials included in systematic reviews and meta-analyses should ideally be of high methodological quality and free of bias

45

such that the differences in outcomes observed between groups of patients can confidently be attributed to the intervention under investigation. The biases that threaten the validity of clinical trials are reviewed in detail in Chapter 5. These relate to systematic differences in the patients' characteristics at baseline (*selection bias*), unequal provision of care apart from the treatment under evaluation (*performance bias*), biased assessment of outcomes (*detection bias*), and bias due to exclusion of patients after they have been allocated to treatment groups (*attrition bias*).[25] Several studies[26-28] have recently attempted to quantify the impact these biases have on the results of controlled clinical trials (see Chapter 5). For example, Schulz et al.[26] assessed the methodological quality of 250 trials from 33 meta-analyses from the Cochrane Pregnancy and Childbirth Database and examined the association between dimensions of trial quality and estimated treatment effects. Compared to trials in which authors reported adequately concealed treatment allocation, failure to prevent foreknowledge of treatment allocation or unclear concealment were associated, on average, with an exaggeration of treatment effects by 30 to 40%. Trials that were not double-blind also yielded larger effects.

The meta-analyses[12,21] of trials comparing LMW heparin with standard heparin for the prevention of postoperative deep-vein thrombosis mentioned earlier are a case in point. Jüni et al.[29] recently showed that in these trials, blinding of outcome assessments is a crucial quality feature: trials that were not double-blind showed a spurious benefit of LMW heparin that disappeared when restricting the analysis to trials with blinded outcome assessment. This is not entirely surprising considering that the interpretation of fibrinogen leg scanning, which is used to detect thrombosis, can be subjective.[30] One of the two reviews summarised in Table 3.1 produced discordant results precisely because the authors chose to ignore the quality of component trials. It is somewhat ironic that the same reviewers were considerably more thorough in their attempt to identify all relevant trials, independent of publication status or language of publication. Although the quality of component trials happened to be more important in this particular situation, the dissemination of findings from clinical trials is known to be biased, and a comprehensive literature search is an essential ingredient of high-quality reviews.

The dissemination of research findings

The dissemination of research findings is not a dichotomous event but a continuum ranging from the sharing of draft papers among colleagues, presentations at meetings, published abstracts to papers in journals that are indexed in the major bibliographic databases.[31] It has long been recognised that only a proportion of research projects ultimately reach publication in an indexed journal and thus become easily identifiable for systematic reviews.[32] Scherer *et al.*[33] showed that only about half of abstracts presented at conferences are later published in full (see Box 3.1). Dickersin and Meinert examined the fate of doctoral theses from the Department of Epidemiology at Johns Hopkins University School of Hygiene and Public Health and found that one-third of graduates had not published a single article from their thesis (see Box 3.2). Similar results were found for trainees in public health in the UK.[44] Four separate studies followed up research

Box 3.1 Full publication of results initially published as abstracts

The dissemination of research findings follows a continuum from oral report to published abstract to full publication in an indexed and accessible journal. Since the main purpose of publication is to report a study in sufficient detail to allow critical appraisal and decision-making on clinical or other questions, neither oral nor "abstract" presentations are considered sufficient to qualify as "complete" dissemination. In a 1994 systematic review, Roberta Scherer and colleagues[33] summarised the results from 11 studies[33-43] describing subsequent full publication of research initially presented in abstract or short report form. To be included, studies had to have followed published abstracts for at least two years to assess full publication. Studies followed a total of 2391 abstracts published in various fields of medicine, including vision research, anaesthesiology, perinatology, and paediatrics. The authors obtained a weighted average rate of full publication of abstracts by weighting by the square root of the total number of abstracts in each report. The average rate of full publication was 51% (95% confidence interval 45% to 57%), and individual study rates ranged from 32% to 66%. Average publication rates were similar for the two studies[33,34] that were confined to randomised controlled trials (50%). The data from eight reports that included data on cumulative rates of publication are summarised in Figure 3.2. The findings from this systematic review are reason for concern. On average, only half of health-related abstracts are published in full, which means that those performing systematic reviews should not omit abstracts from their consideration. While publication in abstract form is better than no publication at all, the format does not allow presentation of methodology or other details that allow the reader to critically assess the findings. And, since investigators change institutions and are often poor responders to mailed or telephoned request, one cannot rely on contact with authors to fill in the details if only abstracts are available. Abstracts are also difficult to locate, as most appear in conference proceedings and these are not typically indexed in bibliographic databases. This situation leads reviewers to focus their analyses mainly on data

47

from full text reports, which may lead to biased and incorrect conclusions (see main text). Scherer is currently undertaking an update of her systematic review for the Cochrane Collaboration.

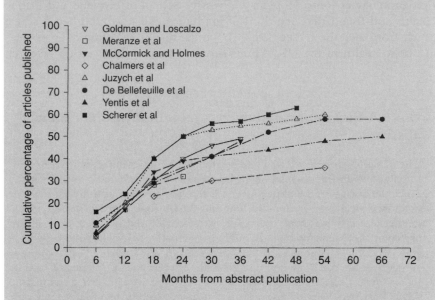

Figure 3.2 Percentages of total abstracts published over time, calculated for eight studies[33,35-40,42] that followed up research presented at meetings and conferences.

proposals approved by ethics committees or institutional review boards in Oxford,[45] Sydney,[46] and at the Johns Hopkins School of Medicine[47] and School of Hygiene and Public Health in Baltimore.[47] For each cohort of research proposals the principal investigators were contacted several years later in order to determine the publication status of each completed study. The rates of full publication as journal articles ranged from 49 to 67% (Table 3.2). Similarly, 20% of trials funded by the National Institutes of Health (NIH) and 45% of trials on HIV infection funded by the National Institute of Allergy and Infectious Diseases (NIAID) were still unpublished several years after completion.[48-50] The fact that a substantial proportion of studies remains unpublished even a decade after the study had been completed and analysed must be of concern as potentially important information remains hidden from reviewers. Making things worse, the dissemination of research findings is not a random process; rather it is strongly influenced by the nature and direction of results. Statistically

Box 3.2 Publication of doctoral dissertations

A study on publication bias, conducted at the Johns Hopkins University Schools of Medicine and Hygiene and Public Health, found that projects associated with thesis work (doctoral and master's level) were less likely than other work to be published.[47] As a follow-up to these findings, Kay Dickersin and Curtis Meinert surveyed 90 graduates of the Department of Epidemiology at Johns Hopkins University School of Hygiene and Public Health who received a doctorate in the years 1967 to 1987 and asked the graduates whether they had published their dissertation work in a full-length report. Work was considered published if it appeared in a journal or book. Eighty-one graduates responded. Overall, 67·9% of respondents published at least one full text report; 8·6% published an abstract only; and 4·9% made a presentation only. Ninety-six per cent of those who published a full-length article did so in a MEDLINE-indexed journal. Publication did not appear to be related to year the degree was granted, current employment status, type of degree (DrPH, PhD, or ScD), or sex of the student. Although numbers were small and differences statistically non-significant, several observations from the study bear testing in future studies of dissertation publication experience. Men and women students published in similar proportions (72·5% versus 60·0%, respectively). Students with women advisors, however, had better publication records compared with those with men advisors (87·5% versus 63·1%). Women students with men for advisors had the lowest publication rate of all combinations (47·6%). The publication rate observed for 1967 to 1987 epidemiology doctoral graduates (67·9%) was similar to that for Johns Hopkins School of Public Health faculty in 1980 (66%), and for British public health trainees (70%).[44] The study represents a special and small population. One might assume, however, that publication rates for graduates of Johns Hopkins are at least as high as those for graduates of other programmes. These findings imply that those performing systematic reviews must include searches of dissertations to assure comprehensive identification of all relevant studies. In addition, it is likely that "positive", statistically significant findings are selectively published from theses. In education research, it has been shown that findings published in journals were more supportive of the hypotheses favoured by the investigators than findings published in theses or dissertations.[51]

significant, "positive" results that indicate that a treatment works are more likely to be published, more likely to be published rapidly, more likely to be published in English, more likely to be published more than once, and more likely to be cited by others. When discussing these *reporting biases*, which are summarised in Table 3.3, we will denote trials with statistically significant (P<0·05) and non-significant results as trials with "positive" and "negative"

49

Table 3.2 Publication status of four cohorts of research projects approved by ethics committees or institutional review boards which had been completed and analysed at the time of follow up (adapted from Dickersin.[50])

	Johns Hopkins University, Baltimore Dickersin et al.[47]		Central Research Ethics Committee Oxford Easterbrook et al.[45]	Royal Prince Alfred Hospital, Sydney Stern and Simes[46]
	Medicine	Public Health		
Reference				
Number approved	342 (100%)	172 (100%)	285 (100%)	321 (100%)
Period of approval	1980	1980	1984–87	1979–88
Year of follow up	1988	1988	1990	1992
Published				
Full publication	230 (67%)	104 (61%)	138 (49%)	189 (59%)
Abstract only	36 (11%)	7 (4%)	69 (24%)	n.a.
Other/unclear	11 (3%)	2 (1%)	0 (0%)	0 (0%)
Unpublished	65 (19%)	59 (34%)	78 (27%)	132 (41%)

n.a. = not assessed.

Table 3.3 Reporting biases: definitions

Type of reporting bias	Definition
Publication bias	The *publication* or *non-publication* of research findings, depending on the nature and direction of the results
Time lag bias	The *rapid* or *delayed* publication of research findings, depending on the nature and direction of the results
Multiple (duplicate) publication bias	The *multiple* or *singular* publication of research findings, depending on the nature and direction of the results
Citation bias	The *citation* or *non-citation* of research findings, depending on the nature and direction of the results
Language bias	The publication of research findings *in a particular language*, depending on the nature and direction of the results
Outcome reporting bias	The *selective reporting* of some outcomes but not others, depending on the nature and direction of the results

results. However, the contribution made to the totality of the evidence by trials with non-significant results is as important as that from trials with statistically significant results.

Publication bias

In a 1979 article on "The 'file drawer problem' and tolerance for null results" Rosenthal described a gloomy scenario where "the journals are filled with the 5 per cent of the studies that show Type I errors, while the file drawers back at the lab are filled with the 95% of the studies that show nonsignificant (e.g., $P>0.05$) results."[52] The file drawer problem has long been recognised in the social sciences: a review of psychology journals found that of 294 studies published in the 1950s, 97·3% rejected the null hypothesis at the 5% level ($P<0.05$).[53] The study was recently updated and complemented with three other journals (*New England Journal of Medicine, American Journal of Epidemiology, American Journal of Public Health*).[54] Little had changed in the psychology journals (95·6% reported significant results) and a high proportion of statistically significant results (85·4%) was also found in the general medical and public health journals. Similar results have been reported for emergency medicine[55] and, more recently, in the area of alternative and complementary medicine.[56,57] It is thus possible that studies which suggest a beneficial treatment effect are published, while an equal mass of data pointing the other way remains unpublished. In this situation, a systematic review of the published trials could identify a spurious beneficial treatment effect, or miss an important adverse effect of a treatment. In

51

the field of cancer chemotherapy such *publication bias* has been demonstrated by comparing the results from studies identified in a literature search with those contained in an international trials registry[58,59] (see Box 3.3). In cardiovascular medicine, investigators who, in 1980, found an increased death rate among patients with acute myocardial infarction treated with a class 1 anti-arrhythmic dismissed it as a chance finding and did not publish

Box 3.3 A demonstration of publication bias

Studies with statistically significant results are more likely to get published than those with non-significant results. Meta-analyses that are exclusively based on published literature may therefore produce biased results. Conversely, the inclusion of a study in a trials register can be assumed not to be influenced by its results: registration generally takes place before completion of the study and the criteria that qualify for registration are exclusively based on design features. The studies enlisted in a register are therefore likely to constitute a more representative sample of all the studies that have been performed in a given area than a sample of published studies. John Simes examined this issue for trials of different cancer chemotherapies by comparing the results from meta-analysis of trials identified in a literature search and of trials registered with the International Cancer Research Data Bank.[58] As shown in Figure 3.3, an analysis restricted to 16 published clinical trials indicates that survival of patients with advanced ovarian cancer is improved with combination chemotherapy as compared to alkylating agent monotherapy (survival ratio 1·16, 95% confidence interval 1·06 to 1·27, P = 0·004). However, an analysis of all registered trials (eight published and five unpublished trials) showed only a modest benefit of combination chemotherapy which was not statistically significant (survival ratio 1·06, 95% confidence interval 0·97 to 1·15, P = 0·17) (adapted from Simes[58]).

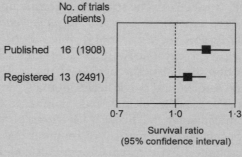

Figure 3.3

their trial at the time.[60] As discussed in Chapter 24 their findings would have contributed to a more timely detection of the increased mortality that has since become known to be associated with the use of class I anti-arrhythmic agents.[19,61]

The proportion of all hypotheses tested for which the null hypothesis is truly false is of course unknown and surveys of published results can therefore only provide indirect evidence of publication bias. Convincing, direct evidence is available from the four cohort studies of proposals submitted to ethics committees mentioned earlier,[45–47] from cohorts of trials funded by the National Institutes of Health,[48] trials submitted to licensing authorities,[62] trials conducted by multicentre trial groups in the domain of human immunodeficiency virus (HIV) infection[49] and from analyses of trial registries.[58] In all these studies publication was more likely if effects were large and statistically significant. A meta-analysis of the four ethics committee cohorts is shown in Figure 3.4. In each study possible predictors of publication were examined in multivariate analyses.[50] The odds of publication were 2·4 times greater if results were statistically significant. Other factors such as the design of the study, its methodological quality, study size and number of study centres, were not consistently associated with the probability of publication.[50] There was some evidence that the source of funding was associated with publication. We will revisit this finding later in the chapter.

Time lag bias

Studies continued to appear in print many years after approval by the ethics committee. Among proposals submitted to the Royal Prince Alfred Hospital Ethics Committee in Sydney, an estimated 85% of studies with significant results as compared to 65% of studies with null results had been published after 10 years.[46] The median time to publication was 4·8 years for studies with significant results and 8·0 years for studies with null results. Similarly, trials conducted by multicentre trial groups in the field of HIV infection in the United States appeared on average 4·2 years after the start of patient enrolment if results were statistically significant but took 6·4 years to be published if the results were negative.[49] As shown in Figure 3.5, trials with positive and negative results differed little in the time they took to complete follow-up. Rather, the time lag was attributable to differences in the time from completion to publication. These findings indicate that *time lag bias*,[49] may be introduced in systematic reviews even in situations when most or all trials will eventually be published. Trials with positive results will dominate the literature and introduce bias for several years until the negative, but equally important, results finally appear.

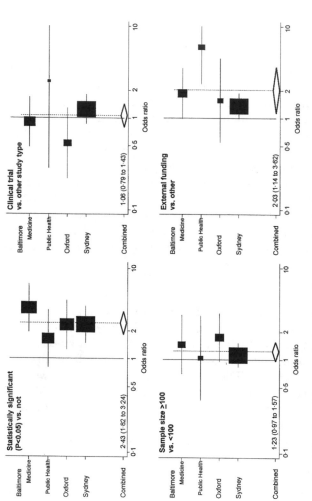

Figure 3.4 Predictors of publication: Meta-analysis of results from four cohort studies of research projects approved by ethics committees or institutional review boards. The analyses of the Johns Hopkins University, Baltimore studies[47,50] were adjusted for all variables shown, plus number of study groups and number of study centres. The Central Oxford Research Ethics Committee study[45] was adjusted for all variables shown, plus number of study groups, pilot study and rating on study importance. The Royal Prince Alfred Hospital, Sydney study[46] was adjusted for all variables shown except sample size, plus study importance for qualitative studies. Meta-analysis was by fixed effects model except for external funding in which case a random effects model was used. Adapted from Dickersin.[50]

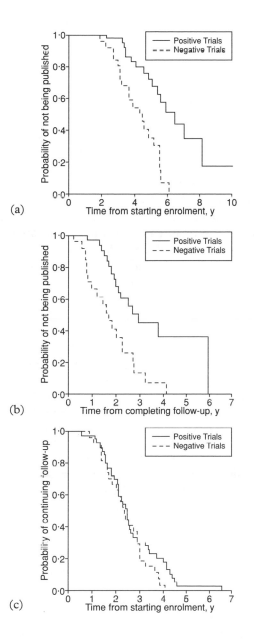

Figure 3.5 Time to publication of 66 clinical trials conducted by multicentre trial groups in HIV infection in the United States: (a) time to publication from start of enrolment, (b) time to publication from completion of follow up, and (c) time to completion from start of enrolment. Reproduced with permission from Ioannidis.[49]

Who is responsible for publication bias: authors, reviewers or editors?

Trials with negative results could remain unpublished because authors fail to write them up and submit to journals, because such trials are reviewed less favourably, or because editors simply don't want to publish negative results. The peer review process is notoriously unreliable and susceptible to subjectivity, bias and conflict of interest.[63,64] Experimental studies in which test manuscripts were submitted to reviewers or journals showed that reviewers are more likely to referee favourably if results were in accordance with their own views.[65-67] For example, when a selected group of authors was asked to review a fictitious paper on transcutaneous electrical nerve stimulation (TENS) they were influenced by their own findings and preconceptions.[67] A similar study using a fabricated trial of a herbal preparation for the treatment of claudication found that a larger, unselected group of reviewers was not influenced by the direction of the results.[68] It thus appears that although reviewers may hold strong beliefs, which will influence their assessments, there is no general bias for or against positive findings.

When authors were directly asked why they had not published their findings, the most frequent answer was that they were not interesting enough to merit publication.[45-47] Rejection of a manuscript by a journal was rarely mentioned as a reason for not publishing. Selective submission of papers by authors rather than selective recommendation by reviewers and selective acceptance by editors thus appears to be the dominant contributor to publication bias. However, that the latter does occur is illustrated by the "instructions to authors" section of one major diabetes journal, which stated that "mere confirmation of known facts will be accepted only in exceptional cases; the same applies to reports of experiments and observations having no positive outcome".[69] Such statements have disappeared from guidelines but authors may rightly be reluctant to submit studies with negative results in anticipation of rejection.

The influence of external funding and commercial interests

External funding was associated with publication independently of the statistical significance of the results. However, results were heterogeneous (Figure 3.3) and the effect appears to depend on the source of funding. Funding by government agencies was significantly associated with publication in three cohorts of proposals submitted to ethics committees[45-47] whereas pharmaceutical industry sponsored studies were less likely to be published in two studies.[45,47] Indeed, a large proportion of clinical trials submitted by drug companies to licensing authorities remain unpublished.[62,70] This is in agreement with a review of publications of clinical trials which separated them into those which were sponsored by the pharmaceutical industry and those supported by other means.[71] The results of 89% of published industry-supported trials favoured the new therapy, as compared to 61% of the other trials. Similar results have been reported for non-steroidal anti-inflammatory drug trials[72] and drug studies published in symposium proceedings.[73] The implication is that the pharmaceutical industry tends to discourage the publication of negative studies which it has funded. For example, a manuscript reporting on a trial comparing the bioequivalence of generic and brand levothyroxine products, which had failed to produce the results desired by the sponsor of the study, Boots Pharmaceuticals, was withdrawn because Boots took legal action against the university and the investigators. The actions of Boots, recounted in detail by one of the editors of *JAMA*, Drummond Rennie,[74] meant that publication of the paper[75] was delayed by about seven years. In a national survey of life-science faculty members in the United States, 20% of faculty members reported that they had experienced delays of more than six months in publication of their work and reasons for not publishing included "to delay the dissemination of undesired results".[76] Delays in publication were associated with involvement in commercialisation and academic–industry research relationship, as well as with male sex and higher academic rank of the investigator.[76]

Should unpublished data be included in systematic reviews?

Publication bias clearly is a major threat to the validity of any type of review, but particularly of unsystematic, narrative reviews. Obtaining and including data from unpublished trials appears to be the obvious way of avoiding this problem. However, the inclusion of data from unpublished studies can itself introduce bias. The trials that can be located may be an unrepresentative sample of all unpublished studies. Unpublished trials may be of lower methodological quality than published trials: a recent study of 60 meta-analyses that included published and unpublished trials found that unpublished trials were less likely to adequately conceal treatment allocation and blind outcome assessments.[77] A further problem relates to the willingness of investigators of located unpublished studies to provide data. This may depend upon the findings of the study, more favourable results being provided more readily. This could again bias the findings of a systematic review. Interestingly, when Hetherington et al.,[78] in a massive effort to obtain information about unpublished trials in perinatal medicine, approached 42 000 obstetricians and paediatricians in 18 countries they identified only 18 unpublished trials that had been completed for more than two years.

A questionnaire assessing the attitudes toward inclusion of unpublished data was sent to the authors of 150 meta-analyses and to the editors of the journals which published them.[79] Support for the use of unpublished material was evident among a clear majority (78%) of meta-analysts.

Journal editors were less convinced – only 47% felt that unpublished data should be included.[79] The condemnation of the inclusion of unpublished trial data by some editors relates to the issue that the data have not been peer reviewed. It should be kept in mind, however, that the refereeing process has not always been a successful way of ensuring that published results are valid.[63] On the other hand, meta-analyses of unpublished data from interested sources is clearly of concern. Such unchallangeable data have been produced in circumstances in which an obvious financial interest exists, as discussed in Box 3.4.

Box 3.4 The controversy over selective serotonin-reuptake inhibitors and depression

Selective serotonin-reuptake inhibitors (SSRIs) are widely used for the treatment of depression, although their clinical advantages over the much less expensive tricyclic antidepressants have not been well established. In their meta-analysis Song et al.,[80] used the drop-out rate among randomised controlled trial participants on SSRIs and those on conventional antidepressants as an indicator of therapeutic success: patients who stop taking their medication because of inefficacy or side-effects are the ones who are not benefiting, and thus the class of drug with the lower drop-out rate can be considered the one with the more favourable effects. There was little difference between SSRIs and the other, usually tricyclic, antidepressants. In response to this analysis, Lilly Industries, the manufacturers of the SSRI fluoxetine, presented a meta-analysis of 14 investigational new drug studies which they stated included every study completed by December 1990.[81] This included what were called (in the usual industry terminology) "unpublished data on file". As shown in Table 3.4, the pooled drop out rates calculated by Lilly Industries differed markedly from the literature-based analysis. Lilly Industries claimed that their analysis was not "subject to biases introduced by selective publication and literature searches" but this is difficult to assess if the trials included represent unpublished "data on file".

Table 3.4

	Trials (n)	Fluoxetine		Tricyclic antidepressant		P
		Patients (n)	Drop-out rate (%)	Patients (n)	Drop-out rate (%)	
Song et al[80]	18*	913	34·5	916	36·7	0·40
Lilly Industries[81]	14	781	36·5	788	47·5	<0·0001

* References 6,12–15,18,29,31,33–35,44,47,63,65–67,69 in Song et al.[80]

Other reporting biases

While publication bias has long been recognised[53] and much discussed, other factors can contribute to biased inclusion of studies in meta-analyses. Indeed, among published studies, the probability of identifying relevant trials for meta-analysis is also influenced by their results. These biases have received much less consideration than publication bias, but their consequences could be of equal importance.

Duplicate (multiple) publication bias

In 1987, Gøtzsche[82] found that among 244 reports of trials comparing non-steroidal anti-inflammatory drugs in rheumatoid arthritis 44 (18%) were redundant, multiple publications, which overlapped substantially with an already published article.[83] Twenty trials were published twice, 10 trials three times and one trial times.[84] The production of multiple publications from single studies can lead to bias in a number of ways.[85] Most importantly, studies with significant results are more likely to lead to multiple publications and presentations,[45] which makes it more likely that they will be located and included in a meta-analysis. The inclusion of duplicated data may therefore lead to overestimation of treatment effects, as recently demonstrated for trials of the efficacy of ondansetron to prevent postoperative nausea and vomiting[86] (Figure 3.6). It is not always obvious that

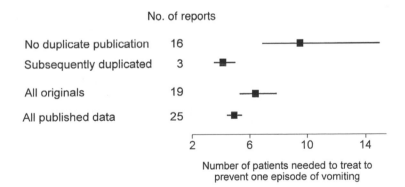

Figure 3.6 The inclusion of duplicated data may lead to overestimation of treatment effects: Tramèr et al.[86] found that of 19 trials that compared prophylactic intravenous ondansetron, data from three large multicentre trials had been duplicated in six further reports. In the 16 reports which were not duplicated, the number needed to treat (NNT) to prevent one episode of vomiting was 9·5 compared to 3·9 in the three reports that were subject to duplication. When all 19 original reports were combined, the NNT was 6·4; when original and duplicate reports were combined, a biased NNT of 4·9 was obtained.

multiple publications come from a single study, and one set of study participants may thus be included in an analysis twice. Huston and Moher[85] and, more recently, Johansen and Gøtzsche[87] vividly described the difficulties and frustration caused by redundancy and the "disaggregation" of medical research when results from a multicentre trial are presented in several publications. Indeed, it may be extremely difficult – if not impossible – for reviewers to determine whether two papers represent duplicate publications of one trial or two separate trials, since examples exist where two articles reporting the same trial do not share a single common author.[84,86]

Citation bias

The perusal of the reference lists of articles is widely used to identify additional articles that may be relevant. The problem with this approach is that the act of citing previous work is far from objective and retrieving literature by scanning reference lists may thus produce a biased sample of studies. There are many possible motivations for citing an article, ranging from decoration to showing up-to-dateness and knowledge. Brooks[88] interviewed academic authors from various faculties at the University of Iowa and asked for the reasons for citing each reference in one of the authors' recent articles. Persuasiveness, the desire to convince peers and substantiate their own point of view emerged as the most important reason for citing articles. Brooks concluded that authors advocate their own opinions and use the literature to justify their point of view: "Authors can be pictured as intellectual partisans of their own opinions, scouring the literature for justification".[88] In Gøtzsche's analysis[82] of trials of non-steroidal anti-inflammatory drugs in rheumatoid arthritis, trials demonstrating a superior effect of the new drug were more likely to be cited than trials with negative results. Similarly, trials of cholesterol lowering to prevent coronary heart disease were cited almost six times more often if they were supportive of cholesterol lowering (see also Box 3.5).[89] Overcitation of unsupportive studies can also occur. Hutchinson et al.[90] examined reviews of the effectiveness of pneumococcal vaccines and found that unsupportive trials were more likely to be cited than trials showing that vaccines worked.

Language bias

Reviews are often exclusively based on trials published in English. For example, among 36 meta-analyses reported in leading English-language general medicine journals from 1991 to 1993, 26 (72%) had restricted their search to studies reported in English.[91] Investigators working in a non-English speaking country will, however, publish some of their work in local journals.[92] It is conceivable that authors are more likely to report in an

Box 3.5 Cholesterol lowering after myocardial infarction: citation bias and biased inclusion criteria

A meta-analysis of trials of cholesterol-lowering after myocardial infarction[93] defined its inclusion criteria as those single-factor randomised trials with at least 100 participants per group, with at least three years of follow up and without the use of hormone treatment to lower cholesterol. Seven trials – one with two treatment arms – were included in this analysis. The pooled odds ratio for all-cause mortality for these trials was reported as 0·91 (95% confidence interval 0·82 to 1·02), indicating a favourable trend. One trial that met all the entry criteria was, however, not included.[94] In this study, the odds ratio for overall mortality was an unfavourable 1·60 (0·95 to 2·70). For the seven trials included in the analysis the mean annual citation count per study for the period up to five years after publication was 20; for the study which was not included it was less than one.[89] It is likely that the latter was missed precisely because it was infrequently quoted. The inclusion criteria relating to study size and length of follow up were somewhat arbitrary: the results of at least 11 other randomised secondary prevention trials of cholesterol lowering were available at the time this analysis was published (references 2a, 3a, 4a, 5a, 9a, 10a, 12a, 13a, 15a, 22a, 35a in Davey Smith *et al.*[95]). The pooled odds ratio for all-cause mortality for these trials is 1·14 (1·03 to 1·26). As shown below, the selective identification of the much-quoted supportive studies, citation bias, and biased inclusion criteria may have distorted the results of this meta-analysis.

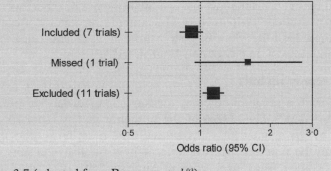

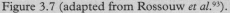

Figure 3.7 (adapted from Rossouw *et al.*[93]).

international, English-language journal if results are positive whereas negative findings are published in a local journal. This has recently been demonstrated for the German language literature.[96] When comparing pairs of articles published by the same first author, 63% of trials published in English had produced significant (P<0·05) results as compared to 35% of

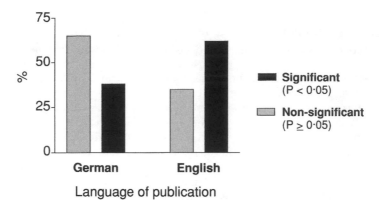

Figure 3.8 Language bias. The proportion of controlled trials with statistically significant results was higher among reports published in English. Analysis based on 40 pairs of trials published by the same author, with one trial published in English and the other in German. Adapted from Egger *et al.*[96]

trials published in German (Figure 3.8). Bias could thus be introduced in meta-analyses exclusively based on English-language reports.[91,97] On the other hand, as with unpublished trials, the lower quality of trials published in languages other than English may in fact introduce bias. Moher *et al.* compared the quality of 133 randomised controlled trials published in English with 96 trials published in French, German, Italian or Spanish.[97] They found no overall difference using a quality score but there were some differences on an item-by-item basis, indicating lower quality of trials published in languages other than English. Sterne *et al.* recently also reported lower methodological quality of non-English trials.[77]

Outcome reporting bias

In many trials a range of outcome measures is recorded but not all are always reported.[98,99] The choice of the outcome that is reported can be influenced by the results: the outcome with the most favourable findings will generally be reported. An example of how published results can be misleading comes from two separate analyses[100,101] of a double-blind placebo-controlled trial assessing the efficacy of amoxicillin in children with non-suppurative otitis media. Opposite conclusions were reached, mainly because different weight was given to the various outcome measures that were assessed in the study. This disagreement was conducted in the public arena, since it was accompanied by accusations of impropriety against the team producing the findings favourable to amoxicillin. The leader of this team had received large monetary sums, both in research grants and as personal honoraria, from the manufacturers of amoxicillin.[102] It is a good example of how reliance upon the data chosen to be presented by the investigators can lead to distortion.[103] Reporting bias may be particularly important for adverse effects. Hemminki[70] examined reports of clinical trials submitted by drug companies to licensing authorities in Finland and Sweden and found that unpublished trials gave information on adverse effects more often than published trials.

Biased inclusion criteria

Once studies have been located and data obtained, there is still potential for bias in setting the inclusion criteria for a meta-analysis. If, as is usual, the inclusion criteria are developed by an investigator familiar with the area under study, they can be influenced by knowledge of the results of the set of potential studies. Manipulating the inclusion criteria could lead to selective inclusion of positive studies and exclusion of negative studies. For example, some meta-analyses of trials of cholesterol-lowering therapy[104,105] have excluded certain studies on the grounds that the treatments used appear to have had an adverse effect that was independent of cholesterol lowering itself. These meta-analyses have, however, included trials of treatments that are likely to favourably influence risk of coronary heart disease, independent of cholesterol lowering. Clearly such an asymmetrical approach introduces the possibility of selection bias, with the criteria for inclusion into the meta-analysis being derived from the results of the studies (see Box 3.5).

The future of unbiased, systematic reviewing

Reporting biases and the inadequate quality of primary research are potentially serious problems for systematic reviews. We need both fair conduct and fair reporting of clinical trials for valid systematic reviews.[106] Important developments have taken place in the last few years which will eventually overcome the problems outlined in this chapter. Firstly, a variety of graphical and statistical methods have been developed for evaluating whether publication and related reporting biases are operating. For example, Hutton and Williamson[107] recently proposed sensitivity analyses to examine the potential impact of biased selection of outcomes. Their approach is similar to the selection models advocated by Copas[108] to examine publication bias which, along with other methods, is discussed in Chapter 11. Secondly, and more importantly, reporting biases are more likely to be prevented nowadays. Only a few years ago searching electronic databases such as MEDLINE or EMBASE was unreliable and reviewers were likely to miss substantial proportions of relevant trials. Indeed, in 1995 only 19 000 reports were readily identifiable as randomised controlled trials in the widely used MEDLINE database, although many more trials were included in that database. As discussed in Chapter 4 this situation is now much improved. The regularly updated Cochrane Controlled Trials Register contains over a quarter of a million of reports of controlled trials and is clearly the best single source of published trials for inclusion in systematic reviews and meta-analyses. The identification of ongoing and unpublished studies has also become more practicable. National research registers, a "Register of Registers", and a "metaRegister" have been set up (see Chapters 4 and 24). One of these registers, Current Controlled Trials (www.controlled-trials.com) will publish trial protocols and full reports of controlled trials. There have also been important initiatives from within the pharmaceutical industry to improve access to information on trials, and to prevent duplicate or selective publication.[109,110] Finally, an "amnesty" for unpublished trials was launched by journal editors.[111]

These initiatives mean that the identification of published and unpublished trials for systematic reviews has become an easier task, but what about the quality of the trials that are identified? There is growing consensus that the methodological quality should routinely be assessed but this is hampered by the quality of reporting, which is often inadequate. With the adoption of the CONSORT (Consolidated Standards of Reporting Trials) guidelines (see http://www.consort-statement.org) by an increasing number of journals this situation is now also improving.[112,113] Considerable progress has thus been made in a short time. This is not to say, however, that in the future unbiased, systematic reviewing will always produce conclusive answers. Many systematic reviews will continue to be based on a small number of trials of doubtful quality. These will have to be inconclusive, even if meta-analysis indicates a statistically significant effect of the intervention. Clearly demonstrating the inadequacy of existing evidence is an important objective of systematic reviews, which should serve as a stimulus for conducting the appropriate and necessary trials.

Acknowledgements

We are grateful to Fujian Song and Sally Hopewell for their help with the literature search, and to Iain Chalmers and Nicola Low for helpful comments on an earlier draft of this chapter.

1 Eysenck HJ. An exercise in mega-silliness. *Am Psychol* 1978;**33**:517.

2 Chalmers I, Enkin M, Keirse M. *Effective care during pregnancy and childbirth*. Oxford: Oxford University Press, 1989.

3 Mann C. Meta-analysis in the breech. *Science* 1990;**249**:476–80.

4 Oakes M. *Statistical inference: a commmentary for the social and behavioural sciences*. Chichester: John Wiley, 1986.

5 Boden WE. Meta-analysis in clinical trials reporting: has a tool become a weapon? *Am J Cardiol* 1992;**69**:681–6.

6 Bailar JC. The promise and problems of meta-analysis. *N Engl J Med* 1997;**337**:559–61.
7 Mann C. Richard Peto: statistician with a mission. *Science* 1990;**249**:479.
8 Chalmers TC, Frank CS, Reitman D. Minimizing the three stages of publication bias. *JAMA* 1990;**263**:1392–5.
9 Egger M, Davey Smith G, Schneider M, Minder CE. Bias in meta-analysis detected by a simple, graphical test. *BMJ* 1997;**315**:629–34.
10 LeLorier J, Grégoire G, Benhaddad A, *et al*. Discrepancies between meta-analyses and subsequent large randomized, controlled trials. *N Engl J Med* 1997;**337**:536–42.
11 Jadad AR, Cook DJ, Browman GP. A guide to interpreting discordant systematic reviews. *Can Med Ass J* 1997;**156**:1411–6.
12 Leizorovicz A, Haugh MC, Chapuis F-R, *et al*. Low molecular weight heparin in prevention of perioperative thrombosis. *BMJ* 1992;**305**:913–20.
13 Yusuf S, Collins R, MacMahon S, Peto R. Effect of intravenous nitrates on mortality in acute myocardial infarction: an overview of the randomised trials. *Lancet* 1988;**i**:1088–92.
14 Gruppo Italiano per lo Studio della Streptochinasi nell'Infarto Miocardico (GISSI). GISSI-3: effects of lisinopril and transdermal glyceryl trinitrate singly and together on 6-week mortality and ventricular function after acute myocardial infarction. *Lancet* 1994;**343**:1115–22.
15 Teo KK, Yusuf S. Role of magnesium in reducing mortality in acute myocardial infarction. A review of the evidence. *Drugs* 1993;**46**:347–59.
16 ISIS-4 Collaborative Group. ISIS-4: A randomised factorial trial assessing early oral captopril, oral mononitrate, and intravenous magnesium sulphate in 58 050 patients with suspected acute myocardial infarction. *Lancet* 1995;**345**:669–87.
17 Stuck AE, Siu AL, Wieland GD, *et al*. Comprehensive geriatric assessment: a meta-analysis of controlled trials. *Lancet* 1993;**342**:1032–6.
18 Reuben DB, Borok GM, Wolde-Tsadik G, *et al*. Randomized trial of comprehensive geriatric assessment in the care of hospitalized patients. *N Engl J Med* 1995;**332**:1345–50.
19 The Cardiac Arrhythmia Suppression Trial (CAST) Investigators. Preliminary report: effect of encainide and flecainide on mortality in a randomized trial of arrhythmia suppression after myocardial infarction. *N Engl J Med* 1989:**321**:406–12.
20 Imperiale TF, Stollenwerk Petrullis A. A meta-analysis of low-dose aspirin for the prevention of pregnancy-induced hypertensive disease. *JAMA* 1991;**266**:261–5.
21 Nurmohamed MT, Rosendaal FR, Bueller HR, *et al*. Low-molecular-weight heparin versus standard heparin in general and orthopaedic surgery: a meta-analysis. *Lancet* 1992;**340**:152–6.
22 Yusuf S. Calcium antagonists in coronary heart disease and hypertension. Time for reevaluation? *Circulation* 1995;**92**:1079–82.
23 Dunnigan MG. The problem with cholesterol. No light at the end of this tunnel? *BMJ* 1993;**306**:1355–6.
24 de Koning HJ. Assessment of nationwide cancer-screening programmes. *Lancet* 2000;**355**:80–1.
25 Altman DG. *Practical statistics for medical research*. London: Chapman and Hall, 1991.
26 Schulz KF, Chalmers I, Hayes RJ, Altman DG. Empirical evidence of bias. Dimensions of methodological quality associated with estimates of treatment effects in controlled trials. *JAMA* 1995;**273**:408–12.
27 Moher D, Pham B, Jones A, *et al*. Does quality of reports of randomised trials affect estimates of intervention efficacy reported in meta-analyses? *Lancet* 1998;**352**:609–13.
28 Jüni P, Tallon D, Egger M. "Garbage in – garbage out?" Assessment of the quality of controlled trials in meta-analyses published in leading journals. *3rd Symposium on Systematic Reviews: beyond the basics*. Oxford, 3–5 July 2000.
29 Jüni P, Witschi A, Bloch R, Egger M. The hazards of scoring the quality of clinical trial for meta-analysis. *JAMA* 1999;**282**:1054–60.
30 Lensing AW, Hirsh J. ^{125}I-fibrinogen leg scanning: reassessment of its role for the diagnosis of venous thrombosis in post-operative patients. *Thromb Haemost* 1993;**69**:2–7.
31 Smith R. What is publication? A continuum. *BMJ* 1999;**318**:142.
32 Dickersin K. The existence of publication bias and risk factors for its occurrence. *JAMA* 1990;**263**:1385–9.

33 Scherer RW, Dickersin K, Langenberg P. Full publication of results initially presented in abstracts. A meta-analysis. *JAMA* 1994;**272**:158–62.
34 Dudley HA. Surgical research: master or servant. *Am J Surg* 1978;**135**:458–60.
35 Goldman L, Loscalzo A. Fate of cardiology research originally published in abstract form. *N Engl J Med* 1980;**303**:255–9.
36 Meranze J, Ellison N, Greenhow DE. Publications resulting from anesthesia meeting abstracts. *Anesth Analg* 1982;**61**:445–8.
37 McCormick MC, Holmes JH. Publication of research presented at the pediatric meetings. Change in selection. *Am J Dis Child* 1985;**139**:122–6.
38 Chalmers I, Adams M, Dickersin K, *et al.* A cohort study of summary reports of controlled trials. *JAMA* 1990;**263**:1401–5.
39 Juzych MS, Shin DH, Coffey JB, Parrow KA, Tsai CS, Briggs KS. Pattern of publication of ophthalmic abstracts in peer-reviewed journals. *Ophthalmology* 1991;**98**:553–6.
40 De Bellefeuille C, Morrison CA, Tannock IF. The fate of abstracts submitted to a cancer meeting: factors which influence presentation and subsequent publication. *Ann Oncol* 1992;**3**:187–91.
41 Juzych MS, Shin DH, Coffey J, Juzych L, Shin D. Whatever happened to abstracts from different sections of the association for research in vision and ophthalmology? *Invest Ophthalmol Vis Sci* 1993;**34**:1879–82.
42 Yentis SM, Campbell FA, Lerman J. Publication of abstracts presented at anaesthesia meetings. *Can J Anaesth* 1993;**40**:632–4.
43 Dirk L. Incidence of acceptance, rejection, re-submission, and nonpublication of full reports of research presented at academic meetings. *Second International Conference on Peer Review.* Chicago, IL, 10 September 1993.
44 Donaldson LJ, Cresswell PA. Dissemination of the work of public health medicine trainees in peer-reviewed publications: an unfulfilled potential. *Public Health* 1996;**110**:61–3.
45 Easterbrook PJ, Berlin J, Gopalan R, Matthews DR. Publication bias in clinical research. *Lancet* 1991;**337**:867–72.
46 Stern JM, Simes RJ. Publication bias: evidence of delayed publication in a cohort study of clinical research projects. *BMJ* 1997;**315**:640–5.
47 Dickersin K, Min YL, Meinert CL. Factors influencing publication of research results. Follow-up of applications submitted to two institutional review boards. *JAMA* 1992;**267**:374–8.
48 Dickersin K, Min YL. NIH clinical trials and publication bias. *Online J Curr Clin Trials* 1993;**2**. Doc No 50:4967.
49 Ioannidis JPA. Effect of the statistical significance of results on the time to completion and publication of randomized efficacy trials. *JAMA* 1998;**279**:281–6.
50 Dickersin K. How important is publication bias? A synthesis of available data. *AIDS Educ Prev* 1997;**9**:15–21.
51 Smith ML. Publication bias and meta-analysis. *Evaluation Education* 1980;**4**:22–4.
52 Rosenthal R. The 'file drawer problem' and tolerance for null results. *Psychological Bulletin* 1979;**86**:638–641.
53 Sterling TD. Publication decisions and their possible effects on inferences drawn from tests of significance – or vice versa. *J Am Stat Assoc* 1959;**54**:30–4.
54 Sterling TD, Rosenbaum WL, Weinkam JJ. Publication decisions revisted: the effect of the outcome of statistical tests on the decision to publish and vice versa. *Am Stat* 1995;**49**:108–12.
55 Moscati R, Jehle D, Ellis D, Fiorello A, Landi M. Positive-outcome bias: comparison of emergency medicine and general medicine literatures. *Acad Emerg Med* 1994; **1**:267–71.
56 Vickers A, Goyal N, Harland R, Rees R. Do certain countries produce only positive results? A systematic review of controlled trials. *Control Clin Trials* 1998;**19**:159–66.
57 Pittler MH, Abbot NC, Harkness EF, Ernst E. Location bias in controlled clinical trials of complementary/alternative therapies. *J Clin Epidemiol* 2000;**53**:485–9.
58 Simes RJ. Confronting publication bias: a cohort design for meta-analysis. *Stat Med* 1987;**6**:11–29.
59 Simes RJ. Publication bias: the case for an international registry of clinical trials. *J Clin Oncol* 1986;**4**:1529–41.

60 Cowley AJ, Skene A, Stainer K, Hampton JR. The effect of lorcainide on arrhythmias and survival in patients with acute myocardial infarction: an example of publication bias. *Int J Cardiol* 1993;**40**:161–6.

61 Teo KK, Yusuf S, Furberg CD. Effects of prophylactic antiarrhythmic drug therapy in acute myocardial infarction. An overview of results from randomized controlled trials. *JAMA* 1993;**270**:1589–95.

62 Bardy AH. Bias in reporting clinical trials. *Br J Clin Pharmacol* 1998;**46**:147–50.

63 Godlee F, Dickersin K. Bias, subjectivity, chance, and conflict of interest in editorial decisions. In Godlee F, Jefferson T, eds. *Peer review in health sciences*, pp. 57–78. London: BMJ Books, 1999.

64 Peters DP, Ceci SJ. Peer review practices of psychology journals: the fate of published articles, submitted again. *Behav Brain Sci* 1982;**5**:187–255.

65 Mahoney MJ. Publication prejudices: An experimental study of confirmatory bias in the peer review system. *Cognit Ther Res* 1977;**1**:161–75.

66 Epstein WM. Confirmational response bias among social work journals. *Sci Tech Hum Values* 1990;**15**:9–37.

67 Ernst E, Resch KL. Reviewer bias: a blinded experimental study. *J Lab Clin Med* 1994;**124**:178–82.

68 Abbot NC, Ernst E. Publication bias: direction of outcome less important than scientific quality. *Perfusion* 1998;**11**:182–4.

69 Anon. Manuscript guideline. *Diabetologia* 1984;**25**:4A.

70 Hemminki E. Study of information submitted by drug companies to licensing authorities. *BMJ* 1980;**280**:833–6.

71 Davidson RA. Source of funding and outcome of clinical trials. *J Gen Intern Med* 1986;**1**:155–8.

72 Rochon PA, Gurwitz JH, Simms RW, *et al.* A study of manufacturer-supported trials of nonsteroidal anti-inflammatory drugs in the treatment of arthritis. *Arch Intern Med* 1994;**154**:157–63.

73 Cho M, Bero L. The quality of drug studies published in symposium proceedings. *Ann Intern Med* 1996;**124**:485–9.

74 Rennie D. Thyroid storms. *JAMA* 1997;**277**:1238–43.

75 Blumenthal BJ, Hauck WW, Gambertoglio JG, *et al.* Bioequivalence of generic and brand-name levothyroxine products in the treatment of hypothyroidism. *JAMA* 1997;**277**:1205–13.

76 Blumenthal D, Campbell EG, Anderson MS, *et al.* Withholding research results in academic life science. Evidence from a national survey of faculty. *JAMA* 1997;**277**:1224–8.

77 Sterne JAC, Bartlett C, Jüni P, Egger M. Do we need comprehensive literature searches? A study of publication and language bias in meta-analyses of controlled trials. *3rd Symposium on Systematic Reviews: beyond the basics.* Oxford, 3–5 July 2000.

78 Hetherington J, Dickersin K, Chalmers I, Meinert CL. Retrospective and prospective identification of unpublished controlled trials: lessons from a survey of obstetricians and pediatricians. *Pediatrics* 1989;**84**:374–80.

79 Cook DJ, Guyatt GH, Ryan G, *et al.* Should unpublished data be included in meta-analyses? Current convictions and controversies. *JAMA* 1993;**269**:2749–53.

80 Song F, Freemantle N, Sheldon TA, *et al.* Selective serotonin reuptake inhibitors: meta-analysis of efficacy and acceptability. *BMJ* 1993;**306**:683–7.

81 Nakielny J. Effective and acceptable treatment for depression. *BMJ* 1993;**306**:1125.

82 Gøtzsche PC. Reference bias in reports of drug trials. *BMJ* 1987;**295**:654–6.

83 Uniform requirements for manuscripts submitted to biomedical journals. International Committee of Medical Journal Editors. *JAMA* 1997;**277**:927–34.

84 Gøtzsche PC. Multiple publication of reports of drug trials. *Eur J Clin Pharmacol* 1989;**36**:429–32.

85 Huston P, Moher D. Redundancy, disaggregation, and the integrity of medical research. *Lancet* 1996;**347**:1024–6.

86 Tramèr MR, Reynolds DJM, Moore RA, McQuay HJ. Impact of covert duplicate publication on meta-analysis: a case study. *BMJ* 1997;**315**:635–40.

87 Johansen HK, Gotzsche PC. Problems in the design and reporting of trials of antifungal agents encountered during meta-analysis. *JAMA* 1999;**282**:1752–9.

67

88 Brooks TA. Private acts and public objects: an investigation of citer motivations. *J Am Soc Information Sci* 1985;**36**:223–9.

89 Ravnskov U. Cholesterol lowering trials in coronary heart disease: frequency of citation and outcome. *BMJ* 1992;**305**:15–19.

90 Hutchison BG, Oxman AD, Lloyd S. Comprehensiveness and bias in reporting clinical trials. *Can Family Physician* 1995;**41**:1356–60.

91 Grégoire G, Derderian F, LeLorier J. Selecting the language of the publications included in a meta-analysis: is there a Tower of Babel bias? *J Clin Epidemiol* 1995;**48**:159–63.

92 Dickersin K, Scherer R, Lefebvre C. Identifying relevant studies for systematic reviews. *BMJ* 1994;**309**:1286–91.

93 Rossouw JE, Lewis B, Rifkind BM. The value of lowering cholesterol after myocardial infarction. *N Engl J Med* 1990;**323**:1112–19.

94 Woodhill JM, Palmer AJ, Leelarthaepin B, McGilchrist C, Blacket RB. Low fat, low cholesterol diet in secondary prevention of coronary heart disease. *Adv Exp Med Biol* 1978;**109**:317–30.

95 Davey Smith G, Song F, Sheldon TA. Cholesterol lowering and mortality: the importance of considering initial level of risk. *BMJ* 1993;**306**:1367–73.

96 Egger M, Zellweger-Zähner T, Schneider M, Junker C, Lengeler C, Antes G. Language bias in randomised controlled trials published in English and German. *Lancet* 1997;**350**:326–9.

97 Moher D, Fortin P, Jadad AR, *et al.* Completeness of reporting of trials published in languages other than English: implications for conduct and reporting of systematic reviews. *Lancet* 1996;**347**:363–6.

98 Pocock S, Hughes MD, Lee RJ. Statistical problems in the reporting of clinical trials. A survey of three medical journals. *N Engl J Med* 1987;**317**:426–32.

99 Tannock IF. False-positive results in clinical trials: multiple significance tests and the problem of unreported comparisons. *J Natl Cancer Inst* 1996;**88**:206–7.

100 Mandel EH, Rockette HE, Bluestone CD, *et al.* Efficacy of amoxicillin with and without decongestant-antihistamine for otitis media with effusion in children. *N Engl J Med* 1987;**316**:432–7.

101 Cantekin EI, McGuire TW, Griffith TL. Antimicrobial therapy for otitits media with effusion ("secretory" otitis media). *JAMA* 1991;**266**:3309–17.

102 Rennie D. The Cantekin affair. *JAMA* 1991;**266**:3333–7.

103 Anon. Subjectivity in data analysis. *Lancet* 1991;**337**:401–2.

104 Peto R, Yusuf S, Collins R. Cholesterol-lowering trial results in their epidemiologic context. *Circulation* 1985;**72** (suppl 3):451.

105 MacMahon S. Lowering cholesterol: effects on trauma death, cancer death and total mortality. *Aust NZ J Med* 1992;**22**:580–2.

106 Rennie D. Fair conduct and fair reporting of clinical trials. *JAMA* 1999;**282**:1766–8.

107 Hutton JL, Williamson RR. Bias in meta-analysis due to outcome variable selection within studies. *Appl Stat* 2000;**49**:359–70.

108 Copas J. What works?: selectivity models and meta-analysis. *J Roy Stat Soc (Series A)* 1999;**162**:95–109.

109 Sykes R. Being a modern pharmaceutical company: involves making information available on clinical trial programmes. *BMJ* 1998;**317**:1172.

110 Wager E, Tumas JA, Field EA, Glazer NB, Schulz G, Grossman L. Improving the conduct and reporting of clinical trials. *JAMA* 2000;**283**:2788–9.

111 Smith R, Roberts I. An amnesty for unpublished trials. *BMJ* 1997;**315**:612.

112 Moher D, Jones A, LePage L, for the CONSORT Group. Does the CONSORT statement improve the quality of reports of randomized trials: a comparative before and after evaluation? *JAMA* (in press).

113 Egger M, Jüni P, Bartlett C, for the CONSORT Group. The value of flow diagrams in reports of randomized controlled trials: bibliographic study. *JAMA* (in press).

4 Identifying randomised trials

CAROL LEFEBVRE, MICHAEL J CLARKE

Summary points

- In 1993, before the establishment of the Cochrane Collaboration, only 19 000 reports of controlled trials were readily identifiable as such in MEDLINE.
- The UK Cochrane Centre and the Baltimore Cochrane Center (now the New England Cochrane Center, Providence Office) have together identified 69 000 additional reports by reading the titles and abstracts of more than 250 000 MEDLINE records.
- The UK Cochrane Centre has identified a further 33 000 reports of controlled trials by reading the titles and abstracts of approximately 100 000 EMBASE records.
- Many tens of thousands of reports of controlled trials have been identified by the handsearching of around 1700 journals within the Cochrane Collaboration.
- All of these records are now available in *The Cochrane Controlled Trials Register*.
- This work is continuing and although the task of identifying controlled trials for systematic reviews has been made much easier in the last five years, many additional sources still remain to be searched, in particular to identify unpublished or ongoing trials.

The chapter entitled "Identifying relevant studies for systematic reviews" in the first edition of this book, published in 1995, was a systematic review of evidence relating to the problems in identifying reports of controlled trials for systematic reviews of the effectiveness of health care interventions.[1] It focussed on a particular difficulty that existed at that time in identifying such studies: only 19 000 reports of randomised controlled trials were readily identifiable as trials in the widely used MEDLINE database,

For more information about the most up to date version of this chapter, please see website: <www.systematicreviews.com>.

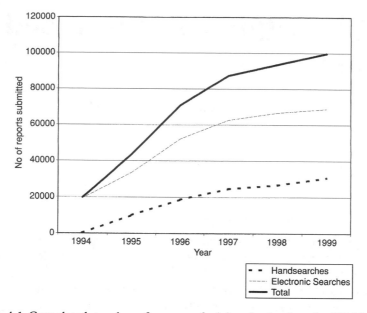

Figure 4.1 Cumulated number of reports of trials submitted to the US National Library of Medicine for re-tagging in MEDLINE since the Cochrane Collaboration began.

although records for many more reports of trials were in that database. This situation is now vastly improved. Since 1994, the Cochrane Collaboration has contributed to the re-tagging of nearly 100 000 additional records in MEDLINE (see Figure 4.1). More importantly, for those wishing to identify trials for systematic reviews, there is now a dedicated register of reports of controlled trials – *The Cochrane Controlled Trials Register* – which is updated quarterly and published electronically in *The Cochrane Library*.[2] At the end of 1999 this register contained records for more than 250 000 reports of controlled trials (see Figure 4.2) and by July 2000 this figure had risen to over 270 000. *The Cochrane Controlled Trials Register* is recognised as the best single source of published trials for inclusion in systematic reviews.[3] It includes all reports of trials which are readily identifiable as such in MEDLINE (with the permission of the database publisher, the US National Library of Medicine (NLM), see Box 4.1), tens of thousands of reports of trials from EMBASE (with the permission of the database publisher, Elsevier, see Box 4.1) and reports identified from searching journals, conference proceedings and other electronic bibliographic databases. It also contains information about unpublished and ongoing studies.

This chapter describes sources which have contributed to *The Cochrane Controlled Trials Register* and the means by which they were searched. It outlines some of the searches which should be done, in addition to a search of

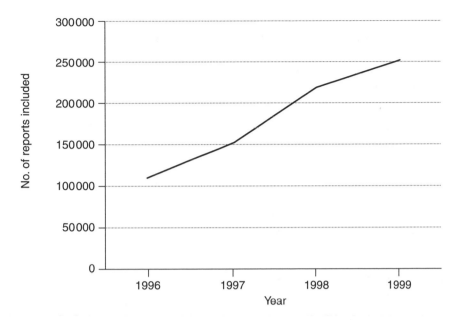

Figure 4.2 Number of reports of controlled trials included in *The Cochrane Controlled Trials Register* in the last issue of *The Cochrane Library* each year, 1996–1999.

The Cochrane Controlled Trials Register, to identify studies for systematic reviews and identifies relevant sources, including those for information about ongoing and unpublished studies. We hope that it will serve as a practical, up-to-date account of issues to keep in mind when searching for randomised controlled trials for systematic reviews.

Project to identify and re-tag reports of controlled trials in MEDLINE

Reports of controlled trials in MEDLINE are indexed with the Publication Type term RANDOMIZED-CONTROLLED-TRIAL or CONTROLLED-CLINICAL-TRIAL. These terms, however, were only introduced to the database in 1991 and 1995 respectively. Tens of thousands of reports of trials were added to MEDLINE prior to the introduction of these terms. Moreover, a 1993 study showed that over 400 reports of randomised controlled trials, which were indexed in the first six months of MEDLINE for 1993, were not tagged with the Publication Type term RANDOMIZED-CONTROLLED-TRIAL, despite its introduction two years previously. This study was presented to staff from the NLM in December 1993 at a conference organised by the US National Institutes of

Box 4.1 Key statistics for the MEDLINE and EMBASE databases

MEDLINE
- contains 10 million references to journal articles
- 400 000 references added annually
- covers 3900 journals in 40 languages
- uses specific thesaurus for indexing (MeSH)
- includes English abstracts for 76% of references
- 1966 to the present
- available online, on CD-ROM, and on the internet
- PubMed internet version available free of charge
- 52% of journals covered are published in the US
- 88% of current references are to English language articles

EMBASE
- contains 8 million references to journal articles
- 415 000 references added annually
- covers 4000 journals from 70 countries
- uses specific thesaurus for indexing (EMTREE)
- includes English abstracts for 80% of references
- 1974 to the present
- available online, on CD-ROM, and on the internet
- no free version available
- 33% of journals covered are published in North America
- 90% of current references are to English language articles
- records on database within 15 days of receipt of journal
- comprehensive inclusion of drug-related information

Health.[4] Agreement was reached that the NLM would re-tag in MEDLINE, with the appropriate Publication Type term, any reports of controlled trials which the Cochrane Collaboration was able to identify. As a consequence, work began in 1994 to identify reports of controlled trials in MEDLINE, which were not already tagged as either RANDOMIZED-CONTROLLED-TRIAL or CONTROLLED-CLINICAL-TRIAL. This made use of a highly sensitive search strategy, consisting of three phases, which had been designed by one of the authors (CL)[5] (see Table 4.1). It was based on knowledge of the NLM Medical Subject Headings (MeSH) and recommendations from clinicians and others who had tried to identify reports of controlled trials in several clinical areas.

Since 1994, phases I and II of this search strategy have been run against MEDLINE for the period 1966–1997. (See below for discussion of phase

III, the final phase of the search strategy). This work was conducted by the UK Cochrane Centre and the Baltimore Cochrane Center/New England Cochrane Center, Providence Office. In total, after excluding reports already tagged as RANDOMIZED-CONTROLLED-TRIAL or CON-TROLLED-CLINICAL-TRIAL, over 250 000 reports were downloaded and printed. The titles and abstracts were read and those records which were judged, on the basis of their title and abstract, to be definitely or possibly a report of a randomised controlled trial or a quasi-randomised

Table 4.1 Highly sensitive search strategy for identifying reports of randomised controlled trials in MEDLINE (SilverPlatter version).

Phase I	1	RANDOMIZED-CONTROLLED-TRIAL in PT
	2	CONTROLLED-CLINICAL-TRIAL in PT
	3	RANDOMIZED-CONTROLLED-TRIALS
	4	RANDOM-ALLOCATION
	5	DOUBLE-BLIND-METHOD
	6	SINGLE-BLIND-METHOD
	7	#1 or #2 or #3 or #4 or #5 or #6
	8	TG=ANIMAL not (TG=HUMAN and TG=ANIMAL)
	9	#7 not #8
Phase II	10	CLINICAL-TRIAL in PT
	11	explode CLINICAL-TRIALS
	12	(clin* near trial*) in TI
	13	(clin* near trial*) in AB
	14	(singl* or doubl* or trebl* or tripl*) near (blind* or mask*)
	15	(#14 in TI) or (#14 in AB)
	16	PLACEBOS
	17	placebo* in TI
	18	placebo* in AB
	19	random* in TI
	20	random* in AB
	21	RESEARCH-DESIGN
	22	#10 or #11 or #12 or #13 or #15 or #16 or #17 or #18 or #19 or #20 or #21
	23	TG=ANIMAL not (TG=HUMAN and TG=ANIMAL)
	24	#22 not (#23 or #9)
Phase III	25	TG=COMPARATIVE-STUDY
	26	explode EVALUATION-STUDIES
	27	FOLLOW-UP-STUDIES
	28	PROSPECTIVE-STUDIES
	29	control* or prospectiv* or volunteer*
	30	(#29 in TI) or (#29 in AB)
	31	#25 or #26 or #27 or #28 or #30
	32	TG=ANIMAL not (TG=HUMAN and TG=ANIMAL)
	33	#31 not (#32 or #24 or #9)
	34	#9 or #24 or #33

Upper case denotes controlled vocabulary and lower case denotes free-text terms. See http://www.cochrane.org/cochrane/hbappend.htm for OVID version. A PubMed version has also been prepared.[6]

73

controlled trial were submitted to the NLM for re-tagging with the appropriate Publication Types in MEDLINE. Definitions for randomised controlled trials and quasi-randomised controlled trials within the Cochrane Collaboration context were agreed in November 1992 (see Box 4.2). Each record submitted for re-tagging in this way was subject to strict quality control procedures. For example, each of the 40 000 records submitted by the UK Cochrane Centre was checked by one of the authors (MC). To date, this exercise has identified nearly 70 000 previously untagged reports of trials in MEDLINE. These reports are included in *The Cochrane Controlled Trials Register* and have been re-tagged in MEDLINE so that they are, therefore, now readily identifiable. The New England Cochrane Center, Providence Office, is continuing this work for the period after 1997, to ensure that all reports of controlled trials in MEDLINE which are identifiable as such from their titles or abstracts, but not already tagged RANDOMIZED-CONTROLLED-TRIAL or CONTROLLED-CLINICAL-TRIAL by the NLM indexers, can be included in *The Cochrane Controlled Trials Register* and re-tagged appropriately in MEDLINE.

The UK Cochrane Centre conducted a pilot study in 1994 on the third and final phase of the highly sensitive search strategy (see Table 4.1). This concluded that these terms were too broad to warrant including them in the project, with the possible exception of the term volunteer*, which was considered adequately precise to warrant its inclusion when the strategy is revised. This revision will follow ongoing research to ascertain how to optimise highly sensitive search strategies in MEDLINE, so as to increase their sensitivity and precision, by textual analysis of a "gold-standard" set of studies previously identified by handsearching.[7] This research is likely to help identify terms which might be added to the strategy and terms which might be removed.

Project to identify reports of controlled trials in EMBASE

It became clear early in the development of the Cochrane Collaboration that it was even more difficult to identify reports of controlled trials in EMBASE than it was in MEDLINE. In January 1993, shortly after the UK Cochrane Centre opened, a meeting was convened to address these issues and to explore some possible solutions. A representative from Elsevier, the producers of EMBASE, confirmed that although the EMBASE thesaurus (EMTREE) contained terms for clinical trials in general, it had no specific term for indexing reports of randomised controlled trials. Elsevier was persuaded of the importance of accurate indexing of clinical trials and of the necessity to differentiate randomised controlled trials from other

Box 4.2 Cochrane definition of randomised and quasi-randomised controlled trials

Criteria for registering studies with the Cochrane Collaboration's International Register of Published RCTs of Health Care

Overarching principle. The highest possible proportion of all reports of RCTs of health care should be included in the International Register. Thus, those searching the literature to identify trials should give reports the benefit of any doubts. Publications which simply mention the possibility of undertaking an RCT should not be included, however.

Eligibility criteria. Reviewers will decide whether to include a particular report in a review. The aim of the Register is to provide reviewers with all possible trials they may wish to include in a review, not to decide whether a report is worthy or relevant for inclusion.

Relevant reports are reports published in any year, of studies comparing at least two forms of health care (medical treatment, medical education, diagnostic tests or techniques, a preventive intervention, etc.) where the study is on either living humans or parts of their body or human parts that will be replaced in living humans (e.g. donor kidneys). Studies on cadavers, extracted teeth, cell lines, etc. are not relevant.

Studies are eligible for inclusion in the Register if allocation to the intervention was random or intended-to-be-random (e.g. alternation), or if a concurrent control group was used in the trial and it is possible that a random or intended-to-be-random method was used to allocate participants to the study groups. Judgements as to the quality of the methods used or whether the authors actually did what they claimed should not be used to decide eligibility for inclusion in the Register.

A trial should thus be included in the Register if, on the basis of the best available information, it is judged that:

- the individuals (or other units) followed in the trial were definitely or possibly assigned prospectively to one of two (or more) alternative forms of health care using:
  - random allocation or
  - some quasi-random method of allocation (such as alternation, date of birth, or case record number).

In addition:

- If one or more outcomes were assessed using "double blinding" or "double masking" such that neither the participant/patient nor the assessor was aware of the intervention received, but randomisation is not mentioned explicitly in the text, a trial should be included.
- Crossover trials, in which patients have been assigned to the first intervention using random or quasi-random allocation, should be included.
- Reports of trials dealing only with animals should not be included.
- Units of randomisation may be individuals, groups (such as communities or hospitals), organs (such as eyes) or other parts of the body (such as teeth).
- A report of a randomised trial should be included even when no results are presented or when results are limited to the analyses of baseline variables.
- Articles describing an intended or ongoing trial or commenting on a trial (such as in an editorial) should be brought to the attention of the Baltimore Cochrane Center but are not eligible for inclusion in the International Register of Published RCTs.

clinical trials. In January 1994, they announced that reports of trials would be more thoroughly indexed in future and introduced a new indexing term specifically for randomised controlled trials.[8]

In 1997, a project was started to identify reports of trials in EMBASE, funded by the Anglia and Oxford Research and Development Programme of the National Health Service in the UK. This project drew on a highly sensitive search strategy, which was developed in 1996, based on the assessment of the EMBASE records for reports of controlled trials identified by handsearching the *BMJ* (*British Medical Journal*) and the *Lancet*.[9] The records identified by the handsearching can be regarded only as a "quasi gold-standard" of known trials, since the handsearching covered only two journals (both of which were English-language general health care journals) and just two years from these journals (1990 and 1994). Consequently, the set contained a relatively small number of studies (384). In contrast, EMBASE indexes a large number of non-English language journals, particularly journals published in other European languages. It is also strong in its coverage of pharmaceutical journals and indexes reports back to 1974. It is, therefore, uncertain to what extent findings based on this study might be generalisable to all reports of randomised controlled trials in EMBASE. The analysis involved assessing how frequently certain free-text terms occurred in the titles or abstracts of the reports in the "quasi gold-standard" and how frequently certain EMTREE terms were used to index these reports. The frequency of these terms within this data set was compared with their frequency across the entire EMBASE database to estimate their sensitivity and precision as means of identifying reports of controlled trials.

These estimates were used to create a hierarchy of terms for identifying reports of trials in EMBASE. As many reports of controlled trials had already been identified through the MEDLINE project, the latter were removed from the result sets of the EMBASE search. To date, approximately 100 000 records from the period 1974 to 1998 not already coded as trials in MEDLINE have been downloaded, using the following search terms: random*, crossover*, cross-over*, factorial*, and placebo*. The titles and abstracts of these records have been read and 33 000 reports of controlled trials have been identified and added to *The Cochrane Controlled Trials Register*.[10] Details have also been sent to Elsevier to enable them to re-tag the relevant records in EMBASE.

Other databases already searched for reports of controlled trials

Other databases have also been searched by the UK Cochrane Centre to identify studies for Cochrane reviews. These include Criminal Justice

Abstracts (1968–1996), the Educational Resources Information Center database (ERIC) (1966–1998), and Sociological Abstracts (1974–1996). The methods involved were similar to those employed for the MEDLINE project. Search strategies were used which included both free-text terms and terms from the thesaurus, where applicable. Records were then processed as for the MEDLINE project. Approximately 1500 reports of controlled trials of health care interventions have been identified from these databases and included in *The Cochrane Controlled Trials Register* with permission of the database publishers, where appropriate.

Identifying reports of controlled trials by handsearching

Despite the considerable efforts described above to identify reports of controlled trials by searching electronic databases, it is still necessary to "handsearch" journals to identify additional reports. For example, MEDLINE and EMBASE only go back to 1966 and 1974 respectively and despite the efforts by NLM to extend MEDLINE back further in time, many earlier reports will never be indexed. Similarly, not all journals published in more recent years are indexed in electronic databases and even for those that are, it is not always possible to tell from the electronic record that the report is a trial.[11,12] Consequently, around the world, approximately 1700 journals have been or are currently being "handsearched" within the Cochrane Collaboration, to identify reports of controlled trials. This activity is co-ordinated by the New England Cochrane Center, Providence Office, which maintains a "Master List of Journals Being Searched" (see Table 4.2 for website). "Handsearching" requires a trained person to check a journal from cover to cover, reading each article until they are satisfied whether or not it is definitely or possibly a report of a randomised controlled trial or a quasi-randomised controlled trial. The principle within the Cochrane Collaboration is that journals are handsearched for *all* reports of controlled trials, irrespective of whether the particular trial is of immediate interest to the individual or group handsearching the journal. In this way, each journal is searched once only, to minimise duplication of effort and maximise the number of controlled trials identified. A recent study confirmed that, although handsearchers will miss some trials, it is generally more efficient for individuals to search different journals than to repeat searches in the same journals.[13] Reports identified by handsearching are submitted to the New England Cochrane Center, Providence Office, for inclusion in *The Cochrane Controlled Trials Register* and, if appropriate, re-tagging in MEDLINE.

The NLM has supported handsearching of American general health care journals. Eighteen journals have been searched and will continue to be

77

Table 4.2 Useful web sites and e-mail addresses (in the order in which they are referred to in the text).

Master list of journals being searched by the Cochrane Collaboration	http://www.cochrane.org/srch.htm
Contact details for the New England Cochrane Center, Providence Office	cochrane@brown.edu
British Library web site, includes British Library Index to Conference Proceedings with information on more than 350 000 conferences world-wide	http://www.bl.uk
Register of trial registers, published as an appendix in *The Cochrane Reviewers' Handbook*	http://www.cochrane.org/cochrane/hbook.htm
UK National Research Register of ongoing health research, which also contains the UK Medical Research Council's Clinical Trials Register, together with details of systematic reviews in progress – updated quarterly	http://www.doh.gov.uk/research/nrr.htm
ClinicalTrials.gov, contains information on controlled trials in the US	http://clinicaltrials.gov
Computer Retrieval of Information on Scientific Projects (CRISP) database, contains information on controlled trials being funded or supported by the US Department of Health and Human Services	http://www-commons.cit.nih.gov/crisp
Glaxo Wellcome register of clinical trials	http://ctr.glaxowellcome.co.uk
Meta-register of controlled trials set up by the publisher Current Science, includes trials from the UK National Research Register, the Medical Editors' Trials Amnesty, the UK Medical Research Council's Clinical Trials Register, and Schering Health Care Ltd and links to other trials registers	http://www.controlled-trials.com
Cancer-specific registers of controlled trials (UK and USA)	http://www.ctu.mrc.ac.uk/ukccr http://cancernet.nci.nih.gov
PubMed – MEDLINE database available free of charge	http://www.ncbi.nlm.nih.gov/PubMed.

searched prospectively. The European Commission has funded two projects under the European Union Biomedical and Health Research Programme (BIOMED), to identify reports of controlled trials in general health care journals published in Western Europe (contract number BMH1-CT94-1289) and in specialised health care journals published in Western Europe (contract number BMH4-CT98-3803). These projects involve Cochrane Centre partners in Denmark, France, Germany, Italy, the Netherlands, Spain, and the UK. During the first project (1994–1997), 120 general health care journals from 18 countries were handsearched, many back to 1948 or to the earliest issue of the journal, if this was more recent, representing a total of 2740 journal years searched.[14] Approximately 22 000 reports of controlled trials were identified. Of these, over 17 000 reports were not previously readily identifiable as trials in MEDLINE – 7000 because the journals had not been indexed in MEDLINE or because they had been published before 1966 when MEDLINE began. The second three-year project started in July 1998. Interim results at the end of June 2000 indicated that 186 specialised health care journals from 12 countries had been or were being handsearched, many back to 1948 as above, representing a total of 3586 journal years searched. Approximately 23 000 reports of controlled trials had been identified. Of these, over 17 000 reports were not previously readily identifiable as trials in MEDLINE.

Whilst it is the responsibility of all Cochrane Centres to handsearch general health care journals within their geographical area of responsibility, it is the responsibility of Cochrane Collaborative Review Groups and Cochrane Fields to search the specialised journals and other publications (including conference proceedings) which fall within their scope and they have already made much progress. This process is described in the Collaborative Review Groups' and Fields' modules, available in *The Cochrane Library*.[15] Their specialized registers of studies for possible inclusion in Cochrane reviews are incorporated in *The Cochrane Controlled Trials Register*, also available in *The Cochrane Library*.

Recommended supplementary searches of databases already searched or in progress

Although *The Cochrane Controlled Trials Register* should usually be the first source searched when looking for reports of randomised controlled trials, there are circumstances under which other databases, including MEDLINE and EMBASE, should still be searched by those wishing to identify controlled trials for inclusion in systematic reviews.

For those prepared to obtain the *full article* of references retrieved to determine the relevance of a study and not just rely on the title and abstract in MEDLINE, (as was done in the re-tagging project), the highly sensitive search strategy (see Table 4.1) may be used in conjunction with appropriate Medical Subject Heading (MeSH) and free-text topic terms. Obtaining the full report of records not already coded as RANDOMIZED-CONTROLLED-TRIAL or CONTROLLED-CLINICAL-TRIAL is likely to identify some additional reports of controlled trials, where it will be clear from the body of the article that it is a report of a trial (but not from the title or abstract). In addition, MEDLINE should be searched for the period since the last re-tagging search was conducted to the current date (i.e. 1998 onwards at the time of writing). Up-to-date information on this can be obtained from the New England Cochrane Center, Providence Office (see Table 4.2). The top two phases of the highly sensitive search strategy should be used, in conjunction with the appropriate Medical Subject Heading (MeSH) and free-text topic terms.

As noted above, a study of the third phase of the highly sensitive search strategy indicated that it would not be worth pursuing across the entire MEDLINE database but individual reviewers may consider it worth combining some of the terms in this phase, particularly the free-text term volunteer*, with appropriate MeSH and free-text topic terms. A recent study evaluated the highly sensitive search strategy against the Publication Type term RANDOMIZED-CONTROLLED-TRIAL for identifying reports of trials in hypertension.[16] This concluded that, in hypertension, RANDOMIZED-CONTROLLED-TRIAL was not sufficiently sensitive, whereas all three phases of the search strategy were, with the exception of the final phase when applied to the years 1991–1996.

Terms not currently in the highly sensitive search strategy but which might be included in an updated version, can also be considered by searchers. Such terms include "crossover" and "versus" and MeSH terms which were introduced after the strategy was devised, for example CROSS-OVER-STUDIES. A recent study has shown that the phrase "latin square", a particular type of study design, might also be included.[6] Finally, reviewers and those conducting searches on their behalf may wish to search MEDLINE and other bibliographic databases for a specific topic or subject, such as a drug name or a technique, without limiting their search by any study design terms. This might identify background material but also additional trials not identifiable through any of the methods listed above.

The project involving the searching and re-coding of EMBASE is ongoing but searchers may wish to search EMBASE and exclude the terms already assessed within the project, as reports identifiable using these terms are already included in *The Cochrane Controlled Trials Register*. To date (July 2000), these terms are random*, factorial*, crossover*, cross-over*, and placebo* but searchers should bear in mind that only titles and abstracts were read and the advice given above in respect of re-searching databases and retrieving and checking the *full article* also applies.

The Australasian Cochrane Centre is undertaking a systematic search of the Australasian Medical Index database for reports of trials. The Brazilian Cochrane Centre is undertaking a similar search for trials in the Latin American and Caribbean Health Sciences Literature database (LILACS), building on work undertaken by Karla Soares on behalf of the Cochrane Schizophrenia Group. The Chinese Cochrane Centre is conducting a similar project on their national bibliographic health care database (Chinese Biomedical Retrieval Literature System). The Japanese informal network for the Cochrane Collaboration is using the Japan Information Centre of Science and Technology File on Science, Technology and Medicine in Japan (JICST-E) to identify reports of trials published in Japan.

Searches of additional databases not currently being searched for *The Cochrane Controlled Trials Register*

The authors are not aware of any bibliographic databases, other than those described above, which have been or are being searched systematically for all reports of controlled trials and these reports of trials being transferred to *The Cochrane Controlled Trials Register* (with the permission of the database producers). Other databases, therefore, need to be considered when aiming to identify as many relevant studies as possible for systematic reviews. Directories of health care databases can be used to assist in the selection of appropriate databases.[17]

Investigations are under way to identify additional databases and other electronic sources which might prove to be rich sources of reports of trials. Meanwhile, reviewers may wish to consider the following databases amongst others for identifying additional studies: Allied and Alternative Medicine (AMED), Biological Abstracts (BIOSIS), CAB Health, Cumulative Index to Nursing and Allied Health Literature (CINAHL), Derwent Drug File, the NLM's pre-1966 equivalent of MEDLINE, Psychological Abstracts (PsycINFO), and Science Citation Index/Current Contents. Each of the above databases will be evaluated to ascertain whether it would be worth doing a MEDLINE/EMBASE-type project globally on behalf of the Cochrane Collaboration as a whole and reviewers more widely. In addition, because a particularly high proportion of controlled trials are only published as meeting abstracts and these trials may have importantly different results from those also published later as full papers,[18] "grey literature" databases are another important source. Thus, searches of products such as the British Library's "Inside" database and the System for Information on Grey Literature in Europe (SIGLE)

81

should also be considered. In addition, patents databases will be investigated. Information about access to and costs of the above databases should be available from your local health care librarian. The publication of journals in full-text electronically might also represent an important new means of identifying trials. Finally, Collaborative Review Groups and Fields within the Cochrane Collaboration are encouraged to identify specialised bibliographic databases which might prove useful sources of trials within their respective areas of health care.

Supplementary searches of journals and conference proceedings

As described above, approximately 1700 journals have been, or are being, searched within the Cochrane Collaboration. Any journal not already searched but likely to contain a high yield of reports of controlled trials in the area of the systematic review might need to be searched. A recent study identified a number of high-yield MEDLINE journals not currently being searched.[19] Alternatively, reviewers may wish to prioritise those journals or parts of journals that are not indexed in MEDLINE or EMBASE.

A recent study assessed the additional yield if a journal were to be searched by more than one person.[13] This study showed that it might occasionally be better to have a very high-yield journal searched by more than one person, rather than have the second person search an additional lower-yield journal. The same would apply to conference proceedings. Potentially relevant conference proceedings can be identified from indexes to conference proceedings such as the "British Library Index to Conference Proceedings", which contains information on more than 350 000 conferences world-wide, irrespective of subject or language. This index can be accessed through the British Library web site (see Table 4.2) by selecting "Online" then "OPAC '97". This website claims that the British Library holds the world's largest collection of conference proceedings. Alternative sources including "grey literature" databases such as SIGLE and discussion with clinicians in the appropriate specialty may also be productive.

Identifying ongoing and/or unpublished studies

Whilst it is difficult to identify published studies, identifying ongoing and/or unpublished studies presents even more of a challenge. If a review is to minimise bias, it is important that unpublished studies are identified (for a discussion of publication bias and related biases see Chapter 11). The least biased way to identify studies is through the registration of ongoing research. Registers of ongoing trials have existed in a number of areas for some years. A "Register of Registers" was set up by Kay Dickersin and colleagues to provide information about these registers, including contact and content information.[20] This is published as an appendix in *The Cochrane Reviewers' Handbook* (see Table 4.2).

There are a number of national initiatives to register ongoing studies. In the UK, the National Research Register aims to hold information on all ongoing research projects funded by, or otherwise of interest to, the National Health Service. Issue 1 2000 contained information on 54 000 research projects. This data set was only partially indexed at the time of publication but of those records indexed, 3159 were indexed as controlled trials (1106 ongoing and 2053 recently completed studies). When indexing is completed, it is expected that the Register will contain more than 10 000 studies indexed as trials. The National Research Register also contains the UK Medical Research Council's Clinical Trials Register, together with details of systematic reviews in progress, collected by the UK National Health Service Centre for Reviews and Dissemination. The National Research Register is updated quarterly and is available on CD-ROM and on the internet (see Table 4.2).

In the US, the Food and Drug Administration Modernization Act (1997) mandated the establishment of a database of government and privately funded clinical trials information for serious or life-threatening conditions. The goal is to provide patients, families, and physicians with easy access to information about clinical research studies and to provide links to additional online health resources. Drug companies will be required by this legislation to submit information on their ongoing trials. In September 1998, it was announced that the NLM would develop this database, in close collaboration with the National Institutes of Health (NIH). The database, ClinicalTrials.gov, was launched in February 2000 and to date (July 2000) contained approximately 5000 clinical trials funded primarily by the NIH (see Table 4.2). Information on controlled trials being funded or supported by the US Department of Health and Human Services is available through the Computer Retrieval of Information on Scientific Projects (CRISP) database (see Table 4.2). This includes not only trials funded by the NIH but also by the Agency for Healthcare Research and Quality, the Centers for Disease Control and Prevention, and the Food and Drug Administration. In May 1999, the database contained 60 000 records, of which over 5000 were indexed as clinical trials.

In Spain, a register of trials known as "Base de Datos Española de Ensayos Clínicos" (Spanish Database of Clinical Trials) was first set up in 1982, following legislation passed in 1978 regulating the conduct of clinical trials. This register has been maintained and updated intermittently since then. The recently appointed Agencia Española del Medicamento (Spanish Drug Agency) is assuming responsibility for updating and maintaining this register.

An international initiative to identify completed trials which have never reached publication was launched in September 1997, when many medical journal editors responded to a proposal by Ian Roberts to announce an amnesty for unpublished trials. Co-ordinated editorials appeared in nearly 100 medical journals to announce The Medical Editors' Trials Amnesty (META), along with an unreported trial registration form to collect a minimum amount of information on each trial.[21] To date, information has been collected on approximately 150 unpublished controlled trials. This is available in *The Cochrane Controlled Trials Register* and the Current Science *meta*Register of Controlled Trials (see below).

There have also been important initiatives from within the pharmaceutical industry to improve access to information on trials. In 1996, Schering Healthcare Ltd, the UK division of the multinational drug company, agreed with the UK Cochrane Centre that they would provide information on all phase III randomised controlled trials with which they had been involved over the past five years (both ongoing and completed), irrespective of publication status. Information on 32 such studies has been made available in *The Cochrane Controlled Trials Register* since January 1997.

Subsequently, in November 1997, Glaxo Wellcome announced that it wished to work with the UK Cochrane Centre to ensure that information on their ongoing trials world-wide was made publicly available.[22] Glaxo Wellcome has since created a Clinical Trials Register which will provide a comprehensive record of all randomised phase II, III and IV studies conducted on their newly registered medicines. The register is still evolving but is currently available to all health care professionals and researchers and contained information on approximately 100 controlled trials in July 2000 (see Table 4.2).

Since the Glaxo Wellcome announcement and subsequent discussions, the publisher Current Science set up a *meta*Register of Controlled Trials (*m*RCT) (see Table 4.2). This was launched in early 1999 and, in July 2000, contained details of more than 6000 trials drawn from 15 separate sources including: the UK National Research Register, the UK Medical Research Council and the NIH ClinicalTrials.gov register. It is hoped that other organisations and individuals will add information about their ongoing trials. Current Science also provides a Controlled Trials Links Register giving direct internet access to an additional 100 trials registers and this is also available on its web site.

Subject-specific registers of controlled trials have been developed and maintained over the years. Examples include the register developed by the UK Co-ordinating Committee on Cancer Research (UKCCCR) and Physicians' Data Query (a US register of controlled trials in cancer).

Conclusions

The inclusion of all relevant studies in systematic reviews is crucial to avoid bias and maximise precision. In this chapter we have discussed the sources, summarised in Box 4.3, which should be searched to identify controlled trials for systematic reviews. Various initiatives, many within the Cochrane Collaboration, mean that the identification of published and unpublished trials for systematic reviews has become an easier task. Ongoing and planned developments will continue to improve the situation.

Box 4.3 Sources to be searched to identify randomised trials for systematic reviews

- *The Cochrane Controlled Trials Register*
- MEDLINE and EMBASE (with the provisos outlined in the text)
- other databases as appropriate
- journals
- conference proceedings
- reference lists
- sources of ongoing and/or unpublished studies

Acknowledgements

The authors would like to acknowledge the following for their contribution to the development of *The Cochrane Controlled Trials Register* and/or their comments on earlier versions of this manuscript: Iain Chalmers, Kay Dickersin, Jeanette Downing-Park, Julie Glanville, Anne Lusher, Eric Manheimer, Steve McDonald, Nina Paul, Karen Robinson, Lois Sims, and Mark Starr. We should like to thank the Trials Search Co-ordinators, Review Group Co-ordinators, and others within the Cochrane Collaboration; the many handsearchers and data processors; those who provided information for this chapter; and those who have provided financial support for the identification of trials. We should also like to thank Katherine Webster and Sarah White for assistance with the preparation of this manuscript and Anne Lusher for assistance with checking the proofs.

Disclaimer

The views expressed in this chapter represent those of the authors and are not necessarily the views or the official policy of the Cochrane Collaboration.

1 Dickersin K, Scherer R, Lefebvre C. Identifying relevant studies for systematic reviews. In: Chalmers I, Altman DG, eds. *Systematic reviews*. London: BMJ Publications, 1995.
2 The Cochrane Controlled Trials Register. In: *The Cochrane Library*. Oxford: Update Software.
3 Egger M, Smith GD. Bias in location and selection of studies. *BMJ* 1998;**316**:61–6.
4 Lefebvre C. Search strategies for finding RCTs in MEDLINE. In: *An evidence-based health care system: the case for clinical trials registries*. Bethesda, MD: National Institutes of Health, Office of Medical Applications of Research, 1994:23–8.
5 Dickersin K, Scherer R, Lefebvre C. Identifying relevant studies for systematic reviews. *BMJ* 1994;**309**:1286–91.
6 Robinson KA, Hinegardner PG, Lansing P. Development of an optimal search strategy for the retrieval of controlled trials using PubMed. *Proc 6th Int Cochrane Colloquium* 1998;**85**:poster B13.
7 Boynton J, Glanville J, McDaid D, Lefebvre C. Identifying systematic reviews in MEDLINE: developing an objective approach to search strategy design. *J Informat Sci* 1998;**24**:137–57.
8 Indexing clinical trials in EMBASE. Profile: *Excerpta Medica Newsl* 1994;**11**(1):2.
9 Lefebvre C, McDonald S. Development of a sensitive search strategy for reports of randomised controlled trials in EMBASE. *Proc 4th Int Cochrane Colloquium* 1996;A-28:abstract 33.
10 Paul N, Lefebvre C. Reports of controlled trials in EMBASE: an important contribution to the Cochrane Controlled Trials Register. *Proc 6th Int Cochrane Colloquium* 1998;**85**:poster B14.
11 McDonald S, Clarke M, Lefebvre C. Should we continue to handsearch MEDLINE-indexed journals prospectively?: some up-to-date empirical evidence. *Proc 5th Ann Cochrane Colloquium* 1997;**296**:poster 294.
12 Reynolds M, Robinson K, Dickersin K. The sensitivity and yield of hand and MEDLINE searching for controlled clinical trials in US general medical journals. *Controlled Clin Trials* 1997;**18**:189S.
13 Clarke M, Westby M, McDonald S, Lefebvre C. How many handsearchers does it take to change a light-bulb – or to find all of the randomised trials? *Proc 2nd Symp Systematic Reviews: beyond the basics* 1999;**43**:poster 6.
14 McDonald S, Lefebvre C, on behalf of the BIOMED General Health Care Journals Project Group. Collaboration to identify controlled trials in general health care journals in Europe. *Proc 5th Ann Cochrane Colloquium* 1997;**288**:poster 277.
15 *The Cochrane Library*. Oxford: Update Software.
16 Brand M, Gonzalez J, Aguilar C. Identifying RCTs in MEDLINE by publication type and through the Cochrane Strategy: the case in hypertension. *Proc 6th Int Cochrane Colloquium* 1988;**89**:poster B22.
17 Armstrong CJ, ed. *World databases in medicine* (2 vols). London: Bowker-Saur, 1993.
18 Scherer RW, Dickersin K, Langenberg P. Full publication of results initially presented in abstracts. A meta-analysis. *JAMA* 1994;**272**:158–62.
19 Villanueva EVS, Robinson K, Dickersin K. Descriptive analysis of current levels of Cochrane Collaboration handsearch activities. *Proc 6th Int Cochrane Colloquium* 1998;**84**:poster B12.
20 Dickersin K. Research registers. In: Cooper H, Hedges LV, eds. *The handbook of research synthesis*. New York: Russell Sage Foundation, 1994.
21 Smith R, Roberts I. An amnesty for unpublished trials. *BMJ* 1997;**315**:622.
22 Sykes, R. Being a modern pharmaceutical company. *BMJ* 1998;**317**:1172.

5 Assessing the quality of randomised controlled trials

PETER JÜNI, DOUGLAS G ALTMAN, MATTHIAS EGGER

Summary points

- Empirical studies show that inadequate quality of studies may distort the results from meta-analyses and systematic reviews.
- The influence of the quality of included studies should therefore routinely be examined in meta-analyses and systematic reviews. This is best done using sensitivity analysis.
- The use of summary scores from quality scales is problematic. Results depend on the choice of the scale, and the interpretation of findings is difficult. It is therefore preferable to examine the influence of individual components of methodological quality.
- Based on empirical evidence and theoretical considerations, concealment of treatment allocation, blinding of outcome assessment, and handling of patient attrition in the analysis should generally be assessed.

The quality of controlled trials is of obvious relevance to systematic reviews. If the "raw material" is flawed, then the conclusions of systematic reviews will be compromised and arguably invalid. Following the recommendations of the Cochrane Collaboration and other experts,[1-3] many reviewers formally assess the quality of the primary trials.[4] However, the methodology for both the assessment of quality and its incorporation into systematic reviews are a matter of ongoing debate.[5 8]

In this chapter we will discuss the concept of "study quality" and review empirical studies that have examined the impact of methodological quality of randomised trials on estimates of treatment effects. Using the example of a meta-analysis comparing low molecular weight heparin with standard heparin for prevention of postoperative thrombosis,[9] we will discuss the potentials and limitations of scoring systems and other methods for assessing study quality.

87

A framework for methodological quality

Quality is difficult to define. It could address the design, conduct and analysis of a trial, its clinical relevance, or the quality of reporting.[10-12] An important dimension of study quality relates to the validity of the findings generated by a study. Campbell proposed a distinction between internal and external validity of clinical trials (Box 5.1).[13-14] Internal validity is defined as the extent to which the results of a study are correct for the circumstances being studied.[15] It applies to the particular "internal" conditions of the trial. In contrast, external validity or generalisability is the extent to which the results of a study provide a correct basis for generalisa-

Box 5.1 Validity of a trial

Internal validity
The extent to which systematic error (bias) is minimised in a clinical trial:

- Selection bias
  - biased allocation to comparison groups

- Performance bias
  - unequal provision of care apart from treatment under evaluation

- Detection bias
  - biased outcome assessment

- Attrition bias
  - biased occurrence and handling of protocol deviations and loss to follow up

Careful design, conduct, and analysis of a trial prevent bias.

External validity
The extent to which the results of a trial provide a correct basis for applicability to other circumstances:

- Patients
  - age, sex
  - severity of disease and risk factors
  - co-morbidity

- Treatment regimens
  - dosage, timing and route of administration
  - type of treatment within a class of treatments
  - concomitant therapies

- Settings
  - level of care (primary to tertiary)
  - experience and specialisation of care provider

- Modalities of outcomes
  - type or definition of outcomes
  - length of follow up

External validity is a matter of judgement.

tions to other circumstances.[15] There is no external validity per se; the term is only meaningful with regard to specified "external" conditions, for example patient populations, treatment regimens, clinical settings, or outcomes not directly examined in the trial. Internal validity is clearly a prerequisite for external validity: the results of a flawed trial are invalid and the question of its external validity becomes redundant.

Dimensions of internal validity

Internal validity implies that the differences observed between groups of patients enrolled in a trial may, apart from random error, be attributed to the intervention under investigation. Internal validity is threatened by bias, which has been defined as "any process at any stage of inference tending to produce results that differ systematically from the true values".[16] In clinical trial research, potential biases fall into four categories. These relate to systematic differences between comparison groups in (i) the patients' characteristics (selection bias), (ii) the provision of care apart from the treatment under evaluation (performance bias), (iii) the assessment of outcomes (detection bias), and (iv) the occurrence and handling of patient attrition (attrition bias) (Box 5.1).[1,17,18]

Selection bias

The aim of randomisation is the creation of groups that are comparable with respect to any known or unknown potential confounding factors.[19] Success depends on two interrelated manoeuvres (Box 5.2).[20,21] First, an unpredictable allocation sequence must be generated, for example by tossing a coin, throwing dice or using a computer algorithm. Second, this sequence must be concealed from investigators enrolling patients. Knowledge of impending assignments, resulting, for example, from the use of a random number table openly posted on a bulletin board, can cause selective enrolment of patients based on prognostic factors.[22] Patients who would have been assigned to a treatment deemed to be "inappropriate" may be rejected, and some patients may deliberately be directed to the "appropriate" treatment by delaying their entry into the trial until the desired assignment becomes available.[17,21] Deciphering of allocation schedules may occur even if an attempt was made to conceal the schedule. For example, assignment envelopes may be opened or held against a very bright light.[23]

Performance and detection bias

Performance bias occurs if additional therapeutic interventions are provided preferentially to one of the comparison groups. Blinding of

Box 5.2 Randomisation consists of two parts

Generation of allocation sequences
- *Adequate* if resulting sequences are unpredictable:
  - computer generated random-numbers
  - table of random-numbers
  - drawing lots or envelopes
  - coin tossing
  - shuffling cards
  - throwing dice

- *Inadequate* if resulting sequences are predictable:
  - according to case record number
  - according to date of birth
  - according to date of admission
  - alternation

Concealment of allocation sequences
- *Adequate* if patients and enrolling investigators cannot foresee assignment:
  - *a priori* numbered or coded drug containers prepared by an independent pharmacy
  - central randomisation (performed at a site remote from trial location)
  - sequentially numbered, sealed, opaque envelopes

- *Inadequate* if patients and enrolling investigators can foresee upcoming assignment:
  - all procedures based on inadequate generation of allocation sequences
  - open allocation schedule
  - unsealed or non-opaque envelopes

patients and care providers prevents this type of bias, and, in addition, safeguards against differences in placebo responses between comparison groups.[18,24] Detection bias arises if the knowledge of patient assignment influences the process of outcome assessment.[24] Detection bias is avoided by blinding of those assessing outcomes, including patients, clinician investigators, radiologists, and endpoint review committees (Box 5.1).

Attrition bias

Protocol deviations and loss to follow-up may lead to the exclusion of patients after they have been allocated to treatment groups, which may introduce attrition bias.[18,25] Possible protocol deviations include the violation of eligibility criteria and non-adherence to prescribed treatments.[26] Loss to follow-up refers to patients becoming unavailable for examinations at some stage during the study period, either because of a patient's conscientious refusal to participate further (also called drop out), because of a clinical decision to stop the assigned intervention, or because the patient cannot be contacted, for example because he or she moved without giving notice.[26]

Patients excluded after allocation are unlikely to be representative of all patients in the study. For example, patients may not be available for follow up because they suffer from an acute exacerbation of their illness, or from the occurrence of severe side effects.[18,27] Patients not adhering to treatments generally differ in respects that are related to prognosis.[28] All randomised patients should therefore be included in the analysis and kept in the originally assigned groups, regardless of their adherence to the study protocol. In other words, the analysis should be performed according to the *intention-to-treat principle*, thus avoiding selection bias.[18,27,29] Naturally, this implies that the primary outcome was in fact recorded for all randomised patients at the pre-specified times throughout the follow-up period.[30,31] If the endpoint of interest is mortality from all causes this can be established most of the time. However, it may be simply impossible retrospectively to ascertain other binary or continuous outcomes and some patients may therefore have to be excluded from the analysis. In this case the proportion of patients not included in the analysis must be reported and the possibility of attrition bias discussed.

Empirical evidence of bias

Numerous case studies demonstrate that the biases described above do occur in practice, distorting the results of clinical trials.[22,24,25,27,29,32] We are aware of seven methodological studies that made an attempt to gauge their relative importance in a sample of systematic reviews or a large population of clinical trials.[33–39] Here we will concentrate on the two studies by Schulz et al.[38] and Moher et al.[39] because these authors avoided confounding by disease or intervention and examined individual dimensions of study quality, such as randomisation and blinding.

In both studies[38,39] inadequate concealment of treatment allocation was, on average, associated with an exaggeration of treatment effects by around 40% (Table 5.1). Inappropriate generation of allocation sequences was not associated with treatment effects.[38,39] However, when only trials with adequate allocation concealment were analysed in one study,[38] those with description of an inadequate generation of allocation sequences again yielded inflated treatment effects. An allocation sequence that is truly random therefore seems to be a necessary but not sufficient condition for the prevention of selection bias. If sequences are predictable, some deciphering can occur even with adequate concealment. The generation of sequences that are truly random, on the other hand, is irrelevant if sequences are not concealed from those involved in patient enrolment.[21]

While Schulz et al.[38] found that lack of double-blinding was, on average, associated with larger treatment effects, Moher and colleagues[39] did not find a significant relationship (Table 5.1). The importance of blinding will

Table 5.1 Summary of the results of two empirical studies relating methodological aspects of controlled trials to their effect estimates.

Study and setting	Domain of methodological quality	Ratio of odds ratios* (95%CI)		Interpretation
Schulz *et al.* (1995)[38]	Allocation concealment			
250 trials from 33 meta-analyses in pregnancy and childbirth	Adequate	1·0	(referent)	
	Unclear	0·67	(0·60 to 0·75)	Exaggerated effects
	Inadequate	0·59	(0·48 to 0·73)	Exaggerated effects
	Sequence generation			
	Adequate	1·0	(referent)	
	Inadequate/unclear	0·95	(0·81 to 1·12)	Similar effects
	Double-blinding			
	No	1·0	(referent)	
	Yes	0·83	(0·71 to 0·96)	Exaggerated effects
	Exclusions after randomisation			
	No	1·0	(referent)	
	Yes	1·07	(0·94 to 1·21)	Similar effects
Moher *et al.* (1998)[39]	Allocation concealment			
127 trials from 11 meta-analyses in circulatory and digestive diseases, mental health, and pregnancy and childbirth	Adquate	1·0	(referent)	
	Inadequate/unclear	0·63	(0·45 to 0·88)	Exaggerated effects
	Sequence generation			
	Adequate	1·0	(referent)	
	Inadequate/unclear	0·89	(0·67 to 1·20)	Similar effects
	Double-blinding			
	No	1·0	(referent)	
	Yes	1·11	(0·76 to 1·63)	Similar effects

* Comparison of effect estimate from trials of inadequate or unclear methodology with effect estimate from trials with adequate methodology.

to some extent depend on the outcomes assessed. In some situations, for example when examining the effect of an intervention on overall mortality, blinding of outcome assessment will be irrelevant. Differences in the type of outcomes examined could thus explain the discrepancy between the two studies. Only Schulz and colleagues[38] addressed attrition bias. Unexpectedly, the authors found a trend towards larger effect estimates in trials apparently free of attrition compared with trials known to have excluded patients after allocation. The authors suggested that this might be explained by the inadequate reporting of exclusions in published reports judged to be of poor quality on other criteria.[38]

Because of empirical studies like these, the aspects of methodology considered in this section – concealment of allocation, blinding, and completeness of data – are emerging as the most often cited key elements of trial quality.

Dimensions of external validity

External validity relates to the applicability of the results of a study to other "populations, settings, treatment variables, and measurement variables".[14] External validity is a matter of judgement which will depend on the characteristics of the patients included in the trial, the setting, the treatment regimens tested, and the outcomes assessed (Box 5.1).[14] In recent years large meta-analyses based on individual patient data have demonstrated that important differences in treatment effects may exist between patient groups and settings. For example, antihypertensive treatment reduces total mortality in middle-aged hypertensive patients[40] but this may not be the case in very old people.[41] The benefits of fibrinolytic therapy in suspected acute myocardial infarction has been shown to decrease linearly with the delay between the start of symptoms and the initiation of treatment.[42] In trials of cholesterol lowering the benefits in terms of reduction of non-fatal myocardial infarction and mortality due to coronary heart disease depends on the reduction in total cholesterol achieved, and the length of follow-up.[43] At the very least, therefore, assessment of the value of a trial requires adequate information about the characteristics of the participants.[44] The application of trial results to the individual patient, which is often problematic, is discussed in more detail in chapter 19.

Quality of reporting

The assessment of the methodological quality is intertwined with the quality of reporting, that is the extent to which a report of a clinical trial provides information about the design, conduct, and analysis of the trial.[6]

93

Trial reports frequently omit important methodological details.[45–48] For example, only 1 of 122 randomised trials of selective serotonin reuptake inhibitors specified the method of randomisation.[49] A widely used approach to this problem consists in assuming that the quality was inadequate unless the information to the contrary is provided (the "guilty until proven innocent" approach). This will often be justified because faulty reporting generally reflects faulty methods.[38,50] However, a well conducted but badly reported trial will of course be misclassified. An alternative approach is to explicitly assess the quality of reporting rather than the adequacy of methods. This is also problematic because a biased but well reported trial will receive full credit.[51] The adoption of guidelines on the reporting of clinical trials[52] has recently improved this situation for a number of journals, but deficiencies in reporting of trials will continue to be confused with deficiencies in design, conduct, and analysis.

Assessing trial quality: composite scales

Composite scales combine information on a range of quality components in a single numerical value. A large number of quality assessment scales is available. In a search of the literature covering the years up to 1993, Moher *et al.* identified 25 different scales (Table 5.2).[6,7] Since then many more have been developed. For example, in a hand search 1993–1997 of five general medicine journals (*Ann Intern Med, BMJ, JAMA, Lancet* and *N Engl J Med*) another 14 instruments were identified.[8]

The problems of composite scales

The use of composite scales is problematic for several reasons. Different scales vary considerably in terms of dimensions covered, size and complexity. Many scales include items for which there is little evidence that they are in fact related to the internal validity of a trial. Some scales include context-specific aspects, which relate to external validity. For example, a scale used in a meta-analysis of trials of the effect of anti-hypertensive therapy on serum lipids used a scale including items related to how the measurements were made and how the samples were stored.[53] Key features of commonly used scales are summarised in Table 5.2.

Unsurprisingly, different scales can lead to discordant results. This has been demonstrated for a meta-analysis[9] of 17 trials comparing low molecular weight heparin to standard heparin for thromboprophylaxis in general surgery patients.[8] Nurmohamed and colleagues[9] found a significant reduction in the risk of deep vein thrombosis with low molecular weight heparin. However, when the analysis was limited to trials of strong methodology, as assessed by a scale consisting of eight criteria, no

Table 5.2 Characteristics of 25 scales for quality assessment of clinical trials identified by Moher et al.[6] Total number of items, range of possible scores, threshold scores for definition of "high quality", and weight allocated to methodological domains most relevant to the control of bias.

Scale	No. of items	Scoring range	Threshold score for definition of "high" quality (%)*	Weight of methodological domain (%)*		
				Randomisation†	Blinding‡	Attrition
Andrew	11	0–22	73	9	9	9
Beckerman	24	–3–25	52	4	12	16
Brown	6	0–21	81	14	5	–
Chalmers I	3	0–9	67	33	33	33
Chalmers TC	30	0–100	–	13	26	7
Cho	24	0–49	–	14	8	8
Colditz	7	0–7	–	29	–	14
Detsky	14	0–15	–	20	7	–
Evans	33	0–100	–	3	4	11
Goodman	34	1–5	60	3	3	6
Gøtzsche	16	0–16	–	6	13	13
Imperiale	5	0–5	80	–	–	–
Jadad	3	0–5	60	40	40	20
Jonas	18	0–36	76	11	11	6
Kleijnen	7	0–100	55	20	20	–
Koes	17	0–100	50	4	20	12
Levine	29	0–100	60	3	3	3
Linde	7	0–7	71	29	29	29
Nurmohamed	8	0–8	88	13	13	13
Onghena	10	–10–100	–	5	10	5
Poynard	14	–2–26	50	8	23	15
Reisch	34	0–34	–	6	6	3
Smith	8	0–40	50	–	25	13
Spitzer	32	0–32	–	3	3	9
ter Riet	18	0–100	50	12	15	5

* Threshold scores and weights expressed as per cent of maximum score. No thresholds were described for nine scales.
† Generation of random sequences and/or concealment of allocation.
‡ Blinding of patients and/or outcome assessors.

significant difference between the two heparins remained. This led the authors to conclude that there was no convincing evidence that low molecular weight heparin was superior to standard heparin.[9] Jüni et al. re-analysed this meta-analysis[8] using the 25 scales shown in Table 5.2 to assess trial quality. As shown in Figure 5.1, the results differed depending on the scale used. Using some scales, relative risks of "high quality" trials were close to unity and statistically not significant, indicating that low molecular weight heparin was not superior to standard heparin, whereas "low quality" trials assessed by these scales showed better protection with the low molecular weight type. With other scales the opposite was the case: "high quality" trials indicated that low molecular weight heparin was superior to standard heparin, whereas "low quality" trials found no significant difference.

Such disagreements may be common. For example, in a meta-analysis of vitamin B6 in the treatment of premenstrual syndrome Wyatt and colleagues[54] assessed the quality of trials using a scale developed by Jadad et al.[55] (see below) and also their own eight point scale. The scores obtained by these two methods were negatively correlated, and not a single trial was rated as of "high quality" by both scores.

When examining the association of effect estimates with quality scores, interpretation of results is difficult. Greenland[56] pointed out that in the absence of an association there are three possible explanations: (i) there is no association with any of the components; (ii) there are associations with one or several components, but these components have so little weight that the effects are drowned in the summary score; or (iii) there are associations with two or more components, but these cancel out so that no association is found with the overall score. On the other hand, if treatment effects do vary with quality scores, meta-analysts will have to identify the component or components that are responsible for this association in order to interpret this finding.

Some of these problems are discussed in more detail below for the two widely used scales developed by TC Chalmers et al.[57] and Jadad et al.[55]

A critique of two widely used quality scales

The scale by Thomas C Chalmers et al.[57] (not to be confused with the scale developed by Iain Chalmers et al.[58,59]), summarised in Box 5.3, includes components of internal validity as well as features related to external validity, data presentation, statistical analysis, and trial organisation. The proportion of the total weight given to aspects which are now accepted dimensions of internal validity is relatively small (Table 5.2). Based on a total of 30 different items, the resulting summary score is difficult to

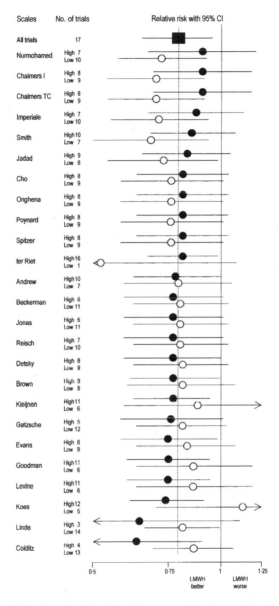

Figure 5.1 Combined results for 17 trials comparing low molecular with standard heparin and results from stratified analyses dividing trials in "high" and "low quality" strata, using 25 different quality assessment scales. Relative risks for deep vein thrombosis with 95% confidence intervals are shown. Black circles indicate estimates from "high quality" trials, open circles indicate estimates from "low quality" trials. The scales are arranged in decreasing order of the relative risks in trials deemed to be of "high quality". Modified from Jüni et al.[8]

97

interpret. Unsurprisingly, it has not been found to be related to effect estimates.[36]

Another widely used scale, developed by Jadad *et al*,[55] is described in Box 5.4. It focuses exclusively on three dimensions of internal validity,

Box 5.3 Issues addressed by TC Chalmers' quality assessment scale (1981)[57]

Internal validity
- Randomisation
  - Allocation sequence adequately concealed?

- Blinding
  - Patients blinded as to assigned treatment?
  - Physicians/outcome assessors blinded as to assigned treatment?
  - Patients/physicians blinded as to ongoing results?
  - Statisticians blinded as to results?
  - Control treatment (e.g. placebo) described as indistinguishable?
  - Blinding of patients and physicians tested?

- Patient attrition
  - Attrition described, proportion smaller than 10–15% of assigned patients?
  - Attrition appropriately analysed (e.g. intention-to-treat analysis)?

- Statistical analysis
  - Appropriate tests used?
  - Adjustments for multiple testing done?

- Avoiding random error
  - Prior power calculations done?
  - Baseline variables tabulated?
  - Baseline distribution tested?
  - *Post hoc* power calculations done for negative trials?

External validity
- Patients
  - Inclusion and exclusion criteria provided?
  - Rejected patients described?

- Treatment
  - Treatment regimens described?
  - Biological availability evaluated?
  - Compliance evaluated?

Other aspects
- Additional statistical tests
  - Life-table or time-series analysis done?
  - Appropriate subgroup analyses done?
  - Regression or correlation analysis done?

- Data presentation
  - Test statistic and P-value provided?
  - Confidence limits provided?
  - Endpoints tabulated?
  - Time to occurrence of endpoints provided (e.g. survival time)?

- Organisational aspects
  - Starting and stopping dates of trial provided?

- Side effects
  - Side effects analysed and discussed?

Box 5.4 Issues addressed by Jadad's quality assessment scale (1996)[55]

- Randomisation
  - Described as randomised?
  - Allocation sequences appropriately generated?

- Blinding
  - Described as double blind?
  - Control treatment (e.g. placebo) described as indistinguishable?

- Patient attrition
  - Attrition described for each group (including the number of patients lost or excluded, along with the reasons)?

randomisation, blinding and withdrawals (Table 5.2), but gives more weight to the quality of reporting than to actual methodological quality. For example, a statement on patient attrition will earn the point allocated to this domain, independently of how many patients were excluded or whether or not the data were analysed according to the intention-to-treat principle. The scale addresses the generation of allocation sequences, a domain not consistently related to bias,[38,39] but it does not assess allocation concealment, which has clearly been shown to be associated with exaggerated treatment effects (Table 5.1).[38,39] Therefore, the use of an open random number table is considered equivalent to concealed randomisation using a telephone or computer system. The authors advocate that a score of 3 should be taken to indicate "high quality"; however, 3 points can be earned by a trial which neither used random nor concealed allocation of patients. It has been noted[6] that this scale, which was evaluated for discrimination, reliability, and construct validity, is the only published instrument that has been constructed according to psychometric principles. While this is true, it does not follow that this particular scale is therefore necessarily better than other instruments.

Note that both scales[55,57] give considerable importance to blinding, but neither allows for the fact that in many trials blinding may not be feasible.

Potential of quality scales

Although the use of composite quality scales to identify trials of apparent "low" or "high quality" in a given meta-analysis is problematic, scales may provide a useful overall assessment when comparing populations of trials or assessing trends in trial quality over time. For example, using Jadad's scale[55] Moher *et al.*[60] found that the quality of reporting was equally inadequate for trials published in English and trials published in other languages: in both groups the total quality score was on average only about 50% of the maximum possible score. Similar results were found by other groups.[61] Using the Jadad scale, Rüther and colleagues examined the reporting quality of 3230 controlled clinical trials published in five German language general medicine journals during the period 1948–95.[62] As shown in Figure 5.2, the quality of reporting clearly improved in more recent decades.

Assessing trial quality: the component approach

The analysis of individual components of study quality overcomes many of the shortcomings of composite scores. This "component approach" takes into account that the importance of individual quality domains, and the direction of potential biases associated with these domains, will vary between the contexts in which trials are performed. In the heparin example (Figure 5.1)[8,9] regression analyses showed that none of the 25 composite scales yielded a statistically significant difference in effect estimates between "high quality" and "low quality" trials. This included the scale used in the original report by Nurmohamed *et al.*[9] Incidentally, Nurmohamed and colleagues' interpretation of the difference in results observed for trials that scored high or low (see above) represents a common, but incorrect, approach to examining heterogeneity.[63–65]

We examined whether there is evidence for an influence of individual dimensions of study quality on estimates of treatment effect. Figure 5.3 shows the results from an analysis stratified by concealment of randomisation, blinding of outcome assessment and handling of patient attrition. The results show similar effect estimates in trials with and without adequate concealment of treatment allocation. In both strata low molecular weight heparin appeared to be more effective than standard heparin. A clearly superior effect of low molecular weight heparin is evident in trials with open assessment of the endpoint deep vein thrombosis, whereas only a small difference is evident in trials with blind outcome assessment. Trials analysed according to the intention-to-treat principle showed a more pronounced difference between the two heparins than trials not analysed in this way. Blinding and the handling of attrition in the analysis thus appear to affect estimates of treatment effects.

We used multivariable regression analysis[66,67] to investigate whether these differences in treatment effects could have been produced by chance alone, and whether confounding between different dimensions of study quality was present (see Chapters 8–11 for discussion of regression techniques in meta-analysis). The results are shown in Table 5.3. Blinding of outcome assessment is the only quality feature significantly associated with

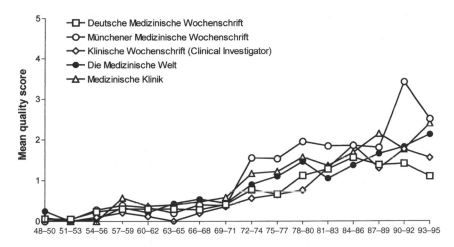

Figure 5.2 Quality of 3230 controlled clinical trials published in five German language general medicine journals, 1948–1995.[62] Mean quality scores from Jadad's scale[55] are shown.

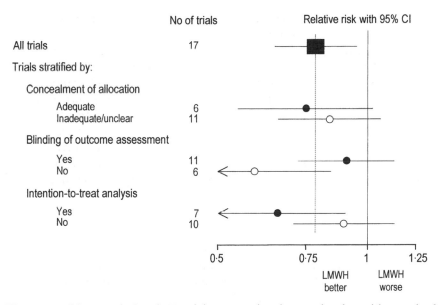

Figure 5.3 Meta-analysis of 17 trials comparing low molecular with standard heparin for the prevention of deep vein thrombosis, stratified by individual components of study quality. Relative risks for deep vein thrombosis with 95% confidence intervals are shown. Black circles indicate estimates of methodologically superior trials, open circles indicate estimates of methodologically inferior trials.

101

Table 5.3 Results from multivariable regression analysis relating methodological key domains to effect sizes in 17 trials comparing heparins for thromboprophylaxis in general surgery.

Methodological domain	Ratio of relative risks* (95% CI)		P
Concealment of allocation			
Adequate	1·00	(referent)	0·25
Inadequate/unclear	1·37	(0·80 to 2·33)	
Blinding of outcome assessment			
Yes	1·00	(referent)	0·03
No	0·56	(0·33 to 0·95)	
Intention-to-treat analysis			
Yes	1·00	(referent)	0·63
No	1·12	(0·70 to 1·82)	

Analysis adjusted for all variables listed.
* A ratio of relative risks of less than one indicates that trials of lower quality exaggerate the benefits of low molecular weight heparins, compared to the referent group of methodologically superior trials; a ratio of relative risks above one indicates the opposite.

estimates of treatment effect, the effect being exaggerated by 44% (P = 0·03), whereas no significant associations were present for the other two domains of study quality. The importance of blinding outcome assessors could have been anticipated because the interpretation of fibrinogen leg scanning, the test used to detect deep vein thrombosis, can be subjective.[68] The lack of an association with allocation concealment was surprising but its importance may to some extent depend on whether strong beliefs exist among investigators regarding the benefits or risks of assigned treatments, or whether equipoise of treatments is accepted by most of the investigators involved.[23] Strong beliefs are probably more common in trials comparing an intervention to placebo than in trials comparing two similar, active interventions.

Scales or components?

There is no consensus on whether scales or components are preferable, although it is generally agreed that trial quality ought to be investigated in systematic reviews.[1-3] Moher et al.[69] reviewed the use of quality assessment in systematic reviews published in medical journals or the Cochrane Database of Systematic Reviews (CDSR). Trial quality was assessed in 78 (38%) of the 204 journal reviews, of which 52/78 (67%) used scales and 20/78 (26%) used components. By contrast, all 36 CDSR reviews assessed quality, of which 33/36 (92%) used components and none used scales.

Incorporating study quality into meta-analysis

It makes intuitive sense to take information on the quality of studies into account when performing meta-analysis. One approach is to simply exclude trials that fail to meet some standard of quality. This may often be justified but runs the danger of excluding studies which could contribute valid information. It may therefore be prudent to exclude only trials with gross design deficiencies, for example those that clearly failed to create comparable groups. The possible influence of study quality on effect estimates should, however, always be examined in a given set of included studies. A number of different approaches have been proposed for this purpose.

Quality as a weight in statistical pooling

The most radical approach is to incorporate directly information on study quality as weighting factors in the analysis. In standard meta-analysis effect estimates of individual trials are weighted by the inverse of their variance.[70] The larger the trial, the smaller the variance of the effect estimate, and the greater the weight the study receives in meta-analysis (see Chapter 15 for a discussion of statistical methods). Study weights can be multiplied by quality scores, thus increasing the weight of trials deemed to be of "high quality" and decreasing the weight of "low quality" studies.[5,39] A trial with a quality score of 40 out of 100 will thus get the same weight in the analysis as a trial with half the amount of information (based on sample size) but a quality score of 80.

For example, Kasiske et al. reviewed 474 studies of the effect of antihypertensive drugs on serum lipids, including double blind, single blind and open randomised trials, non-randomised comparative studies and case series.[53] All 474 studies were pooled in a single analysis. To account for differences in study type and quality the authors developed a quality scale and weighted the analysis by the total score. There was no direct examination of the influence of study type and methodological quality, which makes the results extremely difficult to interpret.

Weighting by quality scores is problematic for several reasons. First, as discussed above, the choice of the scale will influence the weight of individual studies in the analysis, and the combined effect estimate and its confidence interval will therefore depend on the scale used. Second, the width of the confidence interval can readily be modified by transformation of raw scores. Depending on the scale and transformation used, the width of confidence intervals may increase or decrease, but there is no reason why study quality should modify the precision of estimates. Third, in general poor studies are still included. Thus any bias associated with poor methodology is only reduced, not removed. Including both good and poor studies may also increase heterogeneity of estimated effects across trials and may reduce the credibility of a systematic review. As pointed out by Detsky and colleagues,[5] the incorporation of quality scores as weights lacks statistical or empirical justification.

Sensitivity analysis

The robustness of the findings of a meta-analysis to different assumptions should always be examined in a thorough sensitivity analysis (see also Chapter 2). An assessment of the influence of methodological quality should be part of this process. As illustrated for the heparin example, simple stratified analyses and multivariable meta-regression models,[66,67] are useful for exploring associations between treatment effects and multiple study characteristics. Quality summary scores or categorical data on individual components can be used for this purpose. However, for the reasons discussed above, we recommend that sensitivity analysis should be based on the components of study quality that are considered important in the context of a given meta-analysis. Other approaches,[5,71,72] such as plotting effect estimates against quality scores, or performing cumulative meta-analysis (see Chapter 1) in order of quality, are also affected by the problems surrounding composite scales.

Conclusions

The problems associated with measuring methodological quality, which we outlined in this chapter, are not specific to the issue of trial quality. Similar problems have been noted in relation to composite scales used to assess quality of life[73] or scales that purport to measure a range of clinical outcomes. For example, Schneider and Knahr assessed 13 different scoring systems for grading the outcome after forefoot surgery.[74] They found that some of these systems agreed very poorly and in a few cases pairs of scores were negatively correlated.

Nor is the importance of study quality in systematic reviews relevant only to controlled trials. The same basic principles apply to systematic reviews of other types of study, such as diagnostic studies[75] (see Chapters 12–14 on systematic reviews of observational, prognostic and diagnostic studies). For these study designs the key elements of methodological quality are not as well agreed as for randomised trials.

There is ample evidence that many trials are methodologically weak and increasing evidence that deficiencies translate into biased findings of systematic reviews. The assessment of the methodological quality of controlled trials and the conduct of sensitivity analyses should therefore be considered routine procedures in meta-analysis. Although composite quality scales may provide a useful overall assessment when comparing populations of trials, such scales should not generally be used to identify trials of apparent low or high quality in a given meta-analysis. Rather, the relevant methodological aspects should be identified, ideally *a priori*, and assessed individually. This should generally include the key domains of concealment of treatment allocation, blinding of outcome assessment, and handling of attrition.

1 Clarke MJ, Oxman AD (eds). Cochrane Collaboration Handbook [updated September 1997]. In: *The Cochrane Library.* The Cochrane Collaboration. Oxford: Update Software; 1999, issue 4.
2 Cook DJ, Sackett DL, Spitzer WO. Methodologic guidelines for systematic reviews of randomized control trials in health care from the Potsdam consultation on meta-analysis. *J Clin Epidemiol* 1995;**48**:167–71.
3 Pogue J, Yusuf S. Overcoming the limitations of current meta-analysis of randomised controlled trials. *Lancet* 1998;**351**:47–52.
4 Jadad AR, Cook DJ, Jones A, *et al.* Methodology and reports of systematic reviews and meta-analyses. A comparison of Cochrane reviews with articles published in paper-based journals. *JAMA* 1998;**280**:278–80.
5 Detsky AS, Naylor CD, O'Rourke K, McGeer AJ, L'Abbé, KA. Incorporating variations in the quality of individual randomized trials into meta-analysis. *J Clin Epidemiol* 1992;**45**:255–65.
6 Moher D, Jadad AR, Nichol G, Penman M, Tugwell P, Walsh S. Assessing the quality of randomized controlled trials: an annotated bibliography of scales and checklists. *Control Clin Trials* 1995;**16**:62–73.
7 Moher D, Jadad AR, Tugwell P. Assessing the quality of randomized controlled trials. Current issues and future directions. *Int J Technol Assess Health Care* 1996;**12**:195 208.
8 Jüni P, Witschi A, Bloch R, Egger M. The hazards of scoring the quality of clinical trials for meta-analysis. *JAMA* 1999;**282**:1054–60.
9 Nurmohamed MT, Rosendaal FR, Buller HR, *et al.* Low-molecular-weight heparin versus standard heparin in general and orthopaedic surgery: a meta-analysis. *Lancet* 1992;**340**:152–6.
10 Ioannidis JP, Lau J. Can quality of clinical trials and meta-analyses be quantified? *Lancet* 1998;**352**:590–1.
11 Verhagen AP, de Vet HC, de Bie RA, Kessels AG, Boers M, Knipschild PG. The Delphi list: a criteria list for quality assessment of randomized clinical trials for conducting systematic reviews developed by Delphi consensus. *J Clin Epidemiol* 1998;**51**:1235–41.
12 Berlin JA, Rennie D. Measuring the quality of trials: the quality of quality scales. *JAMA* 1999; **282**:1083–5.
13 Campbell DT. Factors relevant to the validity of experiments in social settings. *Psychol Bull* 1957;**54**:297–312.
14 Campbell DT, Stanley JC. Experimental and quasi-experimental designs for research on teaching. In: Gage NL, ed. *Handbook of research on teaching.* Chicago: Rand McNally, 1963:171–246.
15 Fletcher RH, Fletcher SW, Wagner EH. *Clinical epidemiology – the essentials.* Baltimore: Williams & Wilkins, 1982.
16 Murphy EA. *The logic of medicine.* Baltimore: Johns Hopkins University Press, 1976.
17 Chalmers I. Evaluating the effects of care during pregnancy and childbirth. In: Chalmers I, Enkin M, Keirse MJ, eds. *Effective care in pregnancy and childbirth.* Oxford: Oxford University Press, 1989:3–38.
18 Altman DG. *Practical statistics for medical research.* London: Chapman and Hall, 1991.
19 Altman DG, Bland JM. Treatment allocation in controlled trials: why randomise? *BMJ* 1999;**318**:1209.
20 Altman DG. Randomisation. Essential for reducing bias. *BMJ* 1991;**302**:1481–2.

21 Schulz KF. Randomised trials, human nature, and reporting guidelines. *Lancet* 1996;**348**:596–8.
22 Keirse MJ. Amniotomy or oxytocin for induction of labor. Re-analysis of a randomized controlled trial. *Acta Obstet Gynecol Scand* 1988;**67**:731–5.
23 Schulz KF. Subverting randomization in controlled trials. *JAMA* 1995;**274**:1456–8.
24 Noseworthy JH, Ebers GC, Vandervoort MK, Farquhar RE, Yetisir E, Roberts R. The impact of blinding on the results of a randomized, placebo-controlled multiple sclerosis clinical trial. *Neurology* 1994;**44**:16–20.
25 Pocock SJ. *Clinical trials. A practical approach.* Chichester: Wiley, 1983.
26 Meinert CL. *Clinical trials dictionary.* Baltimore: Johns Hopkins Center for Clinical Trials, 1996.
27 Sackett DL, Gent M. Controversy in counting and attributing events in clinical trials. *N Engl J Med* 1979;**301**:1410–12.
28 Coronary Drug Project Research Group. Influence of adherence to treatment and response of cholesterol on mortality in the CDP. *N Engl J Med* 1980;**303**:1038–41.
29 May GS, Demets DL, Friedman LM, Furberg C, Passamani E. The randomized clinical trial: bias in analysis. *Circulation* 1981;**64**:669–73.
30 Lewis JA, Machin D. Intention to treat – who should use ITT? *Br J Cancer* 1993;**68**:647–50.
31 Hollis S, Campbell F. What is meant by intention to treat analysis? Survey of published randomised controlled trials. *BMJ* 1999;**319**:670–4.
32 Peduzzi P, Wittes J, Detre K, Holford T. Analysis as-randomized and the problem of non-adherence: an example from the veterans affairs randomized trial of coronary artery bypass surgery. *Stat Med* 1993;**12**:1185–95.
33 Chalmers TC, Celano P, Sacks HS, Smith H. Bias in treatment assignment in controlled clinical trials. *N Engl J Med* 1983;**309**:1358–61.
34 Colditz GA, Miller JN, Mosteller F. How study design affects outcomes in comparisons of therapy, I: medical. *Stat Med* 1989;**8**:441–54.
35 Miller JN, Colditz GA, Mosteller F. How study design affects outcomes in comparisons of therapy. II: Surgical. *Stat Med* 1989;**8**:455–66.
36 Emerson JD, Burdick E, Hoaglin DC, Mosteller F, Chalmers TC. An empirical study of the possible relation of treatment differences to quality scores in controlled randomized clinical trials. *Control Clin Trials* 1990;**11**:339–52.
37 Ottenbacher K. Impact of random assignment on study outcome: an empirical examination. *Control Clin Trials* 1992;**13**:50–61.
38 Schulz KF, Chalmers I, Hayes RJ, Altman D. Empirical evidence of bias. Dimensions of methodological quality associated with estimates of treatment effects in controlled trials. *JAMA* 1995;**273**:408–12.
39 Moher D, Pham B, Jones A, *et al.* Does quality of reports of randomised trials affect estimates of intervention efficacy reported in meta-analyses? *Lancet* 1998;**352**:609–13.
40 Collins R, Peto R, MacMahon S, *et al.* Blood pressure, stroke, and coronary heart disease. Part 2, short term reduction in blood pressure: overview of randomised drug trials in their epidemiological context. *Lancet* 1990;**335**:827–38.
41 Gueyffier F, Bulpitt C, Boissel JP, *et al.* Antihypertensive drugs in very old people: a sub-group meta-analysis of randomised controlled trials. *Lancet* 1999;**353**:793–6.
42 Fibrinolytic Therapy Trialists' (FTT) Collaborative Group. Indications for fibrinolytic therapy in suspected acute myocardial infarction: collaborative overview of early mortality and major morbidity results from all randomised trials of more than 1000 patients. *Lancet* 1994;**343**:311–22.
43 Thompson SG. Controversies in meta-analysis: the case of the trials of serum cholesterol reduction. *Stat Meth Med Res* 1993;**2**:173–92.
44 Altman DG, Bland JM. Generalisation and extrapolation. *BMJ* 1998;**317**:409–10.
45 Mosteller F, Gilbert JP, McPeek B. Reporting standards and research strategies for controlled trials – agenda for the editor. *Control Clin Trials* 1980;**1**:37–58.
46 DerSimonian R, Charette LJ, McPeek B, Mosteller F. Reporting on methods in clinical trials. *N Engl J Med* 1982;**306**:1332–7.
47 Schulz KF, Chalmers I, Grimes DA, Altman D. Assessing the quality of randomization

from reports of controlled trials published in obstetrics and gynecology journals. *JAMA* 1994;**272**:125–8.

48 Schulz KF, Grimes DA, Altman DG, Hayes RJ. Blinding and exclusions after allocation in randomised controlled trials: survey of published parallel group trials in obstetrics and gynaecology. *BMJ* 1996;**312**:742–4.

49 Hotopf M, Lewis G, Normand C. Putting trials on trial – the costs and consequences of small trials in depression: a systematic review of methodology. *J Epidemiol Community Health* 1997;**51**:354–8.

50 Liberati A, Himel HN, Chalmers TC. A quality assessment of randomized control trials of primary treatment of breast cancer. *J Clin Oncol* 1986;**4**:942–51.

51 Feinstein AR. Meta-analysis: Statistical alchemy for the 21st century. *J Clin Epidemiol* 1995;**48**:71–9.

52 Begg CB, Cho M, Eastwood S, *et al.* Improving the quality of reporting of randomized controlled trials. The CONSORT statement. *JAMA* 1996;**276**:637–9.

53 Kasiske BL, Ma JZ, Kalil RS, Louis TA. Effects of antihypertensive therapy on serum lipids. *Ann Intern Med* 1995;**122**:133–41.

54 Wyatt KM, Dimmock PW, Jones PW, O'Brien PM. Efficacy of vitamin B-6 in the treatment of premenstrual syndrome: systematic review. *BMJ* 1999;**318**:1375–81.

55 Jadad AR, Moore RA, Carrol D, *et al.* Assessing the quality of reports of randomized clinical trials: is blinding necessary? *Control Clin Trials* 1996;**17**:1–12.

56 Greenland S. Quality scores are useless and potentially misleading. *Am J Epidemiol* 1994;**140**:300–2.

57 Chalmers TC, Smith H, Blackburn B, *et al.* A method for assessing the quality of a randomized control trial. *Control Clin Trials* 1981;**2**:31–49.

58 Chalmers I, Hetherington J, Elbourne D, Keirse MJ, Enkin M. Materials and methods used in synthesizing evidence to evaluate the effects of care during pregnancy and childbirth. In: Chalmers I, Enkin M, Keirse MJ, eds. *Effective care in pregnancy and childbirth.* Oxford: Oxford University Press, 1989:39–65.

59 Prendiville W, Elbourne D, Chalmers I. The effects of routine oxytocic administration in the management of the third stage of labour: an overview of the evidence from controlled trials. *Br J Obstet Gynaecol* 1988;**95**:3–16.

60 Moher D, Fortin P, Jadad AR, *et al.* Completeness of reporting of trials published in languages other than English: implications for conduct and reporting of systematic reviews. *Lancet* 1996;**347**:363–6.

61 Egger M, Zellweger-Zähner T, Schneider M, Junker C, Lengeler C, Antes G. Language bias in randomised controlled trials published in English and German. *Lancet* 1997;**350**:326–9.

62 Rüther A, Galandi D, Antes G. Medizinische Entscheidungsfindung: Systematische Erfassung von klinischen Studien in medizinischen Fachzeitschriften. Deutsche Gesellschaft für Innere Medizin, 103. Kongreß für innere Medizin, Wiesbaden. 1997.

63 Altman DG, Matthews JNS. Interaction 1: Heterogeneity of effects. *BMJ* 1996;**313**:486.

64 Matthews JN, Altman DG. Interaction 2: compare effect sizes, not p values. *BMJ* 1996;**313**:808.

65 Matthews JN, Altman DG. Interaction 3: how to examine heterogeneity. *BMJ* 1996;**313**:862.

66 Thompson SG, Sharp S. Explaining heterogeneity in meta-analysis: a comparison of methods. *Stat Med* 1999;**18**:2693–708.

67 Lau J, Ioannidis JP, Schmid CH. Summing up evidence: one answer is not always enough. *Lancet* 1998;**351**:123–7.

68 Lensing AW, Hirsh J. ^{125}I-fibrinogen leg scanning: reassessment of its role for the diagnosis of venous thrombosis in post-operative patients. *Thromb Haemost* 1993;**69**:2–7.

69 Moher D, Cook DJ, Jadad AR, Tugwell P, Moher M, Jones A. Assessing the quality of reports of randomised trials: implications for the conduct of meta-analyses. *Health Technol Assess* 1999;**3**(12).

70 Hedges LV, Olkin I. *Statistical methods for meta-analysis.* Boston: Academic Press, 1985.

71 Linde K, Scholz M, Ramirez G, Clausius N, Melchart D, Jonas WB. Impact of study

quality on outcome in placebo-controlled trials of homeopathy. *J Clin Epidemiol* 1999;**52**:631–6.

72 Tritchler D. Modelling study quality in meta-analysis. *Stat Med* 1999;**18**:2135–45.

73 Sanders C, Egger M, Donovan J, Tallon D, Frankel S. Reporting on quality of life in randomised controlled trials: bibliographic study. *BMJ* 1998;**317**:1191–4.

74 Schneider W, Knahr K. Scoring in forefoot surgery: a statistical evaluation of single variables and rating systems. *Acta Orthop Scand* 1998;**69**:498–504.

75 Lijmer JG, Mol BW, Heisterkamp S, *et al*. Empirical evidence of design-related bias in studies of diagnostic tests. *JAMA* 1999;**282**:1061–6.

6 Obtaining individual patient data from randomised controlled trials

MICHAEL J CLARKE, LESLEY A STEWART

Summary points

- Individual randomised trials in health care are, on their own, rarely able to estimate typical differences between treatments on major outcomes because these differences may be relatively small.
- Such differences may, however, be very important, especially in common diseases where they could result in many life years saved and have an important impact on public health.
- Large scale, unbiased randomised evidence such as that from systematic reviews of randomised trials, is needed to investigate these differences as reliably as possible.
- The central collection of individual patient data (IPD) is perhaps the most resource intensive and time-consuming approach for systematic reviews. It will, however, overcome many of the problems associated with a reliance on published data only, some of the problems associated with a reliance on aggregate data and will add to the analyses and investigations that can be performed.
- The relative contribution of different aspects of the IPD approach and its importance to the reliability of the findings of systematic reviews is the subject of ongoing and future research.

The ultimate aim of any systematic review should be to ensure that relevant data on all randomised patients from all relevant randomised trials are included. Increasing the number of trials or patients will reduce the influence of chance effects and consequently result in more tightly defined and precise estimates of treatment differences. However, it is important that the aim to be all inclusive is not done at the expense of introducing systematic bias. For example, if not all trials can supply data and be included and the availability of particular trials might be related to results, then the reviewer needs to be cautious. This is a well-documented problem in traditional reviews if only data from published trials are included, as we know that studies with significant results are more likely to be published than those with non-significant results (see Chapter 3).[1] On the other hand the same problem can apply if unpublished trials are sought but not all of these trials are made available for inclusion. For example, if trialists have only kept, or are only willing to provide, data from their unpublished trials that showed promising results, then the review will be biased towards the positive. A similar difficulty could arise if not all the subgroups or outcomes of interest are available from all trials. Again, trialists might be more likely to publish or supply only those with the most interesting findings, whereas the reviewer needs to include the relevant data regardless of the result within an individual trial.

This chapter discusses the process of obtaining data for inclusion in systematic reviews, with particular emphasis on those using individual patient data (IPD). These IPD reviews which have been described as the "yardstick" against which other forms of systematic review should be measured,[2] are time consuming but have, in a number of cases, produced definitive answers which might not have been obtained in any other way.[3] Many of the points raised in relation to collecting IPD are also of relevance to systematic reviews using aggregate data supplied directly by the trialists, and the most important issue related to the reliability of a review is not usually whether it used IPD or aggregate data but whether or not it used unpublished data (either IPD or aggregate).

What are individual patient data reviews?

IPD reviews involve obtaining individual information or "raw data" on all patients included in each of the trials directly from those responsible for the trial. This information, which is often brought up to date for the purposes of the review, is collected, checked and re-analysed centrally by the researchers responsible for coordinating the review. As with any systematic review, the first, and perhaps most important, step is to identify all relevant trials and this is discussed elsewhere in this book (see Chapter 4). Then if appropriate, the results of the identified trials are combined in a meta-analysis. The datasets supplied are checked carefully and any apparent inconsistencies or problems are discussed and, hopefully, resolved by communication with the responsible trialists. The finalised data for each trial are analysed separately to obtain summary statistics, which are combined to give an overall estimate of the effect of treatment. In this way, patients in one trial are compared directly only with other patients in the same trial, and each of the trials is analysed in the same way.[4]

The use of IPD in a systematic review shares benefits, resulting from direct contact between reviewers and trialists, with reviews that use updated aggregate data provided by the trialists. For example, both approaches allow the reviewer to incorporate unpublished data which may be the most important hurdle to overcome in minimising bias. In addition, the IPD approach provides a number of further benefits that cannot otherwise be achieved readily. It also has some possible disadvantages. These features are shown in Box 6.1 and the most important are discussed below.

Box 6.1 Possible benefits and disadvantages of IPD reviews

Possible benefits of collecting aggregate data from trialists
- include unpublished trials
- include all randomised, and no non-randomised, patients
- analyse on the basis of allocated treatment
- analyse common outcomes
- analyse common patient subgroups
- improve the overall follow-up
- ensure equal follow-up for the randomised groups

Possible additional benefits of involving the relevant trialists in the conduct of the review
- better identification of trials
- more balanced interpretation of the results of the review
- wider endorsement
- increased possibilities for dissemination of the results of the review
- better clarification of the implications for future research
- possibilities for collaboration in future research

Possible additional benefits of using individual patient data
- analyse by time to event
- increase statistical power
- more flexible analysis of patient subgroups
- more flexible analysis of outcomes
- might be easier for trialists to supply IPD than to prepare tables
- easier for trialists to supply small amounts of additional or new data
- data can be checked and corrected

Possible disadvantages of IPD reviews
- make take longer and cost more
- reviewers need wider range of skills
- inability to include IPD from all relevant trials

111

Improved follow-up

Even in trials where the outcomes of most interest are expected within months or a few years of randomisation, longer follow-up may yield important information. This may confirm that an important benefit only becomes apparent after several years, as discussed below, or identify a late hazard which may overwhelm the early benefit.[5] Most trials do not report long term follow-up and are too small to identify these long term effects which therefore might only come to light through a systematic review. This is unlikely to be possible in a review which relies only on published data, since these remain static and are "frozen-in-time" by the publication process. The problem can be overcome if the trialist has maintained the data in their trial and if the updated results can be obtained for the review (either as IPD or aggregate data). Even if the trialist has not done so or is unable to bring the information up to date themselves, it may be possible for the organisers of the review to track the outcome of patients, for example through national death registries or cancer registries if the trialists can supply sufficient information on each patient. It is similarly important that reviewers consider new evidence and update existing information, as appropriate, and thus ensure that their results do not become "frozen-in-time". In recent years, the establishment of the Cochrane Collaboration (see Chapters 25 and 26) has emphasised the importance of maintaining and updating reviews in this way.

As an example of the importance of updating data, an IPD review[6] of ovarian ablation versus control for breast cancer showed a significant long term survival benefit when data from 10 trials (720 deaths among 1746 women) were combined in the early 1990s (Figure 6.1). However, if a meta-analysis of published data had been done at that time it would have only been able to include data from seven trials (417 deaths among 1644 women) and this would not have shown any significant difference between ovarian ablation and control.[7] The main reason for these contrasting findings were that the statistical power of the review was increased by the inclusion of the unpublished trials, time-to-event analyses could be performed and, perhaps most importantly, considerably improved follow-up information could be used for each trial.[7]

Time-to-event analyses

A major benefit of collecting IPD is the ability to undertake time-to-event analyses which take account of not just whether or not an outcome happened but, also the point in time at which it happened. The period that an individual remains free of an adverse outcome can be of the utmost importance. For example, in chronic diseases such as cancer where cure is rare, we can investigate the important question not only of whether one

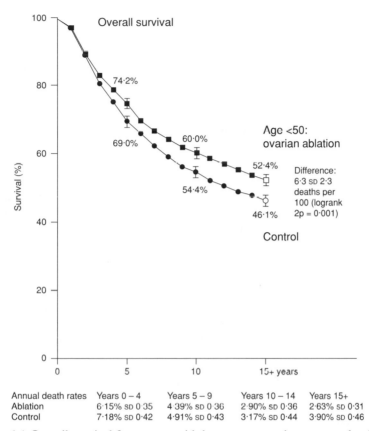

Figure 6.1 Overall survival for women with breast cancer who were randomised to ovarian ablation versus control. Taken from the Early Breast Cancer Trialists' Collaborative Group overview of ovarian ablation, and reproduced with permission from the *Lancet*.[6]

treatment leads to a prolongation of survival, but also the pattern of this prolongation.[8] Other examples where IPD reviews have allowed the investigation of how well different treatments delay adverse events include the effects of exercise in reducing falls in the elderly[9] and the maintenance of vascular patency with anti-platelet therapy.[10] Clearly, this would not be possible if data for a fixed point in time were collected but could – potentially – be estimated from aggregate data as discussed below.

Estimating time-to-event outcomes from published information

Provided that trials are sufficiently well reported or the trialist can provide appropriate statistical information, it may be possible to estimate

113

hazard ratios from a variety of statistical summary measures. These hazard ratios, which give the overall relative chance of an event on a treatment as compared to control or an alternative treatment, account for both "censoring" and time-to-event. This is in contrast to odds ratios, which use only the numbers of events, and which are the most commonly reported outcome measure in this type of meta-analysis. Where log hazard ratios, hazard ratios or log rank observed-minus-expected numbers of events plus log rank variances are presented, these can be used directly in the calculation of an overall hazard ratio. Even when these are not presented, manipulation of the chi-square value, P value, or variance can be used to calculate a hazard ratio indirectly.[11] The particular method used will depend on which information is presented for particular trials and different methods can be used for different trials as appropriate. If there is not sufficient information to obtain an estimated hazard ratio from summary statistics, it might be possible to estimate the hazard ratio by splitting the published survival curves into discrete time intervals, calculating an odds ratio for each of these periods and then combining these over time.

However, even if the required data were provided for each trial and hazard ratios could be estimated as above, IPD offers the additional advantage that the sequence of outcomes can be analysed properly and may well lead to a better understanding of the disease and treatments under investigation.

Effects in patient subgroups and on different outcomes

It is well known that in small trials and reviews, subgroup or multiple outcome analyses may lead to misleading conclusions and should be avoided. The availability of large-scale randomised evidence may be the only situation where it is reasonable to do subgroup analyses to determine – with appropriate caution – whether differences between treatments are smaller or greater for particular pre-defined groups of patients (see also Chapters 8 and 9). Any such analyses should, ideally, be regarded as hypothesis-generating, for testing in future studies. If subgroup analyses are to be done, they need to be as complete as possible and should involve commonly defined subgroups and outcomes across all the trials in a review.

This will rarely be possible for reviews based solely on the published literature since, regardless of the problems associated with not being able to include unpublished trials, the information presented on subgroup analyses is usually incomplete and likely to be biased if only those subgroups with interesting results are reported. Thus for subgroup analysis to be at all possible within the context of a review, additional data will need to be sought from the trialists. In theory, this could be done by asking trialists to complete tables providing separate outcome data for each of the subgroups of interest. For example, to investigate subgroups defined by age, trialists might need to provide aggregate data on the survival of those patients younger than 50 years, between 50 and 60 years and over 60 years, for both treatment and control groups. Where a number of subgroups are explored this might prove practically difficult for many trialists, particularly for those with no data-management or statistical support.

In addition, if the outcome data had also to be supplied for different lengths of follow-up (to allow a time-to-event analysis), the necessary tables could potentially contain more cells than the number of patients in a trial. Further, to complete such a table, trialists would need to adopt the centrally determined definitions for subgroups and outcomes.

In consequence, providing IPD may actually prove simpler for trialists. It also allows the secretariat for the analyses to prepare the necessary files for analysis and to apply consistent subgroup and outcome definitions across the included trials. It is worth remembering, however, that whether or not a particular subgroup or outcome can be analysed depends on both its initial collection in the trial (which could not be biased by the trial's results) and on the willingness of the trialist to supply data on that variable (which could potentially be biased by the observed results in the trial) – a problem that can happen with any of the data or trials in the meta-analysis.

Occasionally subgroup analyses will complement independent research and demonstrate that treatment effects vary so much between different types of patient that this would influence the decision about which treatment to use. In operable breast cancer, the overview of IPD from 37 000 women in 55 trials of tamoxifen versus control showed a moderate but highly significant benefit of tamoxifen for women who were not known to have estrogen receptor (ER) negative disease – one extra survivor at ten years for every twelve such women allocated five years of tamoxifen. In contrast, the benefit was much smaller and non-significant in women reported to have estrogen receptor negative disease (Figure 6.2).[12] This is in keeping with the biological understanding of breast cancer, since the main action of tamoxifen is probably through its blocking of estrogen receptors. In consequence of these findings, estrogen receptor status is increasingly recognised as an important determinant in the decision on how to treat women with early breast cancer.

Subgroup analysis, using large scale randomised evidence, indicating that the effect of treatment does not vary greatly between different types of patient can also be of great practical importance. For example, a meta-analysis of trials comparing standard chemotherapy with more intensive combination chemotherapy regimens for the treatment of myeloma suggested that combination chemotherapy was better for those with poor prognosis, while standard therapy was better for good prognosis patients.[13] A subsequent IPD review of this question, which collected data on twelve baseline variables, found no evidence for a survival benefit of combination chemotherapy either overall or in any prognostic subgroup (Figure 6.3).[14]

115

Recurrence as first event / Mortality (death from any cause)

Nodal status (excludes known ER-poor)	Events/Patients Allocated Tamoxifen	Allocated Control	Tamoxifen events Obs.–Exp. of O–E	Variance of O–E	Ratio of recurrence rates: Reduction (% & SD)	Deaths/Patients Allocated Tamoxifen	Allocated Control	Tamoxifen events Obs.–Exp. of O–E	Variance of O–E	Ratio of death rates: Reduction (% & SD)
(a) Tamoxifen ~1 year										
Node negative ~78% ER+	253/1079 (23.4%)	291/1086 (26.8%)	−23.4	126.2	17% SD 8	285/1079 (26.4%)	318/1086 (29.3%)	−19.7	138.5	13% SD 8
Node positive ~83% ER+	1410/2685 (52.5%)	1617/2687 (60.2%)	−157.6	655.8	21% SD 3	1469/2685 (54.7%)	1588/2687 (59.1%)	−84.3	682.7	12% SD 4
(a) subtotal 82% ER+	1663/3764 (44.2%)	1908/3773 (50.6%)	−181.0	782.1	21% SD 3 (2p < 0.00001)	1754/3764 (46.6%)	1906/3773 (50.5%)	−104.1	821.2	12% SD 3 (2p < 0.0003)
Difference between tamoxifen effects in N− and N+:					$\chi^2_1 = 0.3$; 2p > 0.1: NS					$\chi^2_1 = 0.0$; 2p > 0.1: NS
(b) Tamoxifen ~2 years										
Node negative ~82% ER+	517/3131 (16.5%)	684/3080 (22.2%)	−86.8	266.6	28% SD 5	526/3131 (16.8%)	623/3080 (19.5%)	−30.4	253.1	11% SD 6
Node positive ~88% ER+	1968/4180 (47.1%)	2299/4086 (56.3%)	−317.8	900.0	30% SD 3	1839/4180 (44.0%)	2034/4086 (49.8%)	−178.3	855.5	19% SD 3
(b) subtotal 87% ER+	2486/7311 (34.0%)	2983/7166 (41.6%)	−404.7	1166.7	29% SD 2 (2p < 0.00001)	2365/7311 (32.3%)	2634/7166 (36.8%)	−208.7	1108.6	17% SD 3 (2p < 0.00001)
Difference between tamoxifen effects in N− and N+:					$\chi^2_1 = 0.2$; 2p > 0.1: NS					$\chi^2_1 = 1.5$; 2p > 0.1: NS
(c) Tamoxifen ~5 years										
Node negative ~96% ER+	486/2611 (18.6%)	844/2606 (32.4%)	−213.2	313.7	49% SD 4	475/2611 (18.2%)	604/2606 (23.2%)	−74.3	258.8	25% SD 5
Node positive ~92% ER+	406/1127 (36.0%)	539/1083 (49.8%)	−116.6	205.6	43% SD 5	399/1127 (35.4%)	462/1083 (42.7%)	−62.1	192.7	28% SD 6
(c) subtotal 94% ER+	892/3738 (23.9%)	1383/3689 (37.5%)	−329.8	519.3	47% SD 3 (2p < 0.00001)	874/3738 (23.4%)	1066/3689 (28.9%)	−136.5	451.5	26% SD 4 (2p < 0.00001)
Difference between tamoxifen effects in N− and N+:					$\chi^2_1 = 1.6$; 2p > 0.1: NS					$\chi^2_1 = 1.5$; 2p > 0.1: NS

Ratio Tamoxifen : Con. 0.0 0.5 1.0 1.5 2.0
Tamoxifen better | Tamoxifen worse

■ 99% or ◇ 95% confidence intervals

Figure 6.2 Proportional risk reductions for recurrence and survival among women with breast cancer who were randomised to tamoxifen versus control, subdivided by tamoxifen duration and estrogen receptor status. Taken from the Early Breast Cancer Trialists' Collaborative Group overview of tamoxifen, and reproduced with permission from the *Lancet*.[12]

Parameter	Deaths/Patients CCT	Deaths/Patients MP	Statistics (O−E)	Var.	O.R. & 99% CI (CCT : MP)
Age:					
<50	213/284	175/242	−6.4	85.3	
50–64	837/1098	759/1052	0.7	385.5	
65–74	625/799	637/818	−15.4	296.0	
75+	207/248	198/249	19.6	86.1	
Sex:					
Male	1078/1393	994/1318	−1.9	498.4	
Female	843/1100	822/1104	−12.1	398.7	
Durie–Salmon stage:					
Stage I	112/156	122/159	−6.7	50.5	
Stage II	257/383	269/422	18.8	122.2	
Stage III	1065/1296	927/1183	−29.5	474.3	
Haemoglobin:					
<7.5	227/278	199/253	10.3	96.6	
7.5–10.5	635/812	663/870	−6.4	315.9	
>10.5	662/946	659/949	−16.2	322.7	
Platelets:					
<100	135/151	93/112	−3.0	46.2	
100–199	485/588	496/602	−12.1	231.4	
200+	866/1096	812/1079	−10.7	402.8	
White blood count:					
<5	414/506	416/523	4.6	194.2	
5–10	900/1106	832/1063	−5.9	417.3	
>10	165/192	126/153	−10.0	57.7	

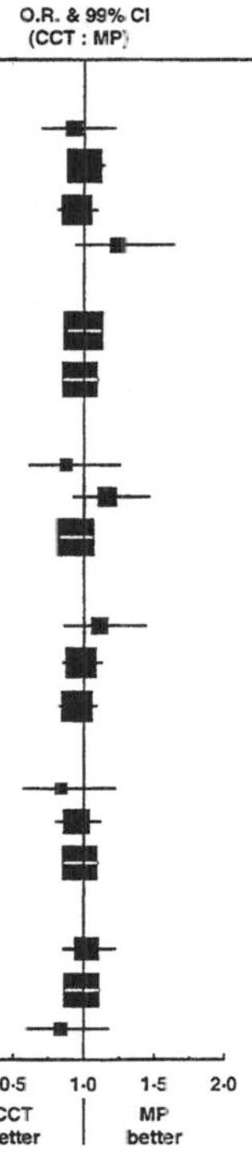

Parameter	Deaths/Patients CCT	Deaths/Patients MP	Statistics (O−E)	Var.	O.R. & 99% CI (CCT : MP)
b2-microglobulin:					
<2.0	107/141	111/137	−3.8	52.2	
2.0–3.9	131/195	128/214	4.5	63.0	
4.0–8.0	189/253	193/259	−10.5	92.9	
>8.0	179/206	151/176	3.2	79.3	
M band type:					
IgA	412/507	359/452	3.0	181.1	
IgG	932/1173	897/1184	−23.2	436.3	
Other	149/186	128/168	1.3	60.4	
Creatinine:					
<130	992/1289	948/1251	−25.2	469.6	
130–200	222/260	211/262	−1.6	101.3	
200+	279/314	241/281	−2.9	114.8	
Calcium:					
<2.6	682/905	637/879	−8.2	317.0	
2.6–2.8	234/286	248/311	1.5	108.2	
>2.8	368/446	295/374	−6.8	153.2	
Bone lesions:					
None	450/551	442/547	−0.8	214.9	
Minimal	517/653	439/604	9.0	225.8	
Multiple	542/683	525/672	−20.9	250.4	
Perform. status:					
Asymptomatic	648/775	568/686	−17.2	285.4	
Minimal symptoms	271/375	269/366	−15.5	131.9	
Restricted activity	422/609	432/653	2.6	206.0	
Confined to bed	488/619	448/595	0.3	224.0	

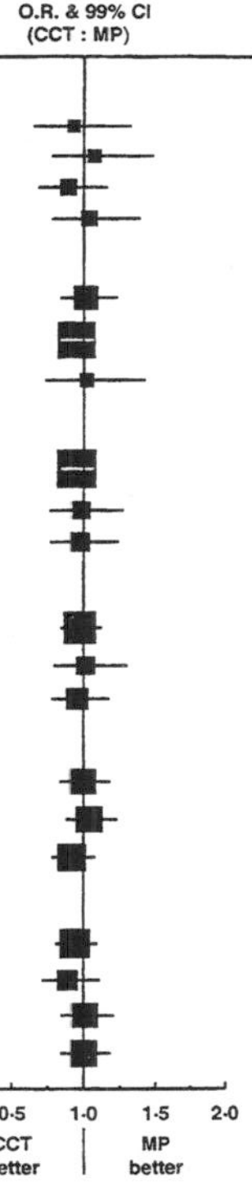

Figure 6.3 Proportional risk reductions for survival among patients with multiple myeloma who were randomised to combination chemotherapy (CCT) versus melphalan plus prednisone (MP), subdivided by various prognostic factors. Taken from the Myeloma Trialists' Collaborative Group overview, and reproduced with permission from *Journal of Clinical Oncology*.[14]

How to obtain data that are as complete as possible

Irrespective of whether the information on the participants in the relevant randomised trials is collected as aggregate data or IPD, data must be collected from as many trials as possible. It is especially important to ensure that any trials which do not contribute data are not so numerous or unrepresentative to introduce important bias into the result of the systematic review. The data collection process may, therefore, present the reviewer with several difficulties. Some trialists may be reluctant to supply their data and there will often be practical difficulties in the preparation of data. In practical terms it is important, therefore, to stress that any data supplied will be treated confidentially and will not be used for any additional purpose without the permission of the responsible trialist. In addition, any publications arising from the meta-analysis should be in the name of all the collaborators and each trialist should have an opportunity to comment on the manuscript before publication. The trialists should also be the first people, other than the statistical secretariat, to see and discuss the results. This is often achieved for IPD reviews by first presenting results at a closed meeting of the collaborative group of the participating trialists.

If there are trialists who initially felt unable to prepare and supply their data, some of these points may help persuade them to do so. In addition, the process of data collection should be as simple and flexible as possible in order to help and encourage trialists to participate. Trialists should be allowed to supply their data in a format and manner that is agreed with them. If a trial group has all of their data on computer, it might be relatively easy for them to send an electronic file. However, if a particular trialist does not store their data electronically and has only limited access to computers it would be inappropriate to expect them to supply data in this way. Likewise, it might be inappropriate to expect a trialist in this situation to prepare aggregate data if this is what was being requested for the review. This can represent an additional advantage for IPD reviews, since it might actually be easier for some trialists to send their raw data than to prepare a tabular version of it. The secretariat for the analyses can help to avoid the possibility that such problems will mean that the data are not supplied at all, by being prepared to accept data in a variety of ways and taking responsibility for computerising, reformatting and recoding it as necessary. Increasingly, though, our experience is that data are likely to be supplied electronically (Table 6.1).

What if IPD are not available?

One potential disadvantage of attempting to do an IPD review is that it may not always be possible to collect IPD from all relevant trials. Some

118

Table 6.1 Ways in which individual patient data were supplied for IPD reviews of treatments for ovarian cancer and soft tissue sarcoma.

	Ovarian cancer (1994)	Soft tissue sarcoma (1997)
Data forms	29%	0%
Computer printout	36%	0%
Computer disk	33%	29%
Electronic mail	2%	71%

trialists may be unwilling or unable to provide data on individual patients but might perhaps be willing to supply updated aggregate data. Others might not wish to collaborate in the project at all and will therefore not supply any material. In some cases it might prove impossible to locate those responsible for some of the identified trials. The approach taken within any one review will depend on how much IPD it has been possible to collect. If the number of trials for which IPD are not available is so small that the proportion of missing data is insufficient to affect the results of the review in any important way, it is probably not worth trying to include results from these trials. It might be preferable to continue trying to obtain the IPD so that they can be used in the future, and to clearly state which trials were unavailable when the review is published. If, however, the proportion of non-IPD material could importantly influence the conclusions of the review then it might be necessary to try to include some data from these trials, and the benefits of the IPD approach may be correspondingly diminished. One way to deal with this situation would be to undertake a sensitivity analysis comparing the results of analyses based on the IPD alone with the results of analyses using all the data. If the results of both analyses are broadly similar, then the reviewer and reader can be more confident about them. If they differ markedly, then we must be cautious about any conclusions that are drawn and additionally diligent in trying to obtain IPD from the missing trials.

Potential disadvantages of IPD reviews

As already noted, IPD reviews may take longer and require more resources than reviews using more conventional approaches such as those restricted to aggregate data from published trials. They are also very dependent on the willingness of trialists to collaborate in the project. However, it is difficult to quantify these disadvantages or to balance them against the advantages outlined above. Instead, any reviewers trying to decide whether or not they should embark on an IPD review and anyone trying to assess whether or not reviewers should have done so, needs to keep in mind that the approach taken should be driven by the therapeutic

119

question that the review is trying to answer. This should determine whether or not the particular features of IPD reviews would be a help or a hindrance to the particular review.

Examples of how the collection of IPD can make a difference to the findings of a review

A number of projects comparing the results of reviews which used IPD with the results that would have been found with reviews based only on data abstracted from trial publications have been reported over the last few years. These are now the subject of a systematic review,[15] but some examples are discussed below.

An IPD review of 1329 patients in 11 trials of platinum-based combination chemotherapy versus single non-platinum drugs for ovarian cancer found little difference between the treatments. In contrast, a review of the published data would have shown a significant survival benefit for combination chemotherapy. The main reasons for the difference were that the IPD review was able to include unpublished data (3 more trials and more than 500 more patients), the follow-up was improved and a time-to-event analysis was possible.[16]

Similarly, the reduction of publication bias and the re-inclusion of additional women from the published trials meant that the results of a published data review of paternal white blood cell immunization versus control for recurrent miscarriage over-estimated what was shown by an IPD review. Using just four trials (202 women), the published data review showed a significant, 29% increase in live births among those allocated immunization. The IPD review, which included a further four trials and a total of 379 women, estimated the increase to be 12% and this was non-significant.[17]

These examples show that IPD reviews can produce importantly different results, generally finding lower estimates of treatment effect and less statistically significant results. Evidence also exists to show that the reverse can happen and this is discussed above in relation to the review of ovarian ablation versus control for breast cancer. This review, primarily because of prolonged follow-up, showed a significant long-term survival benefit that would not have been apparent from a review of the published literature.[7]

Conclusion

The most important first step in any systematic review is ensuring that all, or nearly all, relevant trials are identified. Data from these trials can then be gathered in a variety of ways. The central collection of IPD is perhaps the most resource intensive and time-consuming of these. It will, however, overcome many of the problems associated with a reliance on published data only, some of the problems associated with a reliance on aggregate data and will add to the analyses that can be performed. The relative contribution of different aspects of the IPD approach and its importance to the reliability of the findings of systematic reviews remains a subject for ongoing and future research.

1 Dickersin K, Min YI. Publication bias: the problem that won't go away. *Ann NY Acad Sci* 1993;**703**:135–48.
2 Chalmers I. The Cochrane Collaboration: preparing, maintaining and disseminating systematic reviews of the effects of health care. *Ann NY Acad Sci* 1993;**703**:156–65.
3 Horton R. The information wars. *Lancet* 1999;**353**:164–5.
4 Stewart L, Clarke M, for the Cochrane Collaboration Working Group on meta-analyses using individual patient data. Practical methodology of meta-analyses (overviews) using updated individual patient data. *Stat Med* 1995;**14**:1057–79.
5 Early Breast Cancer Trialists' Collaborative Group. Favourable and unfavourable effects on long-term survival of radiotherapy for early breast cancer: an overview of the randomised trials. *Lancet* 2000;**355**:1757–70.
6 Early Breast Cancer Trialists' Collaborative Group. Ovarian ablation in early breast cancer: overview of the randomised trials. *Lancet* 1996;**348**:1189–96.
7 Clarke M, Godwin J. Systematic reviews using individual patient data: a map for the minefields? *Ann Oncol* 1998;**9**:827–33.
8 Clarke M, Stewart L, Pignon JP, Bijnens L. Individual patient data meta-analyses in cancer. *Br J Cancer* 1998;**77**:2036–44.
9 Province MA, Hadley EC, Hornbrook MC, *et al.* The effects of exercise on falls in elderly patients: a preplanned meta-analysis of the FICSIT trials. *JAMA* 1995;**273**:1341–7.
10 Antiplatelet Trialists' Collaboration. Collaborative overview of randomised trials of antiplatelet therapy II. Maintenance of vascular graft or arterial patency by antiplatelet therapy. *BMJ* 1994;**308**:159–68.
11 Parmar MK, Torri V, Stewart LA. Extracting summary statistics to perform meta-analyses of the published literature for survival endpoints. *Stat Med* 1998;**17**:2815–34.
12 Early Breast Cancer Trialists' Collaborative Group. Tamoxifen for early breast cancer: an overview of the randomised trials. *Lancet* 1998;**351**:1451–67.
13 Gregory WM, Richards MA, Malpas JS. Combination chemotherapy versus melphalan and prednisolone in the treatment of multiple myeloma: an overview of published trials. *J Clin Oncol* 1992;**10**: 334–42.
14 Myeloma Trialists' Collaborative Group. Combination chemotherapy versus melphalan plus prednisone as treatment for multiple myeloma: an overview of 6633 patients from 27 randomized trials. *J Clin Oncol* 1998;**16**:3832–42.
15 Clarke M, Stewart L. Individual patient data or published data meta-analysis: a systematic review [abstract]. *Proc 5th Cochrane Collaboration Colloquium* 1997;**94**: abstract 019.04.
16 Stewart LA, Parmar MKB. Meta-analysis of the literature or of individual patient data: is there a difference? *Lancet* 1993;**341**:418–22.
17 Jeng GT, Scott JR, Burmeiester LF. A comparison of meta-analytic results using literature vs individual patient data: paternal cell immunization for recurrent miscarriage. *JAMA* 1995;**275**:830–6.

7 Assessing the quality of reports of systematic reviews: the QUOROM statement compared to other tools

BEVERLEY SHEA, CATHERINE DUBÉ,
DAVID MOHER

Summary points

- Systematic reviews within health care are conducted retrospectively which makes them susceptible to potential sources of bias.
- In the last few years steps have been taken to develop evidence based methods to help improve the quality of reporting of randomised trials in the hope of reducing bias when trials are included in meta-analysis. Similar efforts are now underway for reports of systematic reviews.
- This chapter describes the development of the QUOROM statement and compares it to other instruments identified through a systematic review.
- There are many checklists and scales available to be used as evaluation tools, but most are missing important evidence based items when compared against the QUOROM checklist, a "gold standard".
- A pilot study suggests considerable room for improvement in the quality of reports of systematic reviews, using four different instruments.
- It is hoped that journals will support the QUOROM statement in a similar manner to the CONSORT statement.

There are approximately 17 000 new biomedical books published every year along with 30 000 biomedical journals, with an annual increase of 7%.[1] This makes it very difficult for health care professionals to keep on top of the most recent advances and research in their field, as they would need to read, on average, 17 original articles each day (see also Chapter 1).[2]

To make this task slightly more manageable health care providers and other decision-makers now have, among their information resources, a form of clinical report called the systematic review. This is a review in which bias has been reduced by the systematic identification, appraisal, synthesis, and, if relevant, statistical aggregation of all relevant studies on a specific topic according to a predetermined and explicit methodology. Theoretically, such reviews can effectively summarise the accumulated research on a topic, promote new questions on the matter and channel the stream of clinical research towards relevant horizons. Consequently, systematic reviews can also be important to health policy planners and others involved in planning effective health care.

If the results of systematic reviews are to be used by health care providers and health care consumers, it is necessary that they are as free as possible of bias (i.e. systematic error). One way to assess the merits of a systematic review is to assess the quality of its report. It is possible that a scientific report may not reflect how the investigators conducted their review but rather their ability to write comprehensively. Although the data addressing this point are sparse, it appears that a scientific report is a reasonable marker for how the project was conducted. In an assessment of the quality of 63 randomised trials in breast cancer, Liberati and colleagues[3] reported that the average quality of reports was 50% (95%CI: 46 to 54 %) of the maximum score. Following these assessments, the investigators interviewed 62 of the corresponding authors to ascertain whether information in the manuscripts submitted to publication consideration was removed prior to its publication. The authors reported that with the additional information obtained from the interviews the quality scores only increased, marginally, to an average score of 57%. These data come from clinical trials. We are unaware of comparable data for systematic reviews.

Choosing an appropriate evaluation tool for critically appraising the report of a systematic review is as difficult as the assessment of quality of reports of randomised trials (see Chapter 5). A systematic review[4] designed to identify and appraise instruments that assess the quality of reports of randomised trials found twenty-five scales and nine checklists. The scales differed considerably from one another in a variety of areas including: how they defined quality; the scientific rigor in which they were developed; the number of items they used; and the time required to use them. When six of the scales were compared to one another for assessing the same randomised trials, divergent scores and rankings were reported.

In attempting to attain consistency in the quality of reporting, the purpose of this chapter is to identify and appraise instruments developed to assess the quality of reports of systematic reviews. It will also evaluate whether different instruments assessing the same systematic review would provide similar evidence regarding its quality.

Throughout this chapter we refer to the reporting of both systematic reviews and meta-analyses. A systematic review may, or may not, include a meta-analysis, a statistical analysis of the results from independent studies (see Chapter 1 for a discussion of terminology).

A systematic review of published checklists and scales

A literature search was performed to take an inventory of published checklists and scales. Potentially relevant articles were chosen and the tools described were reviewed and quality assessment, across a selected few instruments, was tested based on four randomly chosen systematic reviews. A more detailed description of this process can be found in Box 7.1.

The QUOROM Statement

Although guidelines for reporting systematic reviews have been suggested, until recently, a consensus across disciplines about how they should be reported had not been developed. Following a recent initiative to improve the quality of reporting of randomised controlled trials, the CONSORT statement,[5] a conference referred to as the Quality Of Reporting Of Meta-analyses (QUOROM) was held to address these issues, as they relate to systematic reviews of randomised trials. The QUOROM conference participants were clinical epidemiologists, clinicians, statisticians, and researchers who conduct meta-analysis as well as editors from the UK and North America who were interested in systematic reviews. This conference resulted in the creation of the QUOROM Statement, which consists of a checklist (see Table 7.1) and flow diagram (see Figure 7.1).[6] The checklist consists of 18 items, including 8 evidence based ones,[7–20] addressing primarily the Abstract, Introduction, Methods, and Results section of a report of a systematic review of randomised trials. This checklist encourages authors to provide readers with information regarding searches, selection, validity assessment, data abstraction, study characteristics, quantitative data synthesis, and trial flow. The flow diagram provides information about the progress of randomised trials throughout the review process from the number of potentially relevant trials identified, to those retrieved and ultimately included. Items reported in the QUOROM statement that are to be included in a systematic review report were chosen based on evidence whenever possible, which implies the need to include items that can systematically influence estimates of treatment effects. Over the last 18 months the QUOROM group has evaluated the impact of the

QUOROM statement on the editorial process. Ten medical journals have participated in a randomised trial evaluating the impact of applying the QUOROM criteria on journal peer review. At the time of writing (January 2000) accrual had been completed.

Box 7.1 Methodology

Literature search
- MEDLINE: January 1966–February 1999
- three independent searches with keywords: meta-analysis, review literature, systematic or quantitative or methodological review, overview, review, information synthesis, integrative research review, guideline, checklist, tool, scoring, scale, clinimetric, quality, critical reading, methodology
- PubMed "related articles" function to find others

Identification and selection
- initial screening to identify relevance
- potentially relevant articles reviewed independently by each author
- article eligible regardless of language
- article has to be scale or checklist (see Appendix 1) designed to assess quality of systemic reviews and meta-analyses

Data extraction
- checklists and scales assessed for: (1) number of items included in tool; (2) aspects of quality assessed; (3) whether or not article included explicit statement regarding purpose of tool; and (4) time to completion of tool
- data extraction was completed in a group and consensus reached

Quality assessment
- compared items in each quality assessment instrument against QUOROM statement
- three checklists and one scale were conveniently selected to compare stability of quality assessments across instruments
- randomly selected four systematic reviews (from pool of 400 systematic reviews) to be used for quality assessment based on four selected instruments
- quality assessments completed as a group
- quality assessment established in two ways: (1) a quantitative estimate based on one item from a validated scale; and (2) the proportion of items reported (as a function of the number of items included in tool) in the systematic review report

Table 7.1 Quality of reporting of meta-analyses – QUOROM for clinical randomised controlled trials (RCTs).[6]

Heading	Subheading	Descriptor	Reported? Y/N	Page Number
Title		Identify the report as a meta-analysis (or systematic review) of randomised trials[7]		
Abstract		Use a structured format[8] Describe		
	Objectives	The clinical question explicitly		
	Data sources	The databases (i.e. list) and other information sources		
	Review methods	The selection criteria (i.e. population, intervention, outcome, and study design); methods for validity assessment, data abstraction, and study characteristics, and quantitative data synthesis) in sufficient detail to permit replication		
	Results	Characteristics of the randomised trials included and excluded; qualitative and quantitative findings (i.e., point estimates and confidence intervals); and subgroup analyses		
	Conclusion	The main results.		
Text				
Introduction		Describe The explicit clinical problem, biologic rationale for the intervention, and rationale for review		
Methods	Searching	The information sources, in detail[9] (e.g. databases, registers, personal files, expert informants, agencies, hand-searching), and any restrictions (years considered, publication status,[10] language of publication)[11,12]		
	Selection	The inclusion and exclusion criteria (defining population, intervention principal outcomes, and study design)[13]		
	Validity assessment	The criteria and process used (e.g. masked conditions, quality assessment and their findings)[14-17]		
	Data abstraction	The process used (e.g. completed independently, in duplicate)[16]		
	Study characteristics	The type of study design, participants' characteristics, details of intervention, outcome definitions, etc.;[18] and how clinical heterogeneity was assessed		
	Quantitative data synthesis	The principal measures of effect (e.g. relative risk), method of combining results (statistical testing and confidence intervals), handling of missing data, etc.; how statistical heterogeneity was assessed;[19] a rationale for any a priori sensitivity and subgroup analyses; and any assessment of publication bias[20]		
Results	Trial flow	Provide a meta-analysis profile summarising trial flow (see figure)		
	Study characteristics	Present descriptive data for each trial (e.g. age, sample size, intervention, dose, duration, follow-up)		
	Quantitative data synthesis	Report agreement on the selection and validity assessment; present simple summary results (for each treatment group in each trial, for each primary outcome); data needed to calculate effect sizes and confidence intervals in intention-to-treat analyses (e.g., 2×2 tables of counts, means and standard deviations, proportions)		
Discussion		Summarise the key findings; discuss clinical inferences based on internal and external validity; interpret the results in light of the totality of available evidence; describe potential biases in the review process (e.g. publication bias); and suggest a future research agenda		

126

Potentially relevant RCTs identified and screened for retrieval ($n = ...$)

RCTs excluded, with reasons ($n = ...$)

RCTs retrieved for more detailed evaluation ($n = ...$)

RCTs excluded, with reasons ($n = ...$)

Potentially appropriate RCTs to be included in the meta-analysis ($n = ...$)

RCTs included in meta-analysis ($n = ...$)

RCTs excluded from the meta-analysis, with reasons ($n = ...$)

RCTs with usable information, by outcome ($n = ...$)

RCTs withdrawn, by outcome, with reasons ($n = ...$)

Figure 7.1 Progress through the stages of a meta-analysis, including selection of potentially relevant randomised controlled trials (RCTs), included and excluded RCTs with a statement of the reasons, RCTs with usable information, and RCTs withdrawn by outcome with a statement of the reasons for the withdrawal.

QUOROM as the "gold standard"

The QUOROM statement for reporting systematic reviews was created according to evidence and is a comprehensive set of guidelines. Several methods were used to generate the checklist and flow diagram: a systematic review of the reporting of systematic reviews; focus groups of the steering committee; and a modified Delphi approach during an expert panel consensus conference. QUOROM group members were asked to identify items that they thought should be included in a checklist that would be useful for investigators, editors, and peer reviewers. Items included in the checklist were guided by research evidence suggesting that a failure to adhere to the particular checklist item proposed could lead to biased results.

For example, authors are asked (under the "Methods" heading, and "Searching" subheading) to be explicit in reporting whether they have used any restrictions on language of publication. Approximately one third of published systematic reviews have some language restrictions as part of the eligibility criteria for including individual trials.[11] It is not clear why, since there is no evidence to support differences in study quality,[12] and there is evidence supporting that such action may result in a biased summary. The role of language restrictions has been studied in 211 randomised trials included in 18 meta-analyses in which trials published in languages other than English were included in the quantitative summary.[11] Language-restricted meta-analyses, as compared to language-inclusive ones, over-estimated the treatment effect by only 2%, on average. However, the language-inclusive meta-analyses were more precise.[11]

The QUOROM statement was also formally pre-tested with representatives of several constituencies who would use the recommendations, after which modifications were made.

Results

The search identified 318 potentially relevant articles. After eliminating duplicates or previously published instruments and those that were not scales or checklists (see Appendix 1), twenty-four instruments[21-44] were included in our review; 21 checklists and three scales (see Table 7.2). All of the instruments, except one scale (see Appendix 2),[44] have been published and can be used with all types of systematic reviews. The instruments were developed between 1984 and 1997, indicating a fairly recent interest in this area. The number of items in each instrument ranged from 5 to 101, with only two checklists having more than 35 items (see Table 7.3).[22-24] Fourteen checklists and one scale included an explicit statement regarding the purpose of their instrument. The average time required to assess the quality of a systematic review using the checklists and scales was 12 minutes (range: 5–30) and 12 minutes (range: 5–20), respectively (see Table 7.3). two of the checklists took at least 30 minutes to complete.[22,24]

Comparison of QUOROM to other checklists and scales

Checklists

None of the other checklists included all the items recommended by QUOROM (see Table 7.2). The majority of checklists contained items about what the method section of a systematic review should include and

Table 7.2 Number of criteria reported by each checklist and scale (first author named) fulfilling the 17* headings and subheadings included in the QUOROM statement.[6]

Instruments†‡	Title	Abstract					Introduction	Method						Results			Discussion
		Objectives	Data sources	Review methods	Results	Conclusion		Searching	Selection	Validity assessment	Data abstraction	Description of study characteristics	Quantitative data synthesis	Trial flow	Description of study characteristics	Quantitative data synthesis	
Checklist																	
Bletner	NO	NO	NO	NO	NO	NO	YES	YES	YES	NO	YES	YES	YES	NO	YES	YES	NO
Cook	NO	NO	NO	NO	NO	NO	YES	YES	YES	YES	YES	NO	YES	NO	YES	YES	YES
Geller	NO	NO	NO	NO	NO	NO	NO	YES	YES	YES	NO	NO	YES	NO	NO	YES	YES
Goldschmidt	NO	NO	NO	NO	NO	NO	YES	YES	NO	YES	YES	NO	NO	NO	NO	YES	YES
Greenhalgh	NO	NO	NO	NO	NO	NO	NO	YES	NO	YES	NO	YES	NO	NO	NO	NO	YES
Halvorsen	NO	NO	NO	NO	NO	NO	UN	YES	YES	NO	YES	YES	YES	NO	NO	NO	NO
L'Abbé	NO	NO	NO	NO	NO	NO	YES	YES	YES	NO	NO	YES	NO	NO	NO	UN	YES
Light	YES	NO	YES	NO	NO	YES	NO	YES	YES	NO	NO	YES	YES	NO	NO	NO	UN
Meinert	NO	YES	YES	YES	NO	NO	UN	YES	YES	YES	YES	NO	YES	NO	YES	YES	YES
Mullen	NO	NO	NO	NO	NO	NO	YES	YES	YES	YES	NO	UN	NO	NO	UN	YES	YES
Mulrow	NO	NO	NO	NO	NO	YES	YES	YES	YES	YES	YES	YES	UN	NO	YES	YES	UN
Neely	YES	YES	YES	UN	UN	YES	YES	YES	YES	YES	NO	NO	YES	NO	UN	UN	YES
Nony	NO	NO	NO	NO	NO	NO	YES	YES	YES	YES	YES	UN	YES	NO	YES	YES	YES
Ohlsson	NO	NO	NO	NO	NO	NO	NO	YES	YES	YES	NO	YES	YES	NO	NO	YES	UN
Oxman	NO	NO	NO	NO	NO	NO	NO	YES	YES	YES	YES	YES	UN	NO	YES	NO	YES
Oxman	NO	NO	NO	NO	NO	NO	YES	YES	YES	YES	YES	UN	UN	NO	YES	YES	NO
Pogue	NO	NO	NO	NO	NO	NO	NO	YES	YES	NO	YES	YES	YES	NO	YES	YES	YES
Sacks	NO	NO	NO	NO	NO	NO	YES	NO	YES	YES	NO	YES	YES	NO	YES	YES	UN
Smith	NO	NO	NO	NO	NO	NO	NO	YES	YES	YES	YES	YES	NO	NO	UN	NO	YES
Thacker	NO	NO	NO	NO	NO	NO	YES	YES	YES	YES	YES	UN	UN	NO	UN	UN	YES
Wilson	NO	NO	NO	NO	NO	NO	YES	YES	YES	YES	YES	UN	YES	NO	YES	YES	NO
Scale																	
Assendelft[42]	NO	NO	NO	NO	NO	NO	NO	YES	YES	YES	NO	YES	NO	NO	YES	YES	YES
Auperin[43]	NO	NO	NO	NO	NO	NO	NO	YES	YES	YES	YES	YES	YES	NO	UN	YES	YES
Oxman[44]	NO	NO	NO	NO	NO	NO	NO	YES	YES	YES	YES	NO	YES	NO	NO	YES	YES

* The QUORUM statement includes 18 items. One item, under the Abstract heading, "Use a structured format", was not included here as we did not evaluate the presence of this item in the other instruments.
† When items in an instrument were unclear we reviewed the complete text of the article for possible clarification.
‡ For an instrument to be included, the report had to provide a summary form, such as a checklist, of the items discussed in the text of the article.
UN = uncertain as to whether the item was reported.

129

Table 7.3 Descriptive characteristics of published and unpublished checklists and scales used to assess the quality of systematic reviews and meta-analyses of randomised trials.

Instrument	Number of items	Type of quality assessed	Explicit statement regarding the purpose of tool	Time to complete*
Checklist				
Blettner	12	General	Yes	15
Cook	65	General	No	30
Geller	12	General	Yes	20
Goldschmidt	101	General	Yes	30
Greenhalgh	5	General	No	5
Halvorsen	8	General	No	5
L'Abbé	9†	General	Yes	5
Light	10	General	Yes	5
Meinert	35	General	Yes	15
Mullen	12	General	Yes	10
Mulrow	8	General	Yes	5
Neely	5†	General	No	10
Nony	30	General	No	20
Ohlsson	26	General	No	15
Oxman	11	General	Yes	5
Oxman	8	General	Yes	5
Pogue	20	General	Yes	10
Sacks	23	General	Yes	20
Smith	12	General	No	5
Thacker	15	Specific	Yes	15
Wilson	10	General	Yes	10
Scale				
Assendelft	14	Specific	No	10
Auperin	27	General	No	20
Oxman‡	9	General	Yes	5

* Approximate time which may vary depending on the operator.
† There are several sub categories within each of the questions.
‡ Unpublished.

generally neglected the other components of the report: only one (5%) checklist[22] included an item regarding the title and two (10%) addressed the abstract.[29,32] The Abstract items in the QUOROM checklist were the least frequently encountered among the checklists (0–9%). Thirteen (62%) included an item about the introduction, although we could not tell if this criterion was met in two[27,30] of the checklists.

There was considerable overlap between the content of the QUOROM checklist and the method section of the other checklists. All but two checklists (90%) asked about the searching and all but one (95%) asked about the selection criteria. Sixteen (76%) included an item on validity and twelve (57%) asked about data abstraction. Items about data synthesis were definitely present in 13 checklists (62%), and possibly present in three others (see Table 7.2). However, while quantitative data synthesis was clearly identified as a prerequisite in 13 (62%) of the checklists and may possibly have been required in three others, only nine (43%) of them (and possibly four others) included a question on the individual study characteristics in the methods section.

Items concerning the results and discussion sections in the QUOROM statement were definitely reported in 57% of the checklists, respectively, with the exception of the "trial flow" item which was not included in any of the checklists.

Eleven checklists (52%), and possibly four others, stressed the need for the inclusion of a description of the primary study characteristics in the results' section. Again, the need for quantitative data synthesis in the results section was mentioned in the majority of checklists, i.e. thirteen (62%), and possibly in three others. Twelve checklists (57%), and possibly four others, included an item about a discussion section (see Table 7.2).

Scales

Unlike the QUOROM statement none of the scales included a question on the Title, the Introduction, or the Abstract. The Abstract items in the QUOROM checklist were the least frequently encountered among the scales (0%), while those concerning the methods sections are the most frequently encountered, i.e. from 67% to 100% of the time. For example, all three scales included items on searching, selection and validity assessment. Data abstraction, describing the study characteristics of the primary studies and quantitative data synthesis were included in two of the three scales (see Table 7.2).

In the results section no scale suggested producing a trial flow diagram as recommended by the QUOROM statement. All three scales included a quantitative data synthesis and one,[43] possibly two,[44] included an item on describing the characteristics of the primary studies. Again, all three scales included an item about the discussion.

Assessment of quality across instruments

In order to compare the stability of quality assessments across instruments we completed a small pilot study. We conveniently selected three checklists[27,29,38] and one scale,[44] representing a broad spectrum. Out of the four systematic reviews evaluated using the checklists and scales three were paper based[45-47] while the fourth one was a Cochrane review.[48] All four were published in 1992 or later (see Table 7.4). The quality of the report of each review, based on the proportion of items reported in the review, was fairly stable across instruments. The difference in quality scores, between the four instruments, ranged from 26% to 34% of the maximum possible

131

Table 7.4 Quality scores and ranks of each of four meta-analyses of randomised trials, across three published quality assessment instruments and one unpublished one.*

Title of meta-analysis	Year of publication	Oxman and Guyatt	Oxman and Guyatt	L'Abbé	Sacks	Meinert	% Range (difference)	Rank range
		Score	Proportion of items present % (number of items/total); rank					
Effects of psychosocial interventions With adult cancer patients: a meta-analysis of randomised experiments[45]	1995	43 (3/7); 2	56 (5/9); 2	22 (2/9); 2	26 (6/23); 3	49 (17/35); 2	22–56 (34)	2–3
Impact of post menopausal hormone therapy on cardiovascular events and cancer: pooled data from clinical trials[46]	1997	29 (2/7); 3	22 (2/9); 4	11 (1/9); 4	26 (6/33); 3	37 (13/35); 4	11–37 (26)	3–4
How effective are current drugs for Crohn's Disease? A meta-analysis[47]	1992	29 (2/7); 3	56 (5/9); 2	22 (2/9); 2	35 (8/33); 2	43 (15/35); 3	22–56 (34)	2–3
The efficacy of tacrine in Alzheimer's disease[48]	1997	57 (4/7); 1	67 (6/9); 1	33 (3/9); 1	65 (15/23); 1	49 (17/35); 1	33–67 (34)	1

* We have used the Oxman and Guyatt instrument in two different ways; as a score; and as a proportion of items present in the report of a systematic review.

132

evaluation (see Table 7.4). The Cochrane review had the highest quality regardless of the instrument used. When the systematic reviews were ranked based on the quality score obtained from each instrument, it was apparent that one of them consistently ranked highest, independently of the instrument. The rank ranges were also stable across the different instruments used, with the Cochrane review reporting the highest rank across all four instruments (see Table 7.4).

Discussion

The literature search yielded more than two dozen instruments that have been developed to assess various aspects of a systematic review. The scale developed by Oxman and Guyatt (see Appendix 2)[44] meets several important criteria. Here the developers defined the construct they were interested in investigating, measured the discriminatory power of items, and conducted inter observer reliability studies, as part of the development process. A full discussion of the process of instrument development is beyond the scope of this chapter. It is however fair to say that investigators wishing to develop a new instrument should, at the very least, follow published guidelines for instrument development.[49,50]

Regardless of the checklist or scale used the results of this assessment indicate that the quality of reports of systematic reviews are low and there is considerable room for improvement. Similar data have been reported elsewhere. A classic 1987 survey[38] of 86 meta-analyses assessed each publication on 14 items from six content areas thought to be important in the conduct and reporting of meta-analysis of randomised trials: study design, combinability, control of bias, statistical analysis, sensitivity analysis, and problems of applicability. The results showed that only 24 (28%) of the 86 meta-analyses addressed all six content areas. The survey, updated using more recently published systematic reviews, provided similar results.[51] Comparable results have been reported elsewhere.[52-54]

These results highlight that not only systematic reviewers, but also editors and peer reviewers, may not fully appreciate the elements that should be taken into account during the design, conduct, and reporting of reviews.

The exception to the low quality of reports was the quality of the Cochrane review.[48] It was found that the Cochrane review had the highest absolute score and rank regardless of the instrument used. These results lend further evidence suggesting that the quality of reports of Cochrane reviews are of higher quality, in some aspects, to paper based ones. In a review of 36 Cochrane reviews, compared to 39 paper based ones, published in 1995, the authors found that Cochrane reviews, compared to paper based ones, were more likely to include a description of the inclusion and exclusion criteria (35/36 v 18/39; P < 0·001), and assess trial quality

133

(35/36 v 12/39; P < 0·001).[53] No Cochrane reviews had language restrictions (0/36 v 7/39; P < 0·01) as eligibility criteria and they were more frequently updated (18/36 v 1/39; P < 0·001).

The majority of instruments designed to assess the quality of systematic reviews are checklists rather than scales. Among the checklists there is considerable range in the number of items and time required for completion. The scales are somewhat more consistent in terms of the item pool and time required for use. The instruments have been developed to assess systematic reviews in several content areas; psychology, internal medicine, surgery, and rehabilitation health.

We noted a wide variability between the instruments in how questions, covering the same domain, were framed. For example, 19 (of 21) checklists asked about searching for primary studies. However, this might have resulted in a more focused description of the electronic search strategy used to identify relevant studies, or the breadth, in terms of electronic, manual, and content experts, of the search. Alternatively, there were domains, such as publication bias, addressed by some instruments but not others.

Results reported in this chapter suggest that the items included in the checklists and scales focus on aspects of the methodology of systematic reviews. When compared to the QUOROM checklist the most common items on both were in the methods section. However, many of the instruments had next to no items addressing the abstract. Given that many readers will only read the abstract, it was disappointing to see so little attention paid to this aspect of a report.

No instrument was found that asked authors to report on the flow of studies through the various stages of a systematic review. Such information provides some face validity for the reader regarding the process used by the authors to include studies throughout the review process. Some items included in other assessment tools are not covered within the QUOROM checklist, but we do not believe that many evidence based criteria were missed, given the methodology used to develop the QUOROM checklist.

If the quality of reports of systematic reviews is to improve steps must be taken. The Cochrane Collaboration is starting to achieve this objective through a combination of continual peer review throughout the systematic review process and the use of strict criteria that must be included in the process and report. Paper based journals face additional obstacles. However, the use of evidence based criteria, such as those identified in the QUOROM statement, may help to improve the situation. Similar efforts, such as the CONSORT statement, have recently been made to help improve the quality of reports of randomised trials[5] and we are starting to see the benefits of this approach.[55] We hope journals which have endorsed the CONSORT statement might do likewise with the QUOROM statement.

Acknowledgements

We thank Drs Finlay McAlister and Cindy Mulrow for reviewing earlier drafts of this paper. We thank Dr Peter Tugwell for his support throughout the development of this work. We also thank Drs Andy Oxman and Gord Guyatt for permission to include their unpublished scale.

1 Smith R. Where is the wisdom...?: the poverty of medical evidence. *BMJ* 1991;**303**:798–9.
2 Davidoff F, Haynes B, Sackett D, Smith R. evidence based medicine: a new journal to help doctors identify the information they need. *BMJ* 1995;**310**:1085–8.
3 Liberati A, Himel HN, Chalmers TC. A quality assessment of randomized control trials of primary treatment of breast cancer. *J Clin Oncol* 1986;**4**:942–51.
4 Moher D, Jadad AR, Tugwell P. Assessing the quality of randomized controlled trials: current issues and future directions. *Int J Technol Assess Health Care* 1996;**12**(2):195–208.
5 Begg CB, Cho MK, Eastwood S, *et al.* Improving the quality of reporting of randomized controlled trials: the CONSORT statement. *JAMA* 1996;**276**:637–9.
6 Moher D, Cook DJ, Eastwood S, Olkin I, Rennie D, Stroup D. for the QUOROM group. Improving the quality of reporting of meta-analysis of randomized controlled trials: the QUOROM statement. *Lancet* 1999;**354**:1896–900.
7 Dickersin K, Scherer R, Lefebvre C. Identifying relevant studies for systematic reviews. *BMJ* 1994;**309**:1286–91.
8 Taddio A, Pain T, Fassos FF, Boon H, Illersich AL, Einarson TR. Quality of nonstructured and structured abstracts of original research articles in the British Medical Journal, the Canadian Medical Association Journal and the Journal of the American Medical Association. *Can Med Assoc J* 1994;**150**:1611–15.
9 Tramèr M, Reynolds DJM, Moore RA, McQuay HJ. Impact of covert duplicate publication on meta-analysis: a case study. *BMJ* 1997;**315**:635–40.
10 McAuley L, Pham B, Tugwell P, Moher D. Does the inclusion of Grey literature influence the estimates of intervention effectiveness reported in meta-analyses? *The Lancet* (in press).
11 Moher D, Pham B, Klassen TP, *et al.* What contributions do languages other than English make on the results of meta-analyses? In press. *J Clin Epidemiol* 2000 (in press).
12 Egger M, Zellweger-Zähner T, Schneider M, Junker C, Lengeler C, Antes G. Language bias in randomised controlled trials published in English and German. *Lancet* 1997;**350**:326–9.
13 Khan KS, Daya S, Collins JA, Walter S. Empirical evidence of bias in infertility research: overestimation of treatment effect in crossover trials using pregnancy as the outcome measure. *Fertil Steril* 1996;**65**:939–45.
14 Schulz KF, Chalmers I, Hayes RJ, Altman DG. Empirical evidence of bias: dimensions of methodological quality associated with estimates of treatment effects in controlled trials. *JAMA* 1995;**273**:408–12.
15 Moher D, Pham B, Jones A, *et al.* Does the quality of reports of randomised trials affect estimates of intervention efficacy reported in meta-analyses? *Lancet* 1998;**352**:609–13.
16 Jadad AR, Moore RA, Carroll D, *et al.* Assessing the quality of reports of randomized clinical trials: is blinding necessary? *Controlled Clin Trials* 1996;**17**:1–12.
17 Berlin JA and on behalf of the University of Pennsylvania meta-analysis blinding study group. Does blinding of readers affect the results of meta-analyses? *Lancet* 1997;**350**:185–6.
18 Barnes DE, Bero LA. Why review articles on the health effects of passive smoking reach different conclusions. *JAMA* 1998;**279**:1566–70.
19 Thompson SG. Why sources of heterogeneity in meta-analysis should be investigated. *BMJ* 1994;**309**:1351–5.
20 Simes RJ. Publication bias: the case for an international registry of clinical trials. *J Clin Oncol* 1986;**4**:1529–41.
21 Blettner M, Sauerbrei W, Schlehofer B, Scheuchenpflug T, Friedenreich C. Traditional reviews, meta-analyses and pooled analyses in epidemiology. *Int J Epidemiol* 1999;**28**:1–9.

22 Cook DJ, Sackett DL, Spitzer WO. Methodologic guidelines for systematic reviews of randomized control trials in health care from the Potsdam consultation on meta-analysis. *J Clin Epidemiol* 1995;**48**:167–71.
23 Geller NL, Proschan M. Meta-analysis of clinical trials: a consumer's guide. *J Biopharmaceut Stat* 1996;**6**:377-394.
24 Goldschmidt PG. Information synthesis: a practical guide. *Health Serv Res* 1986;**21**:215–37.
25 Greenhalgh T. Papers that summarise other papers (systematic reviews and meta-analyses). In: *How to read a paper – the basics of evidence based medicine.* London: BMJ Publishing Group, London. 1997.
26 Taylor Halvorsen K. The reporting format. In: Edited by Cooper H, Hedges LV, eds. *The handbook of research synthesis.* New York: Russell Sage Foundation, 1994: 425–37.
27 L'Abbé KA, Detsky AS, O'Rourke K. Meta-analysis in clinical research. *Ann Intern Med* 1987;**107**:224–33.
28 Light RJ, Pillemer DB. *The science of reviewing research.* Cambridge, MA: Harvard University Press 1984:160–86.
29 Meinert CL. Meta-analysis: Science or religion? *Controlled Clin Trials* 1989;**10**:257S–263S.
30 Mullen PD, Ramirez G. Information synthesis and meta-analysis. *Advan Health Educat Promot* 1987;**2**:201–39.
31 Mulrow CD. The medical review article: state of the science. *Ann Intern Med* 1987;**106**:485–8.
32 Neely JG. Literature review articles as a research form. *Otolaryngol – Head & Neck Surg* 1993;**108**:743–8.
33 Nony P, Cucherat M, Haugh MC, Boissel JP. Critical reading of the meta-analysis of clinical trials. *Therapie* 1995;**50**:339–51.
34 Ohlsson A. Systematic reviews – theory and practice. *Scand J Clin Lab Invest* 1994;**54**:25–32.
35 Oxman AD. Checklists for review articles. *BMJ* 1994;**309**:648–51.
36 Oxman AD, Guyatt G. Guidelines for reading literature reviews. *Can Med Assoc J* 1988;**138**:697–703.
37 Pogue JM, Yusuf S. Overcoming the limitations of current meta-analysis of randomized controlled trials. *Lancet* 1998;**351**:47–52.
38 Sacks HS, Berrier J, Reitman D, Ancona-Berk VA, Chalmers TC. Meta-analyses of randomized controlled trials. *N Engl J Med* 1987;**316**:450–4.
39 Smith MC, Stullenbarger E. Meta-analysis: an overview. *Nursing Sci Q* 1989;**2**:114–15.
40 Thacker SB, Peterson HB, Stroup DF. Meta-analysis for the obstetrician-gynecologist. *Am J Obstet Gynecol* 1996;**174**:1403–7.
41 Wilson A, Henry DA. Meta-analysis. *Med J Aust* 1992;**156**:173–87.
42 Assendelft WJJ, Koes B, Knipschild PG, Bouter LM. The relationship between methodological quality and conclusions in reviews of spinal manipulation. *JAMA* 1995;**274**:1942–8.
43 Auperin A, Pignon JP, Poynard T. Critical review of meta-analyses of randomized clinical trials in hepatogastroenterology. *Almeth Pharmacol Therapy* 1999;**11**:215–25.
44 Oxman AD, Guyatt GH. Index of the scientific quality of research overviews. Unpublished.
45 Meyer TJ, Mark MM. Effects of psychosocial interventions with adult cancer patients: A meta-analysis of randomized experiments. *Health Psychol* 1995;**14**:101–8.
46 Hemminki E, McPherson K. Impact of postmenopausal hormone therapy on cardiovascular events and cancer: pooled data from clinical trials. *BMJ* 1997;**315**:149–53.
47 Salomon P, Kornbluth A, Aisenberg J, Janowitz HD. How effective are current drugs for Crohn's disease? A meta-analysis. *J Clin Gastroenterol* 1992;**14**:211–15.
48 Qizilbash N, Birks J, Lopez Arrieta J, Lewington S, Szeto S. Tacrine for Alzheimer's disease (Cochrane Review). In: *The Cochrane Library,* Issue 1, 1997. Oxford: Update Software.
49 Norman DL, Streiner D. *Health measurement scales – a practical guide to their development and use,* 2nd edn. Oxford: Oxford University Press, 1995.
50 McDowell I, Newell C. *Measuring health: a guide to rating scales and questionnaires,* 2nd edn. Oxford: Oxford University Press, 1996.

51 Sacks HS, Reitman D, Pagano D, and Kupelnick B. Meta-analysis: an update. *Mt Sinai J Med* 1996;**63**:216–24.
52 Jadad AR, McQuay HJ. Meta-analyses to evaluate analgesic interventions: a systematic qualitative review of their methodology. *J Clin Epidemiol* 1996;**49**:235–43.
53 Jadad AR, Cook DJ, Jones A, *et al.* Methodology and reports of systematic reviews and meta-analyses: A comparison of Cochrane reviews with articles published in paper-based journals. *JAMA* 1998;**280**:278–80.
54 McAlister FA, Clark HD, van Walraven C, *et al.* The medical review article revisited: has the science improved? *Ann Intern Med* 1999;**131**:947–51.
55 Lebeau DL, Steinmann WC, Patel KV. Has the randomized controlled trial literature improved after CONSORT? Conference presentation at the 50 years of randomized trials. Sponsored by the BMJ Publishing group, London, October, 1998.

Appendix 1

Checklists provide a qualitative estimate of the overall quality of a systematic review using itemised criteria for comparing the reviews. As such, checklists items do not have numerical scores attached to each item.

Scales are similar to checklists except that each item of a scale is scored numerically and an overall quality score is generated. To be considered a scale the construct under consideration should be a continuum with an overall summary score.

Appendix 2

Quality of meta-analysis: Oxman and Guyatt's index of the scientific quality of research overviews

The purpose of this index is to evaluate the scientific quality (i.e. adherence to scientific principles) of research overviews (review articles) published in the medical literature. It is not intended to measure literary quality, importance, relevance, originality, or other attributes of overviews.

The index is for assessing overviews of primary ("original") research on pragmatic questions regarding causation, diagnosis, prognosis, therapy or prevention. A research overview is a survey of research. The same principles that apply to epidemiologic surveys apply to overviews: a question must be clearly specified, a target population identified and accessed, appropriate information obtained from that population in an unbiased fashion, and conclusions derived, sometimes with the help of formal statistical analysis, as is done in "meta-analyses". The fundamental difference between overviews and epidemiologic surveys is the unit of analysis, not the scientific issues that the questions in this index address.

Since most published overviews do not include a methods section it is difficult to answer some of the questions in the index. Base your answers, as much as possible, on the information provided in the overview. If the methods that were used are reported incompletely relative to a specific item, score that item as "partially". Similarly, if there is no information provided regarding what was done relative to a particular question, score it as "can't tell", unless there is information in the overview to suggest either that the criterion was or was not met.

1   Were the search methods used to find evidence (original research) on the primary question(s) stated?
   ❑ yes   ❑ partially   ❑ no

2   Was the search for evidence reasonably comprehensive?
   ❑ yes   ❑ can't tell   ❑ no

3   Were the criteria used for deciding which studies to include in the overview reported?
   ❑ yes   ❑ partially   ❑ no

4   Was bias in the selection of studies avoided?
   ❑ yes   ❑ can't tell   ❑ no

5   Were the criteria used for assessing the validity of the included studies reported?
   ❑ yes   ❑ partially   ❑ no

6   Was the validity of all studies referred to in the text assessed using appropriate criteria (either in selecting studies for inclusion or in analysing the studies that are cited)?
   ❑ yes   ❑ can't tell   ❑ no

7   Were the methods used to combine the findings of the relevant studies (to reach a conclusion) reported?
   ❑ yes   ❑ partially   ❑ no

8   Were the findings of the relevant studies combined appropriately relative to the primary question the overview addresses?
   ❑ yes   ❑ can't tell   ❑ no

For question 8, if no attempt was made to combine findings, and no statement is made regarding the inappropriateness of combining findings, check "no". If a summary (general) estimate is given anywhere in the abstract, the discussion or the summary section of the paper, and it is not reported how the estimate was derived, mark "no" even if there is a statement regarding the limitations of combining the findings of the studies reviewed. If in doubt mark "can't tell".

9   Were the conclusions made by the author(s) supported by the data and/or analysis reported in the overview?
    ❑ yes   ❑ partially   ❑ no

For an overview to be scored as "yes" on question 9, data (not just citations) must be reported that supports the main conclusions regarding the primary question(s) that the overview addresses.

10 How would you rate the scientific quality of the overview?

Extensive Flaws		major flaws		minor flaws		minimal flaws
❑	❑	❑	❑	❑	❑	❑
1	2	3	4	5	6	7

The score for question 10, the overall scientific quality, should be based on your answers to the first nine questions. The following guidelines can be used to assist with deriving a summary score. If the "can't tell" option is used one or more times on the preceding questions, a review is likely to have minor flaws at best and it is difficult to rule out major flaws (i.e. a score of 4 or lower). If the "no" option is used on question 2, 4, 6 or 8, the review is likely to have major flaws (i.e. a score of 3 or less, depending on the number and degree of the flaws).

Part II: Investigating variability within and between studies

8 Going beyond the grand mean: subgroup analysis in meta-analysis of randomised trials

GEORGE DAVEY SMITH, MATTHIAS EGGER

Summary points

- Meta-analysis can be used to examine differences in treatment effects across trials; however, the fact that randomised trials are included in meta-analyses does not mean that comparisons between trials are also randomised comparisons.
- Meta-analytic subgroup analyses, like subgroup analyses within trials, are prone to bias and need to be interpreted with caution.
- A more reliable way of assessing differences in treatment effects is to relate outcome to some underlying patient characteristic on a continuous, or ordered, scale.
- The underlying level of risk is a key variable which is often related to a given treatment effect, with patients at higher risk receiving more benefit then low risk patients.
- Individual patient data, rather than published summary statistics, are often required for meaningful subgroup analyses.

The ultimate purpose of a systematic review is generally considered to be the production of an overall estimate of the intervention's effect by combining studies in a meta-analysis. In this chapter we examine extensions of the use of meta-analysis beyond such combination of the results from individual trials. First, we discuss the pros and cons of performing subgroup analyses. Second, we consider the situation in which the differences in effects between individual trials are related in a graded way to an underlying phenomenon, such as the degree of mortality risk of the trial participants.

Subgroup analysis

The main aim of a meta-analysis is to produce an estimate of the average effect seen in trials comparing therapeutic strategies. The direction and magnitude of this average effect is intended to help guide decisions about clinical practice for a wide range of patients. The clinician is thus being asked to treat her patients as though they were well represented by the patients in the clinical trials included in the meta-analysis. This runs against the concerns physicians have for using the specific characteristics of a particular patient to tailor management accordingly.[1,2] Indeed, it is implausible to assume that the effect of a given treatment is identical across different groups of patients – the young versus the elderly, or those with mild versus those with severe disease, for example. It may therefore seem reasonable to base treatment decisions upon the results of those trials which have included participants with similar characteristics to the particular patient under consideration, rather than on the totality of the evidence as furnished by a meta-analysis.

Decisions based on subgroup analyses are often misleading, however. Consider, for example, a physician in Germany being confronted by the meta-analysis of long term beta-blockade following myocardial infarction that we presented in Chapter 2. Whilst there is a robust beneficial effect seen in the overall analysis, in the only large trial recruiting a substantial proportion of German patients, the European Infarction Study (EIS),[3] there was, if anything, a detrimental effect of using beta-blockers (see Figure 2.1 in Chapter 2). Should the physician give beta-blockers to German post-infarct patients? Common sense would suggest that being German does not prevent a patient obtaining benefit from beta-blockade. Thus, the best estimate of the outcome for German patients may actually come through, essentially, discounting the trial carried out in German patients. This may seem paradoxical; indeed the statistical expression of this phenomenon is known as Stein's paradox[4] (see Box 8.1).

Deciding whether to be guided by overall effects or by the results for a particular group of study participants is not just a problem created by meta-analysis; it also applies to the interpretation of individual clinical trials.[5] Authors of trial reports often spend more time discussing the results seen within subgroups of patients included in the trial than on the overall results. Yet frequently the findings of these subgroup analyses fail to be confirmed by later research. The various trials of beta-blockade after myocardial infarction yielded several subgroup findings with apparent clinical significance.[6] Treatment was said to be beneficial in patients under 65 but harmful in older patients; or only beneficial in patients with anterior myocardial infarction. When examined in subsequent studies, or in a formal pooling project,[7] these findings received no support.[6] This is a

Box 8.1 Stein's paradox

Applying the findings of meta-analyses in clinical practice will often mean that the results from a particular trial are essentially disregarded in favour of the overall estimate of the treatment effect (see discussion of the results from the European Infarction Study, EIS, in the main text). This assessment will generally be based on the conjecture that the opposing outcome in one trial represents the play of chance. Even if we observe that the effect in the patients included in a particular trial differs from other patient groups the overall estimate would still provide the best estimate of the effect in that patient group. This situation can be seen in the broader context of a phenomenon known as Stein's paradox.[4] In 1955, Charles Stein of Stanford University showed that it is generally better to estimate a particular quantity by taking into account the results of related surveys, instead of solely basing one's prediction on what was observed in one specific study. Conversely, conventional statistical theory holds that no other estimation rule is uniformly better than estimations based on the observed average. Using Stein's method it can be shown that the prevalence of a given disease in a particular region of a country is, on average, estimated with higher precision if the results from studies conducted in other parts of the country are taken into account. In other words, the estimation is not solely based on the results from the survey in the region of interest but on studies conducted many miles apart. This may seem paradoxical – why should the data from Oxford influence what we believe is true for Bristol? The central principle of Stein's method is the "shrinking" of the individual data points towards the grand mean, the latter being obtained by averaging the results from all studies. Therefore, if the survey in Oxford indicates a higher prevalence than overall in the UK, then the Oxford estimate is reduced. Conversely, if the survey in Bristol shows a lower prevalence, the figure for Bristol is increased. The amount by which the observed figure is adjusted towards the grand mean, the so-called "shrinkage factor", will depend on the precision attached to the observed value. This makes intuitive sense – an extreme result from a small study is more likely to be due to chance than a similar finding from a large trial. An outlying data point which was measured imprecisely is therefore shrunk to a greater extent than an outlier which was measured with considerable precision. Applying Stein's method to the trials of beta-blockers in myocardial infarction discussed in the main text would thus lead to the EIS result, which contributes only 6.5% of the weight in the combined analysis, being shrunk a long way towards the overall estimate of a beneficial effect of beta-blockade. Simple methods for "shrinking" the effects seen in particular, trials towards the overall effect estimate have been proposed.[8]

general phenomenon. It can be shown that if an overall treatment effect is statistically significant at the 5% level (P < 0·05) and the patients are divided at random into two similarly sized groups, then there is a one in three chance that the treatment effect will be large and statistically highly significant in one group but irrelevant and non-significant in the other.[9] Which subgroup "clearly" benefits from an intervention is thus often a chance phenomenon, inundating the literature with contradictory findings from subgroup analyses and wrongly inducing clinicians to withheld treatments from some patients.[2,10–12]

Meta-analyses offer a sounder basis for subgroup analysis, but they are not exempt from producing potentially misleading findings. One of the explanations put forward for the disappointing result seen in the beta-blocker trial in German post-infarct patients was that the agent used, oxprenolol, had intrinsic sympathomimetic activity (ISA).[13] This seemed plausible because the beneficial effect was assumed to be entirely mediated by blockade of the beta-1 receptor, and this interpretation was supported by a meta-analytic subgroup analysis based on 25 trials [14,15] which showed less benefit in trials of patients treated with ISA agents (Figure 8.1). The difference between the two classes of beta-blockers was statistically significant (P = 0·009). However, an updated analysis based on the 33 trials identified by Freemantle et al.[16] shows a smaller difference in the effect of ISA and non-ISA agents which is no longer statistically significant (P = 0·16, Figure 8.1) This illustrates that, far from aiding clinicians, post hoc subgroup analyses may confuse and mislead. Meta-analyses that utilise individual participant data (IPD), rather than simply the overall results of each trial, have greater power to carry out informative subgroup analyses (see Chapter 6). In such IPD meta-analyses subgroup analyses are performed within each trial and therefore differences in outcome between groups can be replicated (or fail to be replicated), allowing a more thorough assessment as to whether differences are spurious or not. In meta-analysis based on published data a more reliable assessment of differences in treatment effects between groups of study participants is to relate outcome to some characteristic (of the treatment or of the study participant) on a continuous, or ordered, scale.[17,18]

Meta-regression: examining gradients in treatment effects

The clinical trials included in a meta-analysis often differ in a way which would be expected to modify the outcome. In trials of cholesterol reduction the degree of cholesterol lowering attained differs markedly between studies, and the reduction in coronary heart disease mortality is

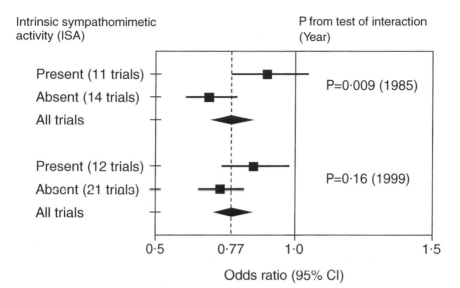

Figure 8.1 Total mortality from trials of beta-blockers in secondary prevention after myocardial infarction. Meta-analysis stratified by whether or not the beta-blocker used had intrinsic sympathomimetic activity (ISA). In 1985 a subgroup analysis based on 25 trials[14] indicated a substantial and statistically significant (P = 0·009 by test of interaction) difference in the reduction of mortality depending on whether ISA was present or absent. This difference was much reduced and became statistically non-significant (P = 0·16 by test of interaction) in an updated 1999 analysis based on 33 trials.[16]

greater in the trials in which larger reductions in cholesterol are achieved[17,19] (see also Chapter 9). Such graded associations are not limited to situations where greater benefits would be expected consequent on greater changes in a risk factor. For example, in the case of thrombolytic therapy after acute myocardial infarction, the greater the delay before therapy is given, the smaller the benefit consequent on thrombolysis.[20,21] Here, the graded association is seen between the outcome and a characteristic of the treatment which is used. The existence of such a gradient allows for a more powerful examination of differences in outcomes, since a statistical test for trend can be performed, rather than the less powerful test for evidence of global heterogeneity. Other attributes of study groups – such as age or length of follow-up – can readily be analysed in this way. As mentioned above, and discussed in detail in Chapter 6, such analyses will often require (or be strengthened by) the use of individual participant data, rather than published summary statistics.

Risk stratification in meta-analysis

A factor which is often related to a given treatment effect is the underlying risk of occurrence of the event the treatment aims to prevent. It makes intuitive sense that patients at high risk are more likely to benefit than low risk patients. In the case of trials of cholesterol lowering, for example, the patient groups have ranged from heart attack survivors with gross hypercholesterolaemia, to groups of healthy asymptomatic individuals with moderately elevated cholesterol levels. The coronary heart disease death rates of the former group have been up to 100 times higher than the death rates of the latter groups. The outcome of treatment in terms of all-cause mortality has been more favourable in the trials recruiting participants at high risk than in the trials involving relatively low-risk individuals.[17] There are two factors contributing to this. First, among the high-risk participants, the great majority of deaths will be from coronary heart disease, the risk of which is reduced by cholesterol reduction. A 30% reduction in coronary heart disease (CHD) mortality therefore translates into a near-equivalent reduction in total mortality. In the low-risk participants, on the other hand, a much smaller proportion – around 40% – of deaths will be from CHD. In this case a 30% reduction in CHD mortality would translate into a much smaller – around 10% – reduction in all-cause mortality. Secondly, if there is any detrimental effect of treatment, it may easily outweigh the benefits of cholesterol reduction in the low-risk group, whereas in high-risk patients among whom a substantial benefit is achieved from cholesterol reduction, this will not be the case. In a recent meta-analysis of cholesterol lowering trials this situation was evident for trials using fibrates but not for trials in which other drugs were used.[22]

A similar association between level of risk and benefit obtained can be seen in meta-analyses carried out for other types of medical treatment.[23] Thus, the use of antiplatelet agents such as aspirin after an acute myocardial infarction produces a 23% reduction in all-cause mortality, whereas in the primary prevention setting there is only a (non-significant) 5% reduction in mortality.[24] This may reflect a small increase in the risk of haemorrhagic stroke consequent on the use of antiplatelet agents which counterbalances the beneficial effects among low-risk individuals, but not among those at higher risk. In the case of the treatment of human immunodeficiency virus (HIV) infection with zidovudine, a large reduction in relative risk of death was seen in the single study which has been reported among patients with AIDS.[25] However, in a meta-analysis of seven trials it was seen that use of zidovudine early in the course of HIV-infection was not associated with any long-term survival benefit[26] (Figure 8.2). In situations where outcomes are very different in groups at different levels of risk, it is inappropriate to perform a meta-analysis in which an overall estimate of the

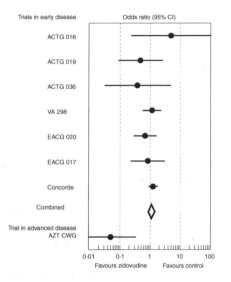

Figure 8.2 Meta-analysis of mortality results of trials of zidovudine in asymptomatic or early symptomatic HIV infection. The results are in stark contrast to the beneficial effect seen in the only trial in high risk patients (AZT Collaborative Working Group). From Egger et al. [26]

effect of treatment is calculated. In the case of the zidovudine trials, for example, an overall effect estimate from all the eight trials (odds ratio 0·96, 95% confidence interval [CI] 0·75 to 1·22) is very different from that seen in the only trial among patients with AIDS (odds ratio 0·04, 95% CI 0·01 to 0·33). If there had been more trials among patients with AIDS the overall effect would appear highly beneficial. Conversely, if there had been more large trials among asymptomatic patients the confidence intervals around the overall effect estimate would exclude any useful benefit, which would be misleading if applied to patients with AIDS.

Problems in risk stratification

When there have been many trials conducted in a particular field, it is possible to perform risk stratification at the level of individual trials. This was carried out in the case of cholesterol lowering,[17] using the CHD mortality rate in the control arm of the trials as the stratification variable. This stratification is of clinical use, since this is the risk of CHD death of patients without treatment, i.e. the risk level which the clinician would want to use for deciding whether or not patients will benefit from therapeutic cholesterol lowering. The analysis can also be performed using control group CHD mortality risk as a continuous variable, through the

149

examination of the interaction between treatment effect and risk in a logistic regression analysis. A significant statistical test for interaction suggests that there is a real difference in outcome at different levels of risk.

The use of control group mortality rates as a stratification variable does introduce a potential bias into the analysis, since control group CHD mortality is included in the calculation of the effect estimate from each trial.[17,27-29] Thus, if through chance variation the CHD death rate in the control group happens to be low, apparently unfavourable effects of the treatment on mortality would be likely, since mortality in the treatment group would apparently be increased. This would itself produce an association between the outcome measure and the level of risk in the control group, with greater benefit (and fewer disbenefits) being seen in those trials in which the play of chance led to a high control group mortality. For example, in a recent meta-regression analysis Hoes et al.[30] examined whether in middle-aged patients with mild-to-moderate hypertension the benefit from drug treatment depends on the underlying risk of death. The scatter plot advocated by L'Abbé et al.[31,32] of event rates in the treated group against control group rates was used (Figure 8.3(a)). This plot is useful for examining the degree of heterogeneity between trials and to identify outliers (see also Chapter 16). If the treatment is beneficial, trials will fall to the right of the line of identity (the no effect line). A set of trials estimating the same reduction in risk will scatter around a line which goes through the origin at 0 and deviates from the diagonal no-effect line. The further the line is from the diagonal line of no effect, the stronger is the treatment effect.

Hoes et al. then computed a linear regression model describing mortality in the treated groups as a function of control group rates.[30] Because the number of deaths and person-years of follow-up varied widely between studies, the analysis was weighted by the inverse of the variance of the rate ratio. The resulting regression line intersects with the null-effect line at a control group rate of 6 per 1000 person-years (Figure 8.3(a)). This was interpreted as indicating "that drug treatment for mild-to-moderate hypertension has no effect on, or may even increase, all-cause mortality in middle-aged patients".[30] In other words, anti-hypertensive treatment was considered to be beneficial only in patients at relatively high risk of death. This interpretation, however, is misleading because it ignores the influence of random fluctuations on the slope of the regression line.[27] If, owing to the play of chance, the control group rate in a trial happens to be particularly low, then the corresponding treatment group rate will, on average, appear to be high. Conversely, if mortality among controls is, by chance, high, then the corresponding rate in the treatment group will appear low. The effect of random error will thus rotate the regression line around a pivot, making it cross the line of identity on the right-hand side of the origin.

This phenomenon, a manifestation of regression to the mean,[28] can be

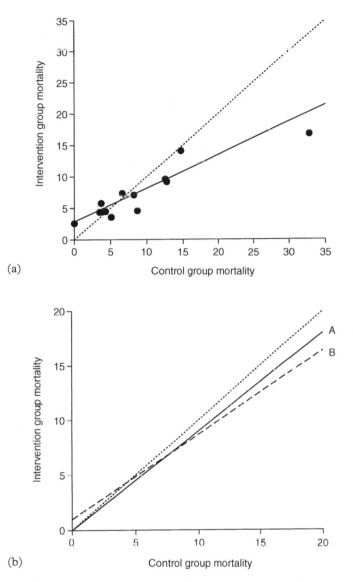

(a)

(b)

Figure 8.3 All cause mortality rates (per 1000 person-years) in the intervention and control groups of clinical trials in mild-to-moderate hypertension. The dotted line represents the no effect line with identical mortality in both groups.
(a) The solid line represents the weighted regression line which intersects the no effect line at a control group mortality risk of 6 per 1000 person-years. From Hoes et al.[30]
(b) A computer simulation based on the same trials. Line A assumes a constant relative risk reduction of 10%. Line B corresponds to Line A after random error was added to the mortality rates. It also intersects the no effect line at a control group mortality rate of around of 6 per 1000 person-years.

151

illustrated in computer simulations. Using the same control group rates and assuming a constant relative reduction of all-cause mortality of 10% in treated groups (relative risk 0·9), we considered the situation both assuming no random fluctuations in rates and allowing random error (Figure 8.3(b)).[27] When adding random error (by sampling 1000 times from the corresponding Poisson distribution) the regression line rotated and crossed the no effect line. Indeed, the intersection is at almost the same point as that found in the earlier meta-analysis, namely at a control group mortality rate of approximately 6 per 1000 person-years. It is thus quite possible that what was interpreted as reflecting detrimental effects of anti-hypertensive treatment[30] was in fact produced by random variation in event rates.

When there is a very wide range of death rates in the control groups or when trials are large, the chance fluctuations which produce spurious associations in the weighted regression of effect size against control group risk will be less important. Alternatively, the analysis can be performed using the combined overall death rate in the control and the treatment arms of the trials as the risk indicator.[17] This will generally, but not always, lead to bias in the opposite direction, diluting any real association between level of risk and treatment effect.[28]

Use of event rates from either the control group or overall trial partici-pants as the stratifying variable when relating treatment effect to level of risk is thus problematic.[27,28] Although more complex statistical methods have been developed which are less susceptible to these biases (see Chapter 10) it is preferable if indicators of risk which are not based on outcome measures are used. In the case of the effect of angiotensin-converting enzyme (ACE) inhibitors on mortality in patients with heart failure use of control group or overall treatment and control group risk demonstrated greater relative and absolute benefit in trials recruiting higher risk partici-pants.[23,33] In a meta-analysis data were available on treatment effects according to clinical indicators.[34] In patients with an ejection fraction at entry equal to or below 0·25, 29% died during the trials, as opposed to 17% of patients with an ejection fraction above 0·25. In the former, higher risk, group there was a substantial reduction in mortality (odds ratio 0·69, 95% CI 0·57 to 0·85) whereas little effect on mortality was seen in the latter, lower risk, group (odds ratio 0·98, 95% CI 0·79 to 1·23). A similar difference was seen if the combination of mortality or hospitalisation for congestive heart failure was used as the outcome measure.

Use of risk indicators in meta-analysis

In several fields risk indicators which do not rely on control group out-comes have been investigated as predictors of outcomes in meta-analyses.

For example an individual participant data meta-analysis of randomised controlled trials of coronary artery bypass grafting (CABG) versus standard medical care demonstrated an overall significant reduction in mortality at 5, 7 and 10 years (for example, at 5 years 10·2% versus 15·8%, P = 0·0001).[35] A modification of the Veterans Administration risk score [36] which is based on the presence of class III/IV angina, ST depression at rest, history of hypertension, and history of myocardial infarction was used in the analyses. This risk score predicts the probability of coronary events occurring in untreated individuals. A clear relation of benefit with the level of risk was evident. As shown in Figure 8.4, no benefit was evident in the lowest risk tertile, which was characterised by a relatively low 5-year mortality of 5·5%. Conversely, a clearly beneficial effect was present for groups of patients at higher risk of death. These findings suggest that targeting treatment at high-risk individuals would produce considerable benefits while extension of treatment to lower risk groups would be expensive – given the much larger number of lower-risk patients – and produce little or no benefit.

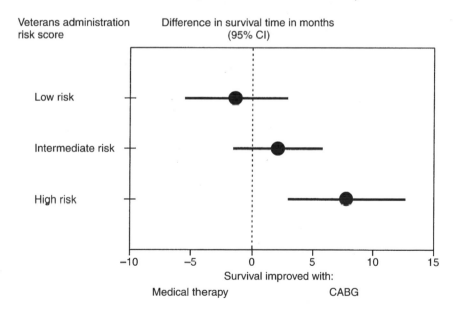

Figure 8.4 Individual participant data meta-analysis of seven randomised trials comparing a strategy of initial coronary artery bypass graft (CABG) surgery with a strategy of initial medical therapy in coronary heart disease. Differences in survival time at ten years are shown by Veterans Administration clinical risk score.[36]

Confounding

The fact that randomised controlled trials are included in meta-analyses does not mean that comparisons being made between trials are randomised comparisons. When relating outcomes to characteristics of the trial participants, or to differences in treatments used in the separate trials, or to the situations in which treatments were given, the associations seen are subject to the potential biases of observational studies. Confounding could exist between one trial characteristic – say drug trials versus diet trials in the case of cholesterol lowering – and another characteristic, such as level of risk of the participants in the trial. In many cases there are simply too few trials, or differences in the average characteristics of participants in the trials are too small, to be able to perform a stratified analysis at the level of the individual trial. It may be possible to consider strata within the trials (e.g. male versus female, or those with or without existing disease), to increase the number of observations to be included in the regression analysis. Increasing the number of data points in this way is of little help if there are strong associations between the factors under consideration. For example, in a meta-regression analysis of total mortality outcomes of cholesterol lowering trials various factors appear to influence the outcome – greater cholesterol reduction leads to greater benefit; trials including participants at a higher level of CHD risk show larger mortality reductions and the fibrate drugs lead to less benefit than other interventions.[19,22] These findings are difficult to interpret, however, since the variables included are strongly related: fibrates tend to have been used in trials recruiting lower risk participants and they lower cholesterol much less than statins. In this situation all the problems of performing multivariable analyses with correlated covariates are introduced.[37,38]

In conclusion, attempting to utilise a meta-analysis to produce more than a simple overall effect estimate is tempting, but needs to be treated cautiously, for the reasons detailed above. The use of individual participant data provides greater power for determining whether differences in effect estimates are real or spurious (see Chapter 6). Finally, one of the more useful extensions of meta-analysis beyond the grand mean relates to the examination of publication and other biases, which is discussed in detail in Chapter 11.

Acknowledgements

We are grateful to Iain Chalmers for helpful comments on an earlier draft of this chapter. This chapter draws on material published earlier in the *BMJ*.[39]

1 Wittes RE. Problems in the medical interpretation of overviews. *Stat Med* 1987;**6**:269–76.
2 Davey Smith G, Egger M. Incommunicable knowledge? Interpreting and applying the results of clinical trials and meta-analyses. *J Clin Epidemiol* 1998;**51**:289–95.
3 The European Infarction Study Group. European Infarction Study (EIS). A secondary prevention study with slow release oxprenolol after myocardial infarction: morbidiy and mortality. *Eur Heart J* 1984;**5**:189–202.
4 Efron B, Morris C. Stein's paradox in statistics. *Sci Am* 1977;**236**:119–27.
5 Oxman AD, Guyatt GH. A consumer's guide to subgroup analyses. *Ann Intern Med* 1992;**116**:78–84.
6 Yusuf S, Wittes J, Probstfield J, Tyroler HA. Analysis and interpretation of treatment effects in subgroups of patients in randomized clinical trials. *JAMA* 1991;**266**:93–8.
7 The Beta-Blocker Pooling Project Research Group. The Beta-Blocker Pooling Project (BBPP): subgroup findings from randomized trials in post infarction patients. *Eur Heart J* 1988; **9**:8–16.
8 Ingelfinger JA, Mosteller F, Thibodeau LA, Ware JH. *Biostatistics in clinical medicine*. New York: McGraw, 1994.
9 Peto R. Statistical aspects of cancer trials. In: Halnan KE, ed. *Treatment of cancer*. London: Chapman and Hall, 1982.
10 Buyse ME. Analysis of clinical trial outcomes: some comments on subgroup analyses. *Contr Clin Trials* 1989;**10**:187S–94S.
11 Mauri F, Gasparini M, Barbonaglia L, et al. Prognostic significance of the extent of myocardial injury in acute myocardial infarction treated by streptokinase (the GISSI trial). *Am J Cardiol* 1989;**63**:1291–5.
12 Peto R. Misleading subgroup analysis in GISSI. *Am J Cardiol* 1990;**64**:771.
13 Schroeder R. Oxprenolol in myocardial infarction survivors: brief review of the European Infarction Study results in the light of other beta-blocker post infarction trials. *Z Kardiol* 1985;**74** (suppl 6):165–72.
14 Yusuf S, Peto R, Lewis J, Collins R, Sleight P. Beta blockade during and after myocardial infarction: an overview of the randomized trials. *Prog Cardiovasc Dis* 1985;**17**:335–71.
15 Peto R. Why do we need systematic overviews of randomized trials. *Stat Med* 1987;**6**:233–40.
16 Freemantle N, Cleland J, Young P, Mason J, Harrison J. Beta blockade after myocardial infarction: systematic review and meta regression analysis. *BMJ* 1999;**318**:1730–7.
17 Davey Smith G, Song F, Sheldon TA. Cholesterol lowering and mortality: the importance of considering initial level of risk. *BMJ* 1993;**306**:1367–73.
18 Bailey K. Generalizing the results of randomized clinical trials. *Contr Clin Trials* 1994;**15**:15–23.
19 Holme I. Relationship between total mortality and cholesterol reduction as found by meta-regression analysis of randomized cholesterol lowering trials. *Contr Clin Trials* 1996;**17**:13–22.
20 Fibrinolytic Therapy Trialists' (FTT) Collaborative Group. Indications for fibrinolytic therapy in suspected acute myocardial infarction: collaborative overview of early mortality and major morbidity results from all randomised trials of more than 1000 patients. *Lancet* 1994;**343**:311–22.
21 Zelen M. Intravenous streptokinase for acute myocardial infarction. *N Engl J Med* 1983;**308**:593.
22 Davey Smith G. Low blood cholesterol and non-atherosclerotic disease mortality: where do we stand? *Eur J Cardiol* 1997;**18**:6–9.
23 Davey Smith G, Egger M. Who benefits from medical interventions? Treating low risk patients can be a high risk strategy. *BMJ* 1994;**308**:72–4.
24 Antiplatelet Trialists' Collaboration. Collaborative overview of randomised trials of antiplatelet therapy – I: prevention of death, myocardial infarction, and stroke by prolonged antiplatelet therapy in various categories of patients. *BMJ* 1994;**308**:81–106.
25 Fischl MA, Richman DD, Grieco MH, et al. The efficacy of azidothymidine (AZT) in the treatment of patients with AIDS and AIDS-related complex. A double-blind, placebo-controlled trial. *N Engl J Med* 1987;**317**:185–91.
26 Egger M, Neaton JD, Phillips AN, Davey Smith G. Concorde trial of immediate versus deferred zidovudine. *Lancet* 1994;**343**:1355.

27 Egger M, Davey Smith G. Risks and benefits of treating mild hypertension: a misleading meta-analysis? *J Hypertens* 1995;**13**:813–15.

28 Sharp SJ, Thompson SG, Altman D. The relation between treatment benefit and underlying risk in meta-analysis. *BMJ* 1996;**313**:735–8.

29 Thompson SG, Smith TC, Sharp SJ. Investigating underlying risk as a source of heterogeneity in meta-analysis. *Stat Med* 1997;**16**:2741–58.

30 Hoes AW, Grobbee DE, Lubsen J. Does drug treatment improve survival? Reconciling the trials in mild-to-moderate hypertension. *J Hypertens* 1995;**13**:805–11.

31 L'Abbé KA, Detsky AS, O'Rourke K. Meta-analysis in clinical research. *Ann Intern Med* 1987;**107**:224–33.

32 Song F. Exploring heterogeneity in meta-analysis: is the L'Abbé plot useful? *J Clin Epidemiol* 1999;**52**:725–30.

33 Eccles M, Freemantle N, Mason J. North of England evidence based development project: guideline for angiotensin converting enzyme inhibitors in primary care management of adults with symptomatic heart failure. *BMJ* 1998;**316**:1369–75.

34 Garg R, Yusuf S. for the Collaborative Group on ACE Inhibitor Trials. Overview of randomised trials of angiotensin-converting enzyme inhibitors on mortality and morbidity in patients with heart failure. *JAMA* 1995;**273**:1450–6.

35 Yusuf S, Zucker D, Peduzzi P, *et al.* Effect of coronary artery bypass graft surgery on survival: overview of 10-year results from randomised trials by the Coronary Artery Graft Surgery Trialists Collaboration. *Lancet* 1994;**344**:563–70.

36 Takaro T, Hultgren HN, Lipton MJ, Detre KM. The VA cooperative randomised study of surgery for coronary arterial occlusive disease II: Subgroup with significant left main lesions. *Circulation* 1976;**54 (suppl 3)**:107–17.

37 Phillips AN, Davey Smith G. How independent are "independent" effects? Relative risk estimation when correlated exposures are measured imprecisely. *J Clin Epidemiol* 1991;**44**:1223–31.

38 Davey Smith G, Phillips AN. Confounding in epidemiological studies: why "independent" effects may not be all they seem. *BMJ* 1992;**305**:757–9.

39 Davey Smith G, Egger M, Phillips AN. Meta-analysis: beyond the grand mean? *BMJ* 1997; **315**:1610–14.

9 Why and how sources of heterogeneity should be investigated

SIMON G THOMPSON

Summary points

- Clinical heterogeneity across the studies included in a meta-analysis is likely to lead to some degree of statistical heterogeneity in their results.
- Investigating potential sources of heterogeneity is an important component of carrying out a meta-analysis.
- Appropriate statistical methods for trial characteristics involve weighted regression and should allow for residual heterogeneity.
- Individual patient data give the greatest scope for useful analyses of heterogeneity.
- Caution is required in interpreting results, especially when analyses have been inspired by looking at the available data.
- Careful investigations of heterogeneity in meta-analysis should increase the scientific and clinical relevance of their results.

The purpose of a meta-analysis of a set of clinical trials is rather different from the specific aims of an individual trial. For example a particular clinical trial investigating the effect of serum cholesterol reduction on the risk of ischaemic heart disease tests a single treatment regimen, given for a specified duration to participants fulfilling certain eligibility criteria, using a particular definition of outcome measures. The purpose of a meta-analysis of cholesterol lowering trials is broader – that is, to estimate the extent to which serum cholesterol reduction, achieved by a variety of means, generally influences the risk of ischaemic heart disease. A meta-analysis also attempts to gain greater objectivity, applicability and precision by including all the available evidence from randomised trials that pertain to the issue.[1] Because of the broader aims of a meta-analysis, the trials included usually

157

encompass a substantial variety of specific treatment regimens, types of patients, and outcomes. In this chapter, it is argued that the influence of these clinical differences between trials, or clinical heterogeneity, on the overall results needs to be explored carefully.

The chapter starts by clarifying the relation between clinical heterogeneity and statistical heterogeneity. Examples follow of meta-analyses of observational epidemiological studies of serum cholesterol concentration, and clinical trials of its reduction, in which exploration of heterogeneity was important in the overall conclusions reached. The statistical methods appropriate for investigating sources of heterogeneity are then described in more detail. The dangers of *post hoc* exploration of results and consequent over-interpretation are addressed at the end of the chapter.

Clinical and statistical heterogeneity

To make the concepts clear, it is useful to focus on a meta-analysis where heterogeneity posed a problem in interpretation. Figure 9.1 shows the

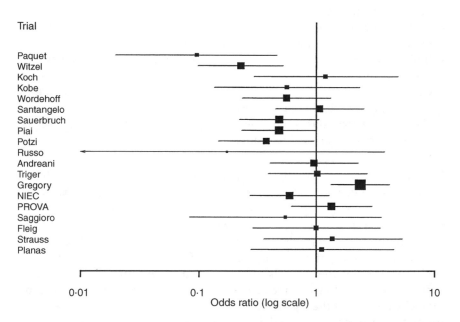

Figure 9.1 Forest plot of odds ratios of death (and 95% confidence intervals) from 19 trials of sclerotherapy. Odds ratios less than unity represent beneficial effects of sclerotherapy. Trials identified by principal author, referenced by Pagliaro *et al.*[2]

results of 19 randomised trials investigating the use of endoscopic sclerotherapy for reducing mortality in the primary treatment of cirrhotic patients with oesophageal varices.[2] The results of each trial are shown as odds ratios and 95% confidence intervals, with odds ratios less than unity representing a beneficial effect of sclerotherapy. The trials differed considerably in patient selection, baseline disease severity, endoscopic technique, management of intermediate outcomes such as variceal bleeding, and duration of follow-up.[2] So in this meta-analysis, as in many, there is extensive clinical heterogeneity. There were also methodological differences in the mechanism of randomisation, the extent of withdrawals, and the handling of losses to follow-up.

It would not be surprising, therefore, to find that the results of these trials were to some degree incompatible with one another. Such incompatibility in quantitative results is termed statistical heterogeneity. It may be caused by known clinical or methodological differences between trials, or may be related to unknown or unrecorded trial characteristics. In assessing the direct evidence of statistical heterogeneity, the imprecision in the estimate of the odds ratio from each trial, as expressed by the confidence intervals in Figure 9.1, has to be taken into account. The statistical question is then whether there is greater variation between the results of the trials than is compatible with the play of chance. As might be surmised from inspection of Figure 9.1, the statistical test (test of homogeneity, see Chapter 15) yielded a highly significant result ($\chi^2_{18} = 43$, $P < 0.001$).

In the example of the sclerotherapy trials, the evidence for statistical heterogeneity is substantial. In many meta-analyses, however, such statistical evidence is lacking and the test of homogeneity is non-significant. Yet this cannot be interpreted as evidence of homogeneity (that is, total consistency) of the results of all the trials included. This is not only because a non-significant test can never be interpreted as direct evidence in favour of the null hypothesis of homogeneity,[3] but in particular because tests of homogeneity have low power and may fail to detect as statistically significant even a moderate degree of genuine heterogeneity.[4,5]

We might be somewhat happier to ignore the problems of clinical heterogeneity in the interpretation of the results if direct evidence of statistical heterogeneity is lacking, and more inclined to try to understand the reasons for any heterogeneity for which the evidence is more convincing. However, the extent of statistical heterogeneity, which can be quantified,[6] is more important than the evidence of its existence. Indeed it is reasonable to argue that testing for heterogeneity is largely irrelevant, because the studies in any meta-analysis will necessarily be clinically heterogeneous.[7] The guiding principle should be to investigate the influences of the specific clinical differences between studies rather than rely on an overall statistical test for heterogeneity. This focuses attention on

159

particular contrasts among the trials included, which will be more likely to detect genuine differences – and more relevant to the overall conclusions. For example, in the sclerotherapy trials, the underlying disease severity was identified as being potentially related to the benefits of sclerotherapy observed (see also Chapter 10).[2]

The quantitative summary of the results, for example in terms of an overall odds ratio and 95% confidence interval, is generally considered the most important conclusion from a meta-analysis. For the sclerotherapy trials, the overall odds ratio for death was given as 0·76 with 95% confidence interval 0·61 to 0·94,[2] calculated under the "fixed effect" assumption of homogeneity.[5] A naive interpretation of this would be that sclerotherapy convincingly decreased the risk of death with an odds reduction of around 25%. However, what are the implications of clinical and statistical heterogeneity in the interpretation of this result? Given the clinical heterogeneity, we do not know to which endoscopic technique, to which selection of patients, or in conjunction with what ancillary clinical management such a conclusion is supposed to refer. It is some sort of "average" statement that is not easy to interpret quantitatively in relation to the benefits that might accrue from the use of a specific clinical protocol. In this particular case the evidence for statistical heterogeneity is also overwhelming and this introduces even more doubt about the interpretation of any single overall estimate of effect. Even if we accept that some sort of average or typical[8] effect is being estimated, the confidence interval given is too narrow in terms of extrapolating the results to future trials or patients, since the extra variability between the results of the different trials is ignored.[5]

The answer to such problems is that meta-analyses should incorporate a careful investigation of potential sources of heterogeneity. Meta-analysis can go further than simply producing a single estimate of effect.[9] For example, in a meta-analysis of trials of thrombolysis in the acute phase of myocardial infarction, the survival benefit has been shown to be greater when there is less delay between onset of symptoms and treatment.[10] Quantifying this relation is important in drawing up policy recommendations for the use of thrombolysis in routine clinical practice. More generally, the benefits of trying to understand why differences in treatment effects occur across trials often outweigh the potential disadvantages.[11] The same is true for differences in exposure-disease associations across epidemiological studies.[12] Such analyses, often called meta-regressions,[13] can in principle be extended, for example in a meta-analysis of clinical trials, to investigate how a number of trial or patient characteristics act together to influence treatment effects (see also Chapters 8, 10 and 11 for more discussion of the use of regression models in meta-analysis). Two examples of the benefits of applying such an approach in published meta-analyses follow.

160

Serum cholesterol concentration and risk of ischaemic heart disease

An extreme example of heterogeneity was evident in a 1994 review[14] of the 10 largest prospective cohort studies of serum cholesterol concentration and the risk of ischaemic heart disease in men, which included data on 19 000 myocardial infarctions or deaths from ischaemic heart disease. The purpose was to summarise the magnitude of the relation between serum cholesterol and risk of ischaemic heart disease in order to estimate the long term benefit that might be expected to accrue from reduction in serum cholesterol concentrations.

The results from the 10 prospective studies are shown in Figure 9.2. These are expressed as proportionate reductions in risk associated with a reduction in serum cholesterol of 0·6 mmol/l (about 10% of average levels in Western countries), having been derived from the apparently log-linear associations of risk of ischaemic heart disease with serum cholesterol concentration in individual studies. They also take into account the under-estimation that results from the fact that a single measurement of serum cholesterol is an imprecise estimate of long term level, sometimes termed

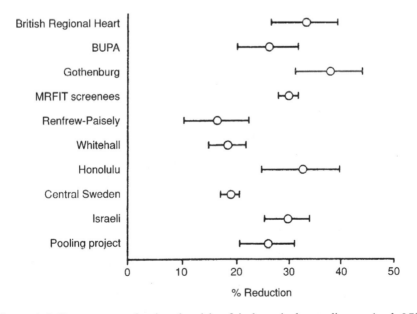

Figure 9.2 Percentage reduction in risk of ischaemic heart disease (and 95% confidence intervals) associated with 0·6 mmol/l serum cholesterol reduction in 10 prospective studies of men. Studies referenced by Law *et al.*[14]

161

regression dilution bias.[15] Although all of the 10 studies showed that cholesterol reduction was associated with a reduction in the risk of ischaemic heart disease, they differed substantially in the estimated magnitude of this effect. This is clear from Figure 9.2, and the extreme value that is obtained from an overall test of homogeneity ($\chi^2_9 = 127$, P < 0·001). This shows that simply combining the results of these studies into one overall estimate is misleading; an understanding of the reasons for the heterogeneity is necessary.

The most obvious cause of the heterogeneity relates to the ages of the participants, or more particularly the average age of experiencing coronary events during follow-up, since it is well known that the relative risk association of ischaemic heart disease with a given serum cholesterol increment declines with advancing age.[16,17] The data from the 10 studies were therefore divided, as far as was possible from published and unpublished information, into groups according to age at entry.[14] This yielded 26 substudies, the results of which are plotted against the average age of experiencing a coronary event in Figure 9.3. The percentage reduction in risk of ischaemic heart disease clearly decreases markedly with age. This relation can be summarised using a quadratic regression of log relative risk

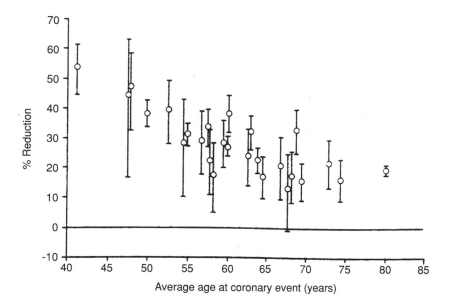

Figure 9.3 Percentage reduction in risk of ischaemic heart disease (and 95% confidence intervals) associated with 0·6 mmol/l serum cholesterol reduction, according to average age of experiencing a coronary event.

reduction on age, appropriately weighted to take account of the different precisions of each estimate. It was concluded that a decrease in cholesterol concentration of 0.6 mmol/l was associated with a decrease in risk of ischaemic heart disease of 54% at age 40, 39% at age 50, 27% at age 60, 20% at age 70, and 19% at age 80. In fact, there remains considerable evidence of heterogeneity in Figure 9.3 even from this summary of results ($\chi^2_{23} = 45$, P = 0·005), but it is far less extreme than the original heterogeneity evident before considering age (Figure 9.2).

The effect on the conclusions brought about by considering age are crucial, for example in considering the impact of cholesterol reduction in the population. The proportionate reductions in the risk of ischaemic heart disease associated with reduction in serum cholesterol are strongly age-related. The large proportionate reductions in early middle age cannot be extrapolated to old ages, at which more modest proportionate reductions are evident. In meta-analyses of observational epidemiological studies, such investigation of sources of heterogeneity may often be a principal rather than subsidiary aim.[18] Systematic reviews of observational studies are discussed in detail in Chapters 12–14.

Serum cholesterol reduction and risk of ischaemic heart disease

The randomised controlled trials of serum cholesterol reduction have been the subject of a number of meta-analyses[14,19,20] and much controversy. In conjunction with the review of the 10 prospective studies just described, the results of 28 randomised trials available in 1994 were summarised;[14] this omits the results of trials of serum cholesterol reduction, notably those using statins, that have become available more recently. The aim was to quantify the effect of serum cholesterol reduction on the risk of ischaemic heart disease in the short term, the trials having an average duration of about five years. There was considerable clinical heterogeneity between the trials in the interventions tested (different drugs, different diets, and in one case surgical intervention using partial ileal bypass grafting), in the duration of the trials (0·3–10 years), in the average extent of serum cholesterol reduction achieved (0·3–1·5 mmol/l), and in the selection criteria for the patients such as pre-existing disease (for example, primary or secondary prevention trials) and level of serum cholesterol concentration at entry. As before it would seem likely that these substantial clinical differences would lead to some heterogeneity in the observed results.

Forest plots such as in Figure 9.1, are not very useful for investigating heterogeneity. A better diagram for this purpose was proposed by Galbraith,[21] and is shown for the cholesterol lowering trials in Figure 9.4. For each trial the ratio of the log odds ratio of ischaemic heart disease to its

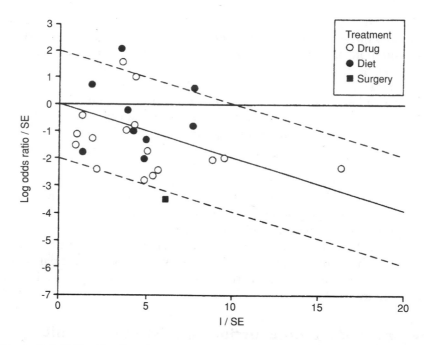

Figure 9.4 Galbraith plot of odds ratios of ischaemic heart disease in 28 trials of serum cholesterol reduction (see text for explanation). Two trials were omitted because of no events in one group.

standard error (the z-statistic) is plotted against the reciprocal of the standard error. Hence the least precise results from small trials appear towards the left of the figure and results from the largest trials towards the right. An overall log odds ratio is represented by the slope of the solid line in the figure; this is an unweighted regression line constrained to pass through the origin. The dotted lines are positioned two units above and below the solid line and delimit an area within which, in the absence of statistical heterogeneity, the great majority (that is, about 95%) of the trial results would be expected to lie. It is thus interesting to note the characteristics of those trials which lie near or outside these dotted lines. For example, in Figure 9.4, there are two dietary trials that lie above the upper line and showed apparently adverse effects of serum cholesterol reduction on the risk of ischaemic heart disease. One of these trials achieved only a very small cholesterol reduction while the other had a particularly short duration.[22] Conversely the surgical trial, below the bottom dotted line and showing a large reduction in the risk of ischaemic heart disease, was both the longest trial and the one that achieved the greatest cholesterol reduction.[22] These observations add weight to the need to investigate heterogeneity of results according to extent and duration of cholesterol reduction.

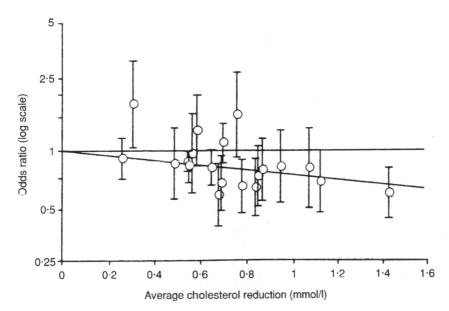

Figure 9.5 Odds ratios of ischaemic heart disease (and 95% confidence intervals) according to the average extent of serum cholesterol reduction achieved in each of 28 trials. Overall summary of results indicated by sloping line. Results of the nine smallest trials have been combined.

Figure 9.5 shows the results according to average extent of cholesterol reduction achieved. There is very strong evidence (P = 0·002) that the proportionate reduction in the risk of ischaemic heart disease increases with the extent of average cholesterol reduction; the appropriate methods for this analysis are explained in the next section. A suitable summary of the trial results, represented by the sloping line in Figure 9.5, is that the risk of ischaemic heart disease is reduced by an estimated 18% (95% confidence interval 13 to 22%) for each 0.6 mmol/l reduction in serum cholesterol concentration.[22] Obtaining data subdivided by time since randomisation[14] to investigate the effect of duration was also informative (Figure 9.6). Whereas the reduction in the risk of ischaemic heart disease in the first two years was rather limited, the reductions thereafter were around 25% per 0·6 mmol/l reduction. After extent and duration of cholesterol reduction were allowed for in this way, the evidence for further heterogeneity of the results from the different trials was limited (P = 0·11). In particular there was no evidence of further differences in the results between the drug and the dietary trials, or between the primary prevention and the secondary prevention trials.[14,22]

This investigation of heterogeneity was again crucial to the conclusions

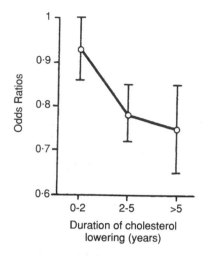

Figure 9.6 Odds ratios of ischaemic heart disease (and 95% confidence intervals) per 0·6 mmol/l serum cholesterol reduction in 28 trials, according to the duration of cholesterol lowering.

reached. The analysis quantified how the percentage reduction in the risk of ischaemic heart disease depends both on the extent and the duration of cholesterol reduction. Meta-analyses ignoring these factors may well be misleading. It also seems that these factors are more important determinants of the proportionate reduction in ischaemic heart disease than the mode of intervention or the underlying risk of the patient.

Statistical methods for investigating sources of heterogeneity

How should analyses such as those described above be carried out? To simplify terminology we consider treatment effects in trials, but the same methods are appropriate for investigating heterogeneity of effects in observational epidemiological studies. We focus on meta-regression, where the aim is to investigate whether a particular covariate or characteristic, with a value defined for each trial in the meta-analysis, is related to the extent of treatment benefit. Figures 9.3 and 9.5 in the meta-analyses discussed above are examples of such analyses. The statistical methods described below are discussed in more detail elsewhere,[23] and can be extended to consider simultaneously the effects of more than one covariate (see also Chapter 11).

The simplest form of analysis assumes that the observed treatment effects in each trial, say log odds ratios, are normally distributed. In the same way that calculating a single overall summary of effect in a meta-analysis takes into account the precision of the estimate in each study,[24] an analysis of a particular covariate as a source of heterogeneity in meta-analysis should be based on weighted regression. The weight that applies to each study is equal to the inverse of the variance of the estimate for that study. This variance has two components: the within-trial variance and the between-trial variance. For example, in the case of log odds ratios, the within-trial variance is simply estimated as the sum of the reciprocal cell counts in the 2×2 table[25] (see Chapter 15). The between-trial variance represents the residual heterogeneity in treatment effects, that is the variability between trial results which is not explained by the covariate. Analyses which assume that the between-trial variance is zero, where weighting is therefore simply according to the within-trial variance, correspond to a "fixed effect" analysis. In general, it is an unwarranted assumption that all the heterogeneity is explained by the covariate, and the between-trial variance should be included as well, corresponding to a "random effects" analysis[26] (see Chapter 15). The same arguments apply here as when estimating a single overall treatment effect, ignoring sources of heterogeneity.[24]

To be explicit, consider the analysis presented in Figure 9.5. Here there are 28 trials, which we index by $i = 1...28$. For the ith trial, we denote the observed log odds ratio of ischaemic heart disease by y_i, its estimated within-trial variance by v_i, and the extent of serum cholesterol reduction in mmol/l by x_i. The linear regression of log odds ratios on extent of cholesterol reduction can be expressed as $y_i = \alpha + \beta x_i$; here we are not forcing the regression through the origin as in Figure 9.5, and α represents the intercept of the regression line. The purpose of the analysis is to provide estimates of α and β, together with their standard errors. An additional point of interest is the extent to which the heterogeneity between results is reduced by including the covariate. The weights for the regression are equal to $1/(v_i + \tau^2)$, where τ^2 is the residual heterogeneity variance. There are a number of ways of estimating τ^2, amongst which a restricted maximum likelihood estimate is generally recommended.[23] Programs to carry out such weighted regression analyses are available in the statistical package STATA[27] (see Chapter 18). Note that these analyses are not the same as usual weighted regression where weights are inversely proportional (rather than equal) to the variances.

Table 9.1 presents results from two weighted regressions, the first assuming that there is no residual heterogeneity ($\tau^2 = 0$) and the second allowing the extent of residual heterogeneity to be estimated. The first analysis provides no evidence that the intercept α is non-zero, and convincing evidence that the slope β is negative (as in Figure 9.5). However the estimate of τ^2 in the second analysis is positive, indicating at least some residual heterogeneity. In fact, about 85% of the heterogeneity variance of results in a simple meta-analysis is explained by considering the extent of

Table 9.1 Estimates of the linear regression relationship between log odds ratio of ischaemic heart disease and extent of serum cholesterol reduction (mmol/l) in 28 randomised trials, obtained by different methods (from Thompson and Sharp[23]).

Method	Residual heterogeneity	Estimates (SEs)		Residual heterogeneity variance (τ^2)
		Intercept (α)	Slope (β)	
Weighted regression:				
	None	0·121 (0·097)	−0·475 (0·138)	0
	Additive[a]	0·135 (0·112)	−0·492 (0·153)	0·005
Logistic regression:				
	None	0·121 (0·097)	−0·476 (0·137)	0
	Additive[b]	0·148 (0·126)	−0·509 (0·167)	0·011

[a] Estimated using restricted maximum likelihood.
[b] Estimated using a random effects logistic regression with second order predictive quasi-likelihood[28] in the software MLwiN[29].

cholesterol reduction as a covariate.[23] The standard errors of the estimates of α and β are quite markedly increased in this second analysis, even though the estimate of τ^2 is small. This exemplifies the point that it is important to allow for residual heterogeneity, otherwise the precision of estimated regression coefficients may be misleadingly overstated and sources of heterogeneity mistakenly claimed. Indeed in examples where the residual heterogeneity is substantial, the effects of making allowance for it will be much more marked than in Table 9.1.

Intuitive interpretation of the estimate of τ^2 is not straightforward. However, consider the predicted odds ratio of ischaemic heart disease if serum cholesterol were reduced, for example, by 1 mmol/l, that is exp $(0·135 − 0·492) = 0·70$. Given the heterogeneity between studies expressed by τ^2, and for a 1 mmol/l cholesterol reduction, the 95% range of true odds ratios for different studies is estimated as exp $(0·135 − 0·492 \pm 2 \times \sqrt{0·005})$, that is 0·61–0·81. The estimated value of τ, $\sqrt{0·005} = 0·07$ or 7%, can thus be interpreted approximately as the coefficient of variation on the overall odds ratio caused by heterogeneity between studies. This coefficient of variation would apply to the predicted odds ratio for any given reduction in serum cholesterol.

The assumption that estimated log odds ratios can be considered normally distributed and that the variances v_i are known may be inadequate for small trials or when the number of events is small. It is possible to frame the analyses presented above as logistic regressions for binary outcome data to overcome these problems.[23] The results assuming no residual heterogeneity were almost identical to the weighted regression results; the estimates from the second analysis were slightly different because a larger estimate of τ^2 was obtained (Table 9.1). Another extension to the analysis, which is appropriate in principle, is to allow for the imprecision in estimating τ^2. This can be achieved in a fully Bayesian analysis, but again results for the cholesterol trials were similar.[23] In general, the use of logistic regression or fully Bayesian analyses, rather than weighted regression, will probably make very little difference to the results. Only when all the trials are small (when the normality assumption will fail, and the results will not be dominated by other larger trials) or the number of trials is limited (when τ^2 is particularly imprecise) might different results be anticipated. Indeed one advantage of the weighted regression approach is that it can easily be used for treatment effects on scales other than log odds ratios, such as log relative risks or absolute risk differences, which are more interpretable for clinical practice.[30]

The relationship between underlying risk and treatment benefit

It is reasonable to ask whether the extent of treatment benefit relates to the underlying risk of the patients in the different trials included in a meta-analysis.[31,32] Underlying risk is a convenient summary of a number of characteristics which may be measurable risk factors but for which individual patient data are not available from some or all of the trials. Here it is atural to plot the treatment effect in each trial against the risk of events observed in the control group. Returning to the sclerotherapy meta-analysis introduced at the beginning of the chapter (Figure 9.1), such a plot is shown in Figure 9.7. Each trial is represented by a circle, the area of which represents the trial precision, so trials which contribute more information are represented by larger circles. A weighted regression line, according to the methods of the previous section, is superimposed and gives strong evidence of a negative association ($P < 0.001$). A naive interpretation of the line would claim that the treatment effect increases (lower odds ratio) with increasing proportion of events in the control group, and that underlying risk is a significant source of heterogeneity. Furthermore, there is a temptation to use the point T in Figure 9.7 to define a cut-off value of risk in the control group and conclude that treatment is effective (odds ratio below 1) only in patients with an underlying risk higher than this value. As discussed in Chapters 8 and 10, these conclusions are flawed and seriously misleading. The reason for this stems from regression to the mean, since the outcome in the control group is being related to the treatment effect, a quantity which itself includes the control group outcome.[31,33–35] Statistical approaches that overcome this problem are described in Chapter 10.

To a clinician, the "underlying risk" of a patient is only known through certain measured characteristics. So a clinically more useful, and statistically less problematic, alternative to these analyses is to relate treatment

169

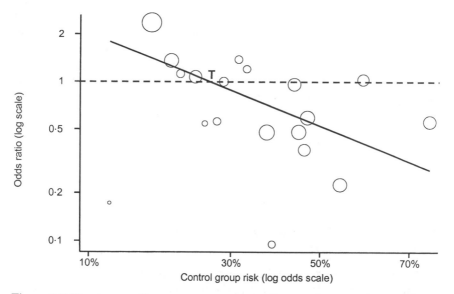

Figure 9.7 Treatment effect versus percentage of events in control group for 19 trials of sclerotherapy. The area of each circle is inversely proportional to the variance of the estimated treatment effect in the trial.

benefit to measurable patient characteristics. This is one of the advantages of individual patient data, as discussed in Chapter 6 and below.

The virtues of individual patient data

Meta-regression using trial-level characteristics can only partially address issues of heterogeneity. The aspects that can be investigated as sources of heterogeneity in such analyses are limited to characteristics of each trial as a whole, for example relating to treatment regimens. Furthermore, analyses using averages of patient characteristics in each trial (such as the mean age of all the patients) can give a misleading impression of the relation for individual patients. This is as a result of the so-called ecological fallacy, whereby the relation with treatment benefit may be different across trials as compared to within trials.[13,36] Clinically more useful information comes from analyses which relate the extent of treatment benefit to individual patient characteristics. As discussed in Chapter 6, meta-analysis based on individual patient data, rather than summary data obtained from publications, has many advantages.[37] Amongst these is the ability to carry out a more thorough and extensive investigation of sources of heterogeneity, since subdivisions according to patients' characteristics can be made within trials and these results combined across trials.

Large individual patient data meta-analyses, undertaken under the auspices of collaborative groups of researchers, have this potential. Even such analyses should allow for the possibility of residual heterogeneity of treatment effects not explained by the patient characteristics available. In practice, however, there may be no great difference between those who advocate a fixed effect approach[8] and those who would be more cautious[5,38,39] when it comes to undertaking particular meta-analyses. For example, a large-scale overview of early breast cancer treatment,[40] carried out ostensibly with a fixed effect approach, included an extensive investigation of heterogeneity according to type and duration of therapy, dose of drug, use of concomitant therapy, age, nodal status, oestrogen receptor status, and outcome (recurrence or mortality).

Exactly how such analyses should be carried out needs further development. For example, assumptions of linearity of covariate effects or normality of the residual variation between trial results can be difficult to assess in practice.[7] The analysis can be viewed as an example of a multilevel model,[41,42] in which information is available at both the trial level and on individuals within trials. Using this structure a general framework for meta-analysis can be proposed, incorporating both trial-level and patient-level covariates, from either a classical or Bayesian viewpoint.[43,44] Some patient characteristics may vary more between trials than within trials; for example, gender would be a within-trial covariate if all the trials in a meta-analysis included both men and women, and a between-trial covariate if trials were either of men alone or of women alone. The strength of inference about how a covariate affects treatment benefit depends on the extent to which it varies within trials. Covariates that vary only between trials have relations with treatment benefit that may be confounded by other trial characteristics. These associations are observational in nature, and do not necessarily have the same interpretation that can be ascribed to treatment comparisons within randomised clinical trials. Covariates that vary within trials are less prone to such biases.

Conclusions

As meta-analysis becomes widely used as a technique for synthesising the results of separate primary studies, an overly simplistic approach to its implementation needs to be avoided. A failure to investigate potential sources of heterogeneity is one aspect of this. As shown in the examples in this chapter, such investigation can importantly affect the overall conclusions drawn, as well as the clinical implications of the review. Therefore the issues of clinical and statistical heterogeneity and how to approach them need emphasis in guidelines and in computer software being developed for conducting meta-analyses, for example by the Cochrane Collaboration.[45]

Although a simple random effects method of analysis[6] may be useful when statistical heterogeneity is present but cannot be obviously explained, the main focus should be on trying to understand any sources of heterogeneity that are present.

There are, however, dangers of over-interpretation induced by attempting to explore possible reasons for heterogeneity, since such investigations are usually inspired, at least to some extent, by looking at the results to hand.[11] Moreover apparent, even statistically significant, heterogeneity may always be due to chance and searching for its causes would then be misleading. The problem is akin to that of subgroup analyses within an individual clinical trial.[46] However the degree of clinical heterogeneity across different trials is greater than that within individual trials, and represents a more serious problem. Guidelines for deciding whether to believe results that stem from investigating heterogeneity depend on, for example, the magnitude and statistical significance of the differences identified, the extent to which the potential sources of heterogeneity have been specified in advance, and indirect evidence and biological considerations which support the investigation.[47] These problems in meta-analysis are greatest when there are many clinical differences but only a small number of trials available. In such situations there may be several alternative explanations for statistical heterogeneity, and ideas about sources of heterogeneity can be considered only as hypotheses for evaluation in future studies.

Although clinical causes of heterogeneity have been focused on here, it is important to recognise that there are other potential causes. For example, statistical heterogeneity may be caused by publication bias[48] whereby, amongst small trials, those with dramatic results may more often be published (see Chapter 3). Statistical heterogeneity can also be caused by defects of methodological quality,[49] as discussed in detail in Chapter 5. For example, poor methodological quality was of concern in the meta-analysis of sclerotherapy trials[2] discussed at the beginning of this chapter. The evidence for publication bias, or other small study biases, can be explored by regression on a Galbraith plot (such as Figure 9.4) without constraining the intercept through the origin.[50] An equivalent analysis can be undertaken using meta-regression of treatment effects against their standard errors, using the methods of this chapter, which also then allow for possible residual heterogeneity.[23] These and other methods are discussed in detail in Chapter 11. Statistical heterogeneity may also be induced by employing an inappropriate scale for measuring treatment effects, for example using absolute rather than relative differences, or even by early termination of clinical trials for ethical or other reasons.[51]

Despite the laudable attempts to achieve objectivity in reviewing scientific data, considerable areas of subjectivity remain in carrying out systematic reviews. These judgments include decisions about which studies are "relevant", which studies are methodologically sound enough to be included in a statistical synthesis, as well as the issue of whether and how to investigate sources of heterogeneity. Such scientific judgements are as necessary in meta-analysis as they are in other forms of medical research, and skills in recognising appropriate analyses and dismissing overly speculative interpretations are required. In many meta-analyses, however, heterogeneity can and should be investigated so as to increase the scientific understanding of the studies reviewed and the clinical relevance of the conclusions drawn.

Acknowledgements

This chapter draws on material published earlier in the *BMJ*.[52]

1 Dickersin K, Berlin J. Meta-analysis: state-of-the-science. *Epidemiol Rev* 1992;**14**:154–76.
2 Pagliaro L, D'Amico G, Sorensen TIA, *et al.* Prevention of first bleeding in cirrhosis: a meta-analysis of randomised trials of non-surgical treatment. *Ann Intern Med* 1992;**117**:59–70.
3 Altman DG. *Practical statistics for medical research*. London: Chapman and Hall, 1991:167–70.
4 Whitehead A, Whitehead J. A general parametric approach to the meta-analysis of randomised clinical trials. *Stat Med* 1991;**10**:1665–77.
5 Thompson SG, Pocock SJ. Can meta-analyses be trusted? *Lancet* 1991;**338**:1127–30.
6 DerSimonian R, Laird N. Meta-analysis in clinical trials. *Controlled Clin Trials* 1986;**7**:177–88.
7 Hardy RJ, Thompson SG. Detecting and describing heterogeneity in meta-analysis. *Stat Med* 1998; **17**:841–56.
8 Peto R. Why do we need systematic overviews of randomised trials? *Stat Med* 1987;**6**:233–40.
9 Chalmers TC. Problems induced by meta-analysis. *Stat Med* 1991;**10**:971–80.
10 Boersma E, Maas ACP, Deckers JW, Simoons ML. Early thrombolytic treatment in acute myocardial infarction: reappraisal of the golden hour. *Lancet* 1996;**348**:771–5.
11 Davey Smith G, Egger M, Phillips AN. Meta-analysis: Beyond the grand mean? *BMJ* 1997;**315**:1610–14.
12 Berlin JA. Benefits of heterogeneity in meta-analysis of data from epidemiologic studies. *Am J Epidemiol* 1995;**142**:383–7.
13 Lau J, Ioannidis JPA, Schmid CH. Summing up evidence: one answer is not always enough. *Lancet* 1998;**351**:123–7.
14 Law MR, Wald NJ, Thompson SG. By how much and how quickly does reduction in serum cholesterol concentration lower risk of ischaemic heart disease? *BMJ* 1994;**308**:367–73.
15 MacMahon S, Peto R, Cutler J, *et al.* Blood pressure, stroke, and coronary heart disease. Part I, prolonged differences in blood pressure: prospective observational studies corrected for the regression dilution bias. *Lancet* 1990;**335**:765–74.
16 Manolio TA, Pearson TA, Wenger NK, Barrett-Connor E, Payne GH, Harlan WR. Cholesterol and heart disease in older persons and women: review of an NHLBI workshop. *Ann Epidemiol* 1992;**2**:161–76.
17 Shipley MJ, Pocock SJ, Marmot MG. Does plasma cholesterol concentration predict mortality from coronary heart disease in elderly people? 18 year follow-up in Whitehall study. *BMJ* 1991;**303**:89–92.
18 Egger M, Schneider M, Davey Smith G. Spurious precision? Meta-analysis of observational studies. *BMJ* 1998;**316**:140–4.

19 Ravnskov U. Cholesterol lowering trials in coronary heart disease: frequency of citation and outcome. *BMJ* 1992;**305**:15–19.
20 Davey Smith G, Song F, Sheldon T. Cholesterol lowering and mortality: the importance of considering initial level of risk. *BMJ* 1993;**306**:1367–73.
21 Galbraith RF. A note on the graphical presentation of estimated odds ratios from several clinical trials. *Stat Med* 1988;7:889–94.
22 Thompson SG. Controversies in meta-analysis: the case of the trials of serum cholesterol reduction. *Stat Meth Med Res* 1993;**2**:173–92.
23 Thompson SG, Sharp SJ. Explaining heterogeneity in meta-analysis: a comparison of methods. *Stat Med* 1999;**18**:2693–708.
24 Thompson SG. Meta-analysis of clinical trials. In: Armitage P, Colton T, eds. *Encyclopedia of Biostatistics*. New York: Wiley, 1998:2570–9.
25 Cox DR, Snell EJ. *Analysis of binary data*, 2nd edn. London: Chapman and Hall, 1989.
26 Berkey CS, Hoaglin DC, Mosteller F, Colditz GA. A random-effects regression model for meta-analysis. *Stat Med* 1995; **14**: 395–411.
27 Sharp SJ. Meta-analysis regression. *Stata Tech Bull* 1998;**42**:16–22.
28 Goldstein H, Rasbash J. Improved approximations for multilevel models with binary responses. *J Roy Statist Soc A* 1996;**159**:505–13.
29 Goldstein H, Rasbash J, Plewis I, *et al. A user's guide to MLwiN*. London: Institute of Education, 1998.
30 McQuay HJ, Moore RA. Using numerical results from systematic reviews in clinical practice. *Ann Intern Med* 1997;**126**:712–20.
31 Sharp SJ, Thompson SG, Altman DG. The relation between treatment benefit and underlying risk in meta-analysis. *BMJ* 1996;**313**:735–8.
32 Schmid CH, Lau J, McIntosh MW, Cappelleri JC. An empirical study of the effect of the control rate as a predictor of treatment efficacy in meta-analysis of clinical trials. *Stat Med* 1998;17:1923–42.
33 Egger M, Davey Smith G. Risks and benefits of treating mild hypertension: a misleading meta-analysis? *J Hypertens* 1995;**13**:813–15.
34 McIntosh M. The population risk as an explanatory variable in research synthesis of clinical trials. *Stat Med* 1996;**15**:1713–28.
35 Thompson SG, Smith TC, Sharp SJ. Investigating underlying risk as a source of heterogeneity in meta-analysis. *Stat Med* 1997;**16**:2741–58.
36 Morgenstern H. Uses of ecological analysis in epidemiologic research. *Am J Public Health* 1982;**72**:127–30.
37 Stewart LA, Clarke MJ. Practical methodology of meta-analysis (overviews) using updated individual patient data. *Stat Med* 1995;**14**:2057–79.
38 Meier P. Meta-analysis of clinical trials as a scientific discipline [commentary]. *Stat Med* 1987;**6**:329–31.
39 Bailey KR. Inter-study differences: how should they influence the interpretation and analysis of results? *Stat Med* 1987;**6**:351–8.
40 Early Breast Cancer Trialists' Collaborative Group. Systemic treatment of early breast cancer by hormonal, cytotoxic, or immune therapy. *Lancet* 1992;**339**:1–15, 71–85.
41 Goldstein H. *Multilevel statistical models*, 2nd edn. London: Edward Arnold, 1995.
42 Stram DO. Meta-analysis of published data using a linear mixed-effects model. *Biometrics* 1996;**52**:536–44.
43 Turner RM, Omar RZ, Yang M, Goldstein H, Thompson SG. A multilevel model framework for meta-analysis of clinical trials with binary outcomes. *Stat Med* 2000, in press.
44 Pauler DK, Wakefield J. Modeling and implementation issues in Bayesian meta-analysis. In: Stangl DK, Berry DA, eds. *Meta-analysis in medicine and policy health*. New York: Marcel Dekker 2000, 205–30.
45 Oxman A. Preparing and maintaining systematic reviews. In: Sackett D, ed. *Cochrane Collaboration Handbook*, Sect. *VI*. Oxford: The Cochrane Collaboration, 1998.
46 Yusuf S, Wittes J, Probstfield J, Tyroler HA. Analysis and interpretation of treatment effects in subgroups of patients in randomised clinical trials. *JAMA* 1991;**266**:93–8.
47 Oxman AD, Guyatt GH. A consumer's guide to subgroup analyses. *Ann Intern Med* 1992;**116**:78–84.

174

48 Easterbrook PJ, Berlin JA, Gopalan R, Matthews DR. Publication bias in clinical research. *Lancet* 1991;**337**:867–72

49 Schulz KF, Chalmers I, Hayes RJ, Altman DG. Empirical evidence of bias: dimensions of methodologic quality associated with estimates of treatment effects in controlled trials. *JAMA* 1995;**273**:408–12.

50 Egger M, Davey Smith G, Schneider M, Minder C. Bias in meta-analysis detected by a simple, graphical test. *BMJ* 1997;**315**:629–34.

51 Hughes MD, Freedman LS, Pocock SJ. The impact of stopping rules on heterogeneity of results in overviews of clinical trials. *Biometrics* 1992;**48**:41–53.

52 Thompson SG. Why sources of heterogeneity in meta-analysis should be investigated. *BMJ* 1994;**309**:1351–5.

10 Analysing the relationship between treatment benefit and underlying risk: precautions and recommendations

STEPHEN J SHARP

Summary points

- Variations in the effect of treatment found in a meta-analysis might be explained by differences in the patients' underlying risk of adverse outcome.
- Such an association would have important implications in the evaluation of the treatment.
- Conventional analysis methods are based on relating the observed treatment effect to observed control group risk or the observed average risk in the control and treatment group.
- Such methods are flawed in most situations and can lead to seriously misleading conclusions.
- At least two statistically valid approaches for the analysis have been developed.
- The methodology and software required to implement these approaches are freely available.

In the previous chapter, a strong case has been developed for investigating potential sources of heterogeneity across trials in meta-analysis, with the aim of increasing the scientific and clinical relevance of the results. Within such an investigation, it is reasonable to ask whether the extent of treatment benefit is related to the underlying risk of the patients in the different trials. The existence of such a relationship would have potential implications for the interpretation of the results of a meta-analysis, both in terms of determining which patients are likely to benefit most, and also for economic considerations.[1]

If the results of a meta-analysis are to affect future clinical practice, the clinician needs to know primarily how the net treatment benefit varies according to certain measurable characteristics of the patient. The "underlying risk" can be understood to be a summary of a number of patient characteristics, which may be measurable risk factors, but for which, as may frequently be the case, the individual patient data are not available in some or all of the trials. Analyses which attempt to investigate the relationship between treatment effect and underlying risk have now been undertaken in a variety of medical areas – for example in trials of cholesterol reduction and mortality,[2] of tocolysis using β-mimetics in pre-term delivery,[3] and of antiarrhythmic drugs after acute myocardial infarction.[4,5] Differences in the underlying risk of patients have also been proposed as an explanation for the differences between the results of meta-analysis and a subsequent mega-trial of magnesium therapy after acute myocardial infarction.[6] Unfortunately, the conventional approaches to the analysis which have been adopted suffer from potentially serious statistical pitfalls, which have already been alluded to in Chapters 8 and 9.

This chapter has two aims: first, to describe in detail the conventional approaches and their pitfalls, and second, to make the reader aware of the existence of at least two recently proposed approaches which overcome the statistical problems of the conventional approaches. The issues in both sections are exemplified using data from a meta-analysis of 19 trials of endoscopic sclerotherapy,[7] introduced in the previous chapter. There were two principal outcomes in the trials of that meta-analysis: death (see Figure 9.1 of Chapter 9) and bleeding, the results for which are shown in Figure 10.1. For the bleeding outcome, as for mortality, there was substantial evidence of statistical heterogeneity across trials (χ^2 on 18 degrees of freedom is 81.5, $P < 0.001$). As discussed in the previous chapter, this is probably due to the substantial clinical differences between the trials which led to the statistical heterogeneity between the odds ratios for death.

Relating treatment effect to underlying risk: conventional approaches

Observed treatment effect versus observed control group risk

A natural measure of underlying risk in a trial population is the observed risk of events in the control group. Figure 10.2 shows graphs of the treatment effect (log odds ratio) against the control group risk (control group log odds) for (a) death and (b) bleeding in the sclerotherapy trials. Each trial on each graph is represented by a circle, the area of which represents the trial precision, so trials which contribute more information are represented by larger circles. Each graph also includes the line of predicted values obtained from a weighted regression. The estimated slopes from these regressions are −0·61 (95% CI −0·99 to −0·23) for death and −1·12 (95% CI −1·45 to −0·79) for bleeding. To understand a slope of −0·61, consider a group of patients who are at average risk of death (35%, or an odds of 0·54 in these trials). The estimated treatment effect for these patients is an odds ratio of 0·77 (i.e. a 23% reduction in odds of death comparing sclerotherapy with placebo). Now consider patients who are at half the average risk (18%, or an odds of 0·22); the estimated treatment effect for these patients is an odds ratio of 1·33 (i.e. a 33% increase in odds of death comparing sclerotherapy with placebo). On the other hand, for patients who are at double average risk (70%, or an odds of 2·3), the estimated treatment effect is an odds ratio of 0·31 (i.e. a 69% decrease in odds of death comparing sclerotherapy with placebo). In other words, higher risk patients are more likely to benefit from sclerotherapy than those at lower risk, in whom sclerotherapy may have a harmful effect. Because the

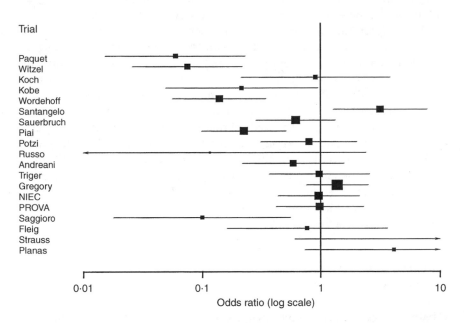

Figure 10.1 Forest plot of odds ratios of bleeding (and 95% confidence intervals) from 19 trials of sclerotherapy. Odds ratios less than unity represent beneficial effects of sclerotherapy. Trials are identified by principal author, referenced by Pagliaro.[7] The area of the box represents the trial precision, so trials which contribute more information are represented by larger boxes.

178

slope is even more negative (−1·12) for bleeding, the conclusion from this analysis would be that for both death and bleeding, there is strong evidence of an association between treatment effect and "underlying risk" (as represented by the observed control group log odds), with the benefit of sclerotherapy increasing (lower log odds ratio, and hence lower odds ratio) with increasing levels of "underlying risk".

Two aspects of the above analysis make the interpretation potentially seriously flawed. The first is that the expression for underlying risk (here control group log odds) also appears in the expression for treatment effect (here log odds ratio, which is treatment group log odds minus control group log odds). This "structural dependence", combined with the second aspect, the fact that both the observed log odds ratio and the observed control group log odds are measured with error, presents a problem associated with regression to the mean, also known as regression dilution bias.[8,9] Such a bias means that a relationship between the two observed quantities may be seen even if the true treatment effect and underlying risk are unrelated, or, if the true quantities are related, the magnitude of the relationship may be artificially exaggerated by the above analysis. To illustrate this bias, consider a situation where there is actually no association between true treatment effect and true underlying risk. A trial with a high observed control group risk (log odds) will lead to a large observed treatment effect (low log odds ratio) because of the structural dependence, while conversely a trial with a low observed control group risk (log odds) will lead to a high observed treatment effect (high log odds ratio), and hence an artificial negative relationship between observed treatment effect (log odds ratio) and observed control group risk (log odds) will be induced.

The extent to which this approach yields misleading conclusions depends on a number of factors. Algebra has shown that the approach will always be biased, with the bias being smallest if the trials are mostly large, or the variation in true underlying risks is large.[10] However, this work is limited to the (usually) unrealistic situation where all the trials in the meta-analysis estimate the treatment effect with the same degree of precision (i.e. the trials are all roughly the same size). A general statement about the extent of the bias where different trials have different precisions cannot be made, because the biases due to regression to the mean are different for each component trial.

Observed treatment effect versus observed average risk

Figure 10.3 shows graphs of the treatment effect (log odds ratio) against the average risk (average of control group log odds and treatment group log odds) for (a) death and (b) bleeding in the sclerotherapy trials, together with weighted regression lines as in Figure 10.2. The estimated slopes from these regressions are −0·16 (95% CI −0·73 to +0·42) for death and −0·82

179

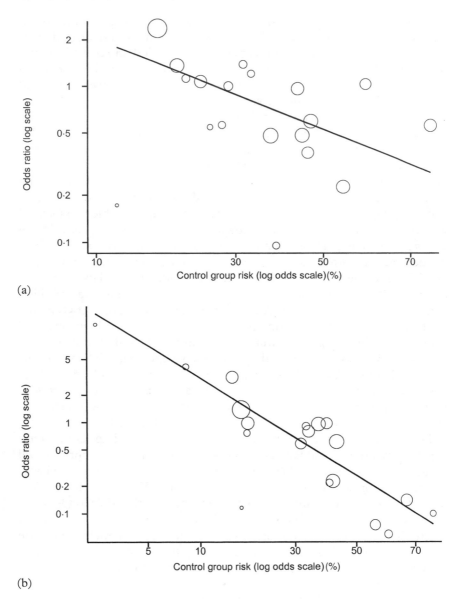

Figure 10.2 Observed treatment effect (log odds ratio) versus observed control group risk (log odds) for (a) death, (b) bleeding, including weighted regression lines. Each trial is represented by a circle, the area of which represents the trial's precision. Larger circles represent trials that contribute more information.
Regression equations:
   (a) Log odds ratio = 0·64–0·61×(control group log odds)
   (b) Log odds ratio = 1·34–1·12×(control group log odds)

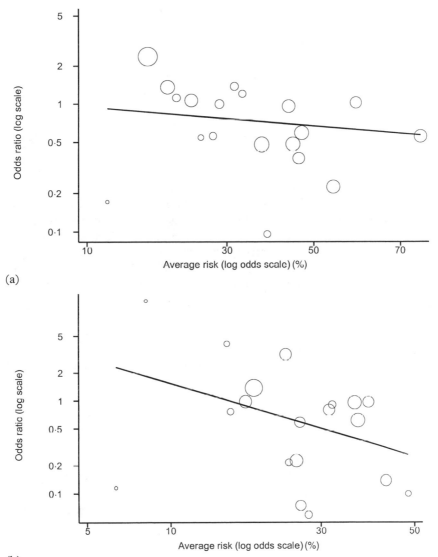

(a)

(b)

Figure 10.3 Observed treatment effect (log odds ratio) versus observed average risk (average of control and treatment group log odds) for (a) death, (b) bleeding, including weighted regression lines. Larger circles represent trials that contribute more information.

Regression equations:

(a) Log odds ratio = 0·40–0·16×(control group log odds + treatment group log odds)/2

(b) Log odds ratio = 1·39–0·82×(control group log odds + treatment group log odds)/2

(95% CI $-1\cdot82$ to $+0\cdot18$) for bleeding. The conclusion from this analysis is very different from the analysis based on control group risk: for both death and bleeding there is now only a slight increase in treatment effect (reduction in log odds ratio) as the level of "underlying risk" increases, with unconvincing evidence for a relationship, as shown by the confidence intervals on the two slopes both including 0.

Unfortunately the above analysis may still be flawed. It is well known in statistics that if x and y represent sets of single observations (e.g. sets of systolic blood pressure measurements on two occasions), then relating $y - x$ to $(x + y)/2$ overcomes the problem of regression to the mean arising from relating $y - x$ to x.[11] However, this does not apply in the case of meta-analysis, where trials are of different sizes and hence the control and treatment group risks are measured with different degrees of precision in the different trials. It is not possible to make general statements about how much a relationship between observed treatment effect and observed average risk is biased, or whether the bias is in a positive or negative direction from the truth, because the bias will depend on the relative magnitudes of the biases incurred from measuring the control group risk and treatment group risk within each trial, and on the relative precisions with which these risks are measured across trials.[10]

Observed treatment group risk versus observed control group risk

The L'Abbé plot of observed treatment group risk against observed control group risk was proposed as a graphical means of exploring possible heterogeneity.[12] If the trials are fairly homogeneous, the points would lie around a line corresponding to the pooled treatment effect parallel to the line of identity – large deviations would indicate possible heterogeneity.

Figure 10.4 shows L'Abbé plots for (a) death and (b) bleeding in the sclerotherapy trials, and in addition, weighted regression lines. The estimated slopes of these regression lines are $+0\cdot39$ (95% CI $+0\cdot01$ to $+0\cdot77$) for death and $-0\cdot12$ (95% CI $-0\cdot45$ to $+0\cdot21$) for bleeding. Notice that these slopes and confidence limits are 1 unit greater than those in the approach "treatment effect versus observed control group risk", which is to be expected, because of the structural relationship between the two equations. The conclusion from this analysis of a L'Abbé plot is therefore the same as that from approach "treatment effect versus observed control group risk", but it also suffers from the same problems of regression to the mean.[8,9] L'Abbé plots may be useful as an exploratory graphical device (their original purpose), for example to identify an unusual or outlying trial, but they cannot be used in conjunction with a regression analysis to determine the relationship between treatment effect and underlying risk. One example where a L'Abbé plot was used in this misleading way was after a

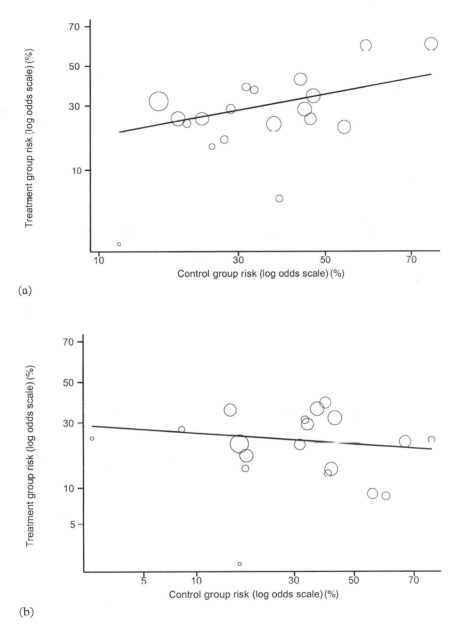

(a)

(b)

Figure 10.4 L'Abbé plot for (a) death, (b) bleeding, including weighted regression lines. Larger circles represent trials that contribute more information.
Regression equations:
   (a) Treatment group log odds = 0·61 + 0·39×(control group log odds)
   (b) Treatment group log odds = 1·29 + 0·12×(control group log odds)

183

meta-analysis of drug trials in mild hypertension.[13,14] This example is described in Chapter 8.

Relating treatment effect to underlying risk: recently proposed approaches

Two approaches have recently been published in the statistical literature,[15,16] both with the specific aim of estimating the true relationship between treatment effect and underlying risk while avoiding the biases inherent in the conventional approaches. Here, the two approaches are described briefly, then one is applied to the death and bleeding data in the sclerotherapy trials, followed by some comments about using the approaches in practice.

The full statistical details of the two approaches are beyond the scope of this article, so the aim of this and the following paragraph is to give the interested reader a flavour of the approaches; these two paragraphs can be skipped without loss of continuity! The approach due to Thompson,[15] extends a Bayesian procedure for performing random effects meta-analysis.[17] The observed number of events in the control group of each trial i, r_i^C is assumed to be from a binomial distribution, defined by a parameter π_i^C which represents the true underlying probability of an event in the control group, and a similar binomial distribution with parameter π_i^T is assumed for the observed number of events r_i^T in the treatment group of trial i. The true treatment effect (here the log odds ratio) parameter δ_i and true underlying risk parameter μ_i (here on a log odds scale) are then constructed as functions of π_i^C and π_i^T, and a regression-type relationship is formed between these true parameters: $\delta_i = \delta_i' + \beta\mu_i$. The δ_i' are assumed to follow a Normal distribution, a similar assumption to that made in a conventional random effects meta-analysis.[18] To estimate the values of the various parameters, their joint probability distribution is formed by combining their prior distributions with the likelihood given the observed data (using Bayes' theorem[19]), and then a numerical algorithm called Gibbs sampling[20] is used to obtain samples from this joint "posterior distribution" for any particular parameter. The estimated value of the parameter is usually the median value from a number of samples (e.g. 5000 samples), and a 95% confidence interval on the estimate is given by the 2·5 and 97·5 percentiles of the sample distribution. In the derivation of the joint "posterior distribution", any unknown parameters, such as β here, are assumed to have a prior distributions which are "non-informative", i.e. the choice of prior distribution does not influence the final estimate of the parameter.

The approach due to McIntosh[16] essentially only differs from the Thompson approach[15] in two respects. First, the data are not entered as the observed number of events from a binomial distribution in each group of each trial, but instead as the observed log odds ratio and control group log odds in each trial. These quantities are then assumed to be from Normal distributions with known variances (given by a standard formula[19]), within each trial. The second difference relates to the underlying model assumptions: while the Thompson approach assumes no particular distribution for the true underlying risks μ_i across trials, the McIntosh approach assumes these parameters are drawn from a Normal distribution, with mean and variance to be estimated from the overall joint distribution. The ability to enter the data as binomial observations is clearly advantageous compared with making an approximating assumption of a Normal distribution for observed log odds ratio and log odds; however, the most appropriate way to handle the μ_i in the model is less obvious, and which of the approaches is more appropriate in this respect remains a question open for debate in the statistical literature.[21,22]

Re-analysis of the sclerotherapy data

Because the approach due to Thompson[15] makes fewer assumptions, the results from this approach, labelled (C), are compared with the conventional approaches (A) and (B) in Table 10.1. For bleeding, the estimated slope and confidence interval from (C) are very close to those from conventional approach (A); however, this is not the case for death, where (A) gives a spuriously convincing and too large negative relationship. While (B) would have correctly identified a non-significant negative relationship for

Table 10.1 Estimated relationship between treatment effect and "underlying risk" obtained from applying two conventional approaches and one recently proposed approach to the death and bleeding data from 19 sclerotherapy trials.

	Slope for relationship between treatment effect and "underlying risk" (95% CI)
Death	
(A) Conventional approach based on observed control group risk	−0·61 (−0·99 to −0·23)
(B) Conventional approach based on observed average risk	−0·16 (−0·73 to +0·41)
(C) Approach due to Thompson[15]	−0·40 (−0·80 to +0·03)
Bleeding	
(A) Conventional approach based on observed control group risk	−1·12 (−1·45 to −0·79)
(B) Conventional approach based on observed average risk	−0·82 (−1·82 to +0·18)
(C) Approach due to Thompson[15]	−1·05 (−1·36 to −0·77)

185

death, it would have missed the convincing negative relationship for bleeding. Even for this one example, it is therefore clear that neither of the conventional approaches is consistently reliable, and it is only in retrospect, with the results from approach (C) available, that one can see which of the conventional approaches is "more correct" in each case. One further observation from Table 10.1 is that the confidence intervals from (C) are wider than those from (A) and (B); this is because the model in approach (C) includes a parameter which represents the heterogeneity across trials that remains unexplained by the underlying risk (the "residual heterogeneity"), allowing more variability than the models in (A) and (B).

The recently proposed approaches overcome the problems of the conventional approaches by modelling the relationship between true parameters, rather than observed quantities. Both approaches can be implemented in the freely available BUGS software,[23] details of which are given in Chapter 17. However, unlike the conventional approaches, their application requires understanding of Bayesian methods, in particular the specifics of Bayesian meta-analysis,[17] the details of which are beyond the scope of this article. A full description of the appropriate models and BUGS code to fit them are provided in my paper reviewing the various recently proposed methods,[24] and this information should enable the analyses to be performed by a reasonably experienced statistician.

Conclusions

An investigation of whether treatment benefit is related to underlying risk can have an important role in a meta-analysis. Unfortunately, while the question posed is simple, it turns out that there is no simple statistical method to provide a valid answer. A similar problem occurs in several guises in medicine, perhaps most commonly the issue of the possible relation between change and initial value.[25]

The search for an approach which avoids the statistical pitfalls described was stimulated by an investigation of 14 controlled trials of β-mimetics for the prevention of preterm birth,[3] in which approach (A) above was used to suggest a negative association between treatment effect and "underlying risk", and there followed a subsequent discussion about the validity of the conclusions based on this analysis.[26,27] Apart from the two recently proposed approaches described in this article, there are other theoretical papers which address the issue,[28-30] but for which doubts remain about the underlying model assumptions, or the ability to apply the methods in practice.[24]

Underlying risk is not a measurable quantity, and hence finding that the treatment effect varies by levels of risk is only of practical value provided that risk can be assessed using measurable characteristics.[10] Where individual patient data are available in all the trials of a meta-analysis, an alternative strategy would be to relate treatment effects to individual patient characteristics to investigate heterogeneity, as mentioned in the previous chapter (see also Chapter 6). Such an analysis would be more directly useful to the clinician considering treatment for an individual patient (see Chapter 19).

In conclusion, where individual patient data are not available for some or all trials in the meta-analysis, an examination of whether the treatment effects observed in the trials are related to the underlying risks of the different patient groups is a potentially important component of an investigation into the sources of heterogeneity. Statistically valid methods are now freely available for such an analysis.

1 Davey Smith G, Egger M. Who benefits from medical interventions? *BMJ* 1994;**308**:72–4.
2 Davey Smith G, Song F, Sheldon T. Cholesterol lowering and mortality: the importance of considering initial level of risk. *BMJ* 1993;**206**:1367–73.
3 Brand R, Kragt H. Importance of trends in the interpretation of an overall odds ratio in the meta-analysis of clinical trials. *Stat Med* 1992;**11**:2077–82.
4 Boissel J-P, Collet J, Lièvre M, Girard P. An effect model for the assessment of drug benefit: example of antiarrhythmic drugs in postmyocardial infarction patients. *J Cardiovasc Pharmacol* 1993;**22**:356–63.
5 Antman EM, Lau J, Kupelnick B, Mosteller F, Chalmers TC. A comparison of results of meta-analyses of randomized control trials and recommendations of clinical experts. Treatments for myocardial infarction. *JAMA* 1992;**268**:240–8.
6 Lau J, Ioannidis JPA, Schmid CH. Summing up evidence: one answer is not always enough. *Lancet* 1998;**351**:123–7.
7 Pagliaro L, D'Amico G, Sørensen T, *et al.* Prevention of first bleeding in cirrhosis – a meta-analysis of randomized trials of nonsurgical treatment. *Ann Intern Med* 1992;**117**:59–70.
8 Bland JM, Altman DG. Regression towards the mean. *BMJ* 1994;**308**:1499.
9 Bland JM, Altman DG. Some examples of regression to the mean. *BMJ* 1994;**309**:780.
10 Sharp SJ, Thompson SG, Altman DG. The relation between treatment benefit and underlying risk in meta-analysis. *BMJ* 1996;**313**:735-8.
11 Hayes R. Methods for assessing whether change depends on initial value. *Stat Med* 1988;**7**:915–27.
12 L'Abbé K, Detsky A, O'Rourke K. Meta-analysis in clinical research. *Ann Intern Med* 1987;**107**:224–33.
13 Hoes AW, Grobbee DE, Lubsen J. Does drug treatment improve survival? Reconciling the trials in mild-to-moderate hypertension. *J Hypertens* 1995;**13**:805–11.
14 Egger M, Davey Smith G. Risks and benefits of treating mild hypertension: a misleading meta-analysis? *J Hypertens* 1995;**13**:813–15.
15 Thompson SG, Smith TC, Sharp SJ. Investigating underlying risk as a source of heterogeneity in meta-analysis. *Stat Med* 1997;**16**:2741–58.
16 McIntosh M. The population risk as an explanatory variable in research synthesis of clinical trials. *Stat Med* 1996;**15**:1713–28.
17 Smith TC, Spiegelhalter DJ, Thomas A. Bayesian approaches to random effects meta-analyses: a comparative study. *Stat Med* 1995;**14**:2685–99.
18 DerSimonian R, Laird N. Meta-analysis in clinical trials. *Controlled Clin Trials* 1986;**7**:177–88.
19 Armitage P, Berry G. In: *Statistical Methods in Medical Research*, 3rd edn. Oxford: Blackwell Science, 1994:288–90.

20 Gilks WR, Clayton DG, Spiegelhalter DJ, *et al.* Modelling complexity: applications of Gibbs sampling in medicine (with discussion). *J Roy Stat Soc* 1993;**55**:39–102.
21 Van Houwelingen H., Senn, S. Letter to the editor: investigating underlying risk as a source of heterogeneity in meta-analysis. *Stat Med* 1999;**18**:107–13.
22 Thompson SG, Prevost (née Smith) TC, Sharp SJ. Author's reply: investigating underlying risk as a source of heterogeneity in meta-analysis. *Stat Med* 1999;**18**:113–15.
23 Gilks WR, Thomas A, Spiegelhalter DJ. A language and program for complex Bayesian modelling. *Statistician* 1994;**43**:169–77.
24 Sharp SJ, Thompson SG. Analysing the relationship between treatment effect and underlying risk in meta-analysis: comparison and development of approaches. *Stat Med* (in press).
25 Blomqvist N. On the relation between change and initial value. *J Am Stat Assoc* 1977;**72**:746–9.
26 Senn S. Letter to the editor. *Stat Med* 1994;**13**:293–6.
27 Brand R. Importance of trends in the interpretation of an overall odds ratio in a meta-analysis of clinical trials (author's reply). *Stat Med* 1994;**13**:295–6.
28 Walter SD. Variation in baseline risk as an explanation of heterogeneity in meta-analysis. *Stat Med* 1997;**16**:2883–900.
29 Van Houwelingen H, Zwinderman K, Stijnen T. A bivariate approach to meta-analysis. *Stat Med* 1993;**12**:2272–84.
30 Cook RJ, Walter SD. A logistic model for trend in $2 \times 2 \times K$ tables with applications to meta-analyses. *Biometrics* 1997;**53**:352–7.

11 Investigating and dealing with publication and other biases

JONATHAN A C STERNE, MATTHIAS EGGER,
GEORGE DAVEY SMITH

Summary points

- Asymmetrical funnel plots may indicate publication bias, or be due to exaggeration of treatment effects in small studies of low quality.
- Bias is not the only explanation for funnel plot asymmetry. Funnel plots should be seen as a means of examining "small study effects" (the tendency for the smaller studies in a meta-analysis to show larger treatment effects) rather than a tool to diagnose specific types of bias.
- When markers of adherence to treatment or of the biological effects of treatment are reported, these may be used to examine bias without assuming a relationship between treatment effect and study size.
- Statistical methods may be used to examine the evidence for bias, and to examine the robustness of the conclusions of the meta-analysis in sensitivity analyses. "Correction" of treatment effect estimates for bias should be avoided, since such corrections may depend heavily on the assumptions made.
- Multivariable models may be used, with caution, to examine the relative importance of different types of bias.

Studies that show a statistically significant effect of treatment are more likely to be published,[1,2,3] more likely to be published in English,[4] more likely to be cited by other authors[5,6] and more likely to produce multiple publications[7,8] than other studies. Such "positive" studies are therefore more likely to be located for and included in systematic reviews, which may introduce bias. Trial quality has also been shown to influence the size of treatment effect estimates, with studies of lower methodological quality showing the larger effects.[9,10] These biases, reviewed in detail in Chapters 3 and 5, are more likely to affect small rather than large studies. The smaller a study, the larger the treatment effect necessary for the results to be declared statistically significant. In addition, the greater investment of money and time in larger studies means that they are more likely to be of high methodological quality and published even if their results are negative. Bias in a systematic review may therefore become evident through an association between treatment effect and study size.

In this chapter we examine how we may check a meta-analysis for evidence of such bias, using graphical and statistical methods. We also examine methods for quantifying the possible impact of bias on overall treatment effect estimates, and for correcting effect estimates for bias.

Funnel plots

First used in educational research and psychology,[11] funnel plots are simple scatter plots of the treatment effects estimated from individual studies on the horizontal axis against some measure of study size on the vertical axis. The name "funnel plot" is based on the fact that the precision in the estimation of the underlying treatment effect will increase as the sample size of component studies increases. Effect estimates from small studies will therefore scatter more widely at the bottom of the graph, with the spread narrowing among larger studies. In the absence of bias, the plot will resemble a symmetrical inverted funnel (see Figure 11.1(a)).

Choice of axes

Relative measures of treatment effect (risk ratios or odds ratios) are plotted on a logarithmic scale. This is important to ensure that effects of the same magnitude but opposite directions, for example risk ratios of 0·5 and 2, are equidistant from 1·0.[12] There are a number of possible choices for the measure of study size to be used as the vertical axis in funnel plots. Treatment effects have generally been plotted against sample size, or log sample size. However, the statistical power of a trial is determined both by the total sample size and the number of participants developing the event of interest. For example, a study with 100 000 patients and 10 events is less powerful than a study with 1000 patients and 100 events. Measures based on the standard error or variance of the effect estimate (or their inverse) rather than total sample size, have therefore been increasingly used in funnel plots. Plotting against standard error may generally be a good choice because it emphasizes differences between studies of smaller size for which biases are most likely to operate. In contrast, plotting against precision (1/standard error) will emphasize differences between larger studies. Using standard error is also consistent with statistical tests for funnel plot asymmetry,[13,14] discussed below, which look for associations between the treatment effect size and its standard error. A disadvantage of using standard error is that the

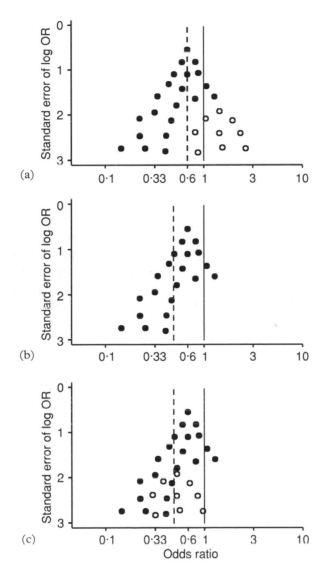

Figure 11.1 Hypothetical funnel plots: (a) symmetrical plot in the absence of bias (open circles indicate smaller studies showing no statistically significant effects); (b) asymmetrical plot in the presence of publication bias (smaller studies showing no statistically significant effects are missing); (c) asymmetrical plot in the presence of bias due to low methodological quality of smaller studies (open circles indicate small studies of inadequate quality whose results are biased towards larger effects). The dashed line is the pooled odds ratio, the solid line is the null effect. The estimated treatment effects are exaggerated in the presence of bias.

vertical axis must be inverted (smallest standard errors at the top) in order to produce the conventional inverted funnel graph.

Bias as a source of funnel plot asymmetry

Bias may lead to asymmetry in funnel plots. For example, if smaller studies showing no statistically significant effects (open circles in Figure 11.1) remain unpublished, then such publication bias[1,2,15] will lead to an asymmetrical appearance of the funnel plot with a gap in the right bottom side of the graph (Figure 11.1(b)). In this situation the combined effect from meta-analysis will overestimate the treatment's effect.[13,16] The more pronounced the asymmetry, the more likely it is that the amount of bias is substantial.

Trials of lower quality also tend to show larger effects. In particular, studies with inadequate concealment of treatment allocation or studies which are not double blind have been shown to result in inflated estimates of treatment effect[9,10] (see also Chapter 5). Smaller studies are, on average, conducted and analysed with less methodological rigour than larger studies. Trials that, if conducted and analysed properly, would have given no evidence for a treatment effect may thus become "positive", as shown in (Figure 11.1(c)), again leading to asymmetry. Thus the funnel plot should be seen as a generic means of examining "small study effects" (the tendency for the smaller studies in a meta-analysis to show larger treatment effects) rather than a tool to diagnose specific types of bias.

Asymmetry is not proof of bias: alternative sources of funnel plot asymmetry

The trials displayed in a funnel plot may not always estimate the same underlying effect of the same intervention and such heterogeneity between results may lead to asymmetry in funnel plots if the true treatment effect is larger in the smaller trials. For example, if a combined outcome is considered then substantial benefit may be seen only in patients at high risk for the component of the combined outcome which is affected by the intervention.[17,18] A cholesterol-lowering drug which reduces coronary heart disease (CHD) mortality will have a greater effect on all cause mortality in high risk patients with established cardiovascular disease than in young, asymptomatic patients with isolated hypercholesterolaemia.[19] This is because a consistent relative reduction in CHD mortality will translate into a greater relative reduction in all-cause mortality in high-risk patients in whom a greater proportion of all deaths will be from CHD. Trials conducted in high-risk patients will also tend to be smaller, because of the difficulty in recruiting such patients and because increased event rates mean that smaller sample sizes are required to detect a given effect.

Small trials are generally conducted before larger trials are established. In the intervening years standard (control) treatments may have improved, thus reducing the relative efficacy of the experimental treatment. Changes in standard treatments could also lead to a modification of the effect of the experimental treatment. Such a mechanism has been proposed as an explanation for the discrepant results obtained in clinical trials of the effect of magnesium infusion in myocardial infarction.[20] It has been argued that magnesium infusion may not work if administered after reperfusion has occurred. By the time the ISIS-4 trial[21] (which gave no evidence of a treatment effect) was performed, thrombolysis had become routine in the management of myocardial infarction. However this argument is not supported by subgroup analysis of the ISIS-4 trial, which shows no effect of magnesium even among patients not receiving thrombolysis.[22]

Some interventions may have been implemented less thoroughly in larger trials, thus explaining the more positive results in smaller trials. This is particularly likely in trials of complex interventions in chronic diseases, such as rehabilitation after stroke or multifaceted interventions in diabetes mellitus. For example, an asymmetrical funnel plot was found in a meta-analysis of trials examining the effect of inpatient comprehensive geriatric assessment programmes on mortality.[13,23] An experienced consultant geriatrician was more likely to be actively involved in the smaller trials and this may explain the larger treatment effects observed in these trials.[13,23]

Odds ratios are more extreme (further from 1) than the corresponding risk ratio if the event rate is high. Because of this, a funnel plot which shows no asymmetry when plotted using risk ratios could still be asymmetric when plotted using odds ratios. This would happen if the smaller trials were consistently conducted in high-risk patients, and the large trials in patients at lower risk, although differences in underlying risk would need to be substantial. Finally it is, of course, possible that an asymmetrical funnel plot arises merely by the play of chance. Mechanisms which can lead to funnel plot asymmetry are summarised in Table 11.1.

Table 11.1 Potential sources of asymmetry in funnel plots.

1. *Selection biases*
   Publication bias and other reporting biases (see Chapter 3)
   Biased inclusion criteria

2. *True heterogeneity*: size of effect differs according to study size
   Intensity of intervention
   Differences in underlying risk

3. *Data irregularities*
   Poor methodological design of small studies (see Chapter 5)
   Inadequate analysis
   Fraud

4. *Artefact*: heterogeneity due to poor choice of effect measure (see Chapter 16)

5. *Chance*

Funnel plot asymmetry thus raises the possibility of bias but it is not proof of bias. It is important to note, however, that asymmetry (unless produced by chance alone) will always lead us to question the interpretation of the overall estimate of effect when studies are combined in a meta-analysis.

Other graphical methods

Examining biological plausibility

In some circumstances, the possible presence of bias can be examined via markers of adherence to treatment, such as metabolites of a drug in patients' urine, or of the biological effects of treatment such as the achieved reduction in cholesterol in trials of cholesterol-lowering drugs, which, as discussed in Chapter 9, predicts the reduction in clinical heart disease[24,25] and mortality.[25]

If patients' adherence to an effective treatment were measured (for example as the percentage of patients actually taking the assigned medication), and varied across trials, then this should result in corresponding variation in treatment effects. Scatter plots of treatment effect (vertical axis) against adherence (horizontal axis) can be a useful means of examining this relationship. The scatter plot should be compatible with there being no treatment effect at 0 per cent adherence, and so a simple linear regression line should intercept the y-axis at zero treatment effect (Figure 11.2(a)). If a scatter plot indicates a treatment effect even when no patients adhere to treatment then bias is a possible explanation (Figure 11.2(b)). Similar considerations apply to scatter plots of treatment effect against change in biological markers believed to be closely associated with effects on clinical outcome. The advantage of such plots is that they provide an analysis that is independent of study size.

In a meta-analysis of trials examining the effect of reducing dietary sodium on blood pressure, Midgley et al.[26] plotted reduction in blood pressure (clinical outcome) against reduction in urinary sodium (biological marker) for each study and performed a linear regression analysis (Figure 11.3). The plot of difference in diastolic blood pressure (treatment effect) against change in urinary sodium (marker) suggests the possibility of bias. However, the assumption that the marker fully captures the treatment's effect on the clinical outcome may not always be appropriate: effects of the intervention not captured by the marker may account for the residual effect.[27,28] For example, dietary changes leading to a reduction in sodium intake may also lead to weight loss and hence to a reduction in blood pressure.

It should be noted that error in estimating the effect of the treatment on

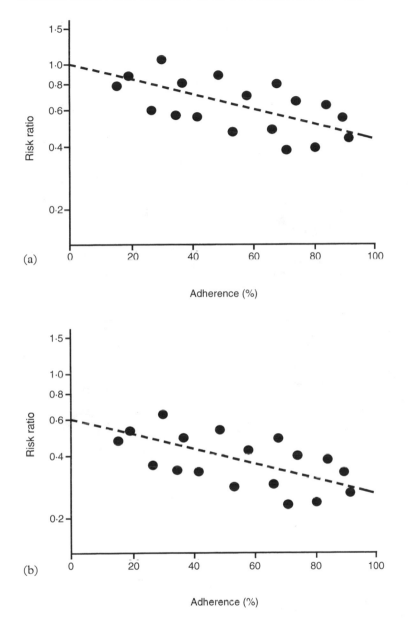

Figure 11.2 Linear regression plot of treatment effects from 18 hypothetical trials against the proportion of patients adhering to the experimental treatment. In the absence of bias the regression line intercepts the vertical axis at zero treatment effect (a). If the plot indicates a treatment effect even when no patients adhere to treatment (b) then bias is a likely explanation.

195

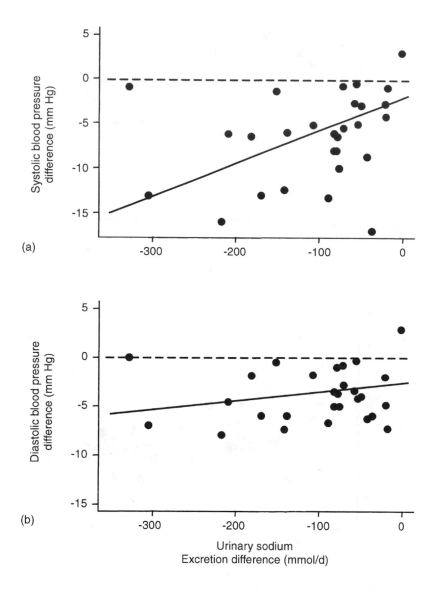

(a)

(b)

Figure 11.3 Regression lines, adjusted for the number of sodium excretion measurements, of the predicted change in blood pressure for a change in urinary sodium excretion from randomised controlled trials of dietary sodium reduction. Note that intercepts indicate a decline in blood pressure even if the diets in intervention and control groups were identical, which may indicate the presence of bias. Modified from Midgley et al.[26]

the marker could lead both to underestimation of its association with treatment, and to the estimated intercept being biased away from zero. In this situation a non-zero intercept could be misinterpreted as evidence of bias. We discuss how to use regression models to overcome this problem below.

Statistical methods to detect and correct for bias

Fail-safe N

Rosenthal[29] called publication bias the "file drawer problem", whose extreme version he described as "that the journals are filled with the 5% of the studies that show Type I errors, while the file drawers back at the lab are filled with the 95% of the studies that show nonsignificant (e.g. P >0·05) results." Rosenthal proposed that the potential for publication bias to have influenced the results of a meta-analysis can be assessed by calculating the 'fail-safe N': the number of 'negative' studies (studies in which the treatment effect was zero) that would be needed to increase the P value for the meta-analysis to above 0·05. Iyengar and Greenhouse[30] noted that the estimate of fail-safe N is highly dependent on the mean treatment effect that is assumed for the unpublished studies. The method also runs against the widely accepted principle that in medical research in general, and systematic reviews in particular, one should concentrate more on the size of the estimated treatment effect and the associated confidence intervals, and less on whether the strength of the evidence against the null hypothesis reaches a particular, arbitrary, threshold.

Selection models

A number of authors have proposed methods to detect publication bias, based on the assumption that an individual study's results (for example the P value) affect its probability of publication. These methods model the selection process that determines which results are published and which are not, and hence are known as "selection models". However, as explained earlier, publication bias is only one of the reasons that will lead to associations between treatment effects and study size (small study effects). Since an unexpected distribution of study results is likely to imply an association between treatment effect size and study size, selection models should perhaps be seen as examining small study effects in general rather than publication bias in particular.

Iyengar and Greenhouse[30] assumed that publication was certain if the study P value was <0·05 (i.e. "statistically significant"). If the study P value was >0·05 ("non-significant") then publication probability might be a constant (less than 1) or might decrease with decreasing treatment effect. Dear and Begg[31] and Hedges[32] extended this approach by assuming that different ranges of study P value (for example 0·01 to 0·05, 0·005 to 0·01 and so on) correspond to different publication probabilities. The observed distribution of P values is compared to the expected distribution assuming no publication bias, so that a reduced proportion of P values in (for example) the range 0·1 to 1 provides evidence of publication bias. These latter methods avoid strong assumptions about the nature of the selection mechanism but require a large number of studies so that a sufficient range of study P values is included.

Figure 11.4 (adapted from Dear and Begg[31]) shows the estimated publication probabilities from a meta-analysis of studies of the effect of open versus traditional education on creativity. Note that the apparent reduction in the probability of publication bias does not appear to coincide with the traditional cutoff of P = 0·05. These methods can be extended to estimate treatment effects, corrected for the estimated publication bias.[33] This approach was recently used in a meta-analysis of placebo-controlled trials of homoeopathy, an example discussed in more detail below.[34] A Bayesian approach in which the number and outcomes of unobserved studies are simulated has also been proposed as a means of correcting treatment estimates for publication bias.[35] For a meta-analysis examining

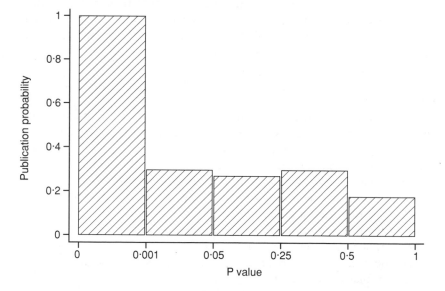

Figure 11.4 Publication probabilities according to study P value, estimated from a meta-analysis of 10 studies using a semi-parametric selection model (modified from Dear and Begg[31]).

the association between passive smoking and lung cancer, the relative risk was 1·22 (95% confidence interval 1·08 to 1·37) before and 1·14 (1·00 to 1·28) after allowing for publication bias.

The complexity of the statistical methods, and the large number of studies needed, probably explain why selection models have not been widely used in practice. In order to avoid these problems, Duval and Tweedie[36-38] have proposed "trim and fill": a method based on adding studies to a funnel plot so that it is symmetrical. The method works by omitting small studies until the funnel plot is symmetrical (trimming), using the trimmed funnel plot to estimate the true "centre" of the funnel, and then replacing the omitted studies and their missing "counterparts" around the centre (filling). As well as providing an estimate of the number of missing studies, an adjusted treatment effect is derived by performing a meta-analysis including the filled studies. Like other selection models, the method depends on the assumption that the association between treatment effect and trial size arises only because of publication bias, and not for the other reasons listed earlier in this chapter. Sutton et al.[39] used the trim and fill method to assess publication bias in 48 meta-analyses from the *Cochrane Database of Systematic Reviews*. They found that 56% of Cochrane meta-analyses had at least one missing study and may therefore be subject to publication bias, while in 10 the number of missing studies was statistically significant. However simulation studies have found that the trim-and-fill method detects "missing" studies in a substantial proportion of meta-analyses, even in the absence of bias.[40] There is thus a danger that uncritical application of the method could mean adding and adjusting for non-existent studies in response to funnel plot asymmetry arising from nothing more than random variation.

The 'correction' of effect estimates when publication bias is assumed to be present is problematic and a matter of ongoing debate. Results may be heavily dependent on the modelling assumptions used. Many factors may affect the probability of publication of a given set of results and it will be difficult if not impossible to model these adequately. It is therefore prudent to restrict the use of statistical methods which model selection mechanisms to the identification of bias rather than correcting for it.[41]

Copas[42] developed a model in which the probability that a study is included in a meta-analysis depends on its standard error. Because it is not possible to estimate all model parameters precisely, he advocates sensitivity analyses in which the value of the estimated treatment effect is computed under a range of assumptions about the severity of the selection bias. Rather than a single estimate treatment effect "corrected" for publication bias, the reader can see how the estimated effect (and confidence interval) varies as the assumed amount of selection bias increases. Application of the method to epidemiological studies of environmental tobacco smoke and lung cancer suggests that publication bias may explain some of the association observed in meta-analyses of these studies.[43]

Statistical analogues of the funnel plot

An alternative approach, which does not attempt to define the selection process leading to publication or non-publication, is to use statistical methods to examine associations between study size and estimated treatment effects, thus translating the graphical approach of the funnel plot into a statistical model. Begg and Mazumdar[14] proposed an adjusted rank correlation method to examine the association between the effect estimates and their variances (or, equivalently, their standard errors). Egger et al.[13] introduced a linear regression approach in which the standard normal deviate (θ/s) is regressed against precision ($1/s$). This latter approach can be shown to correspond to a weighted regression of effect size θ on standard error s ($\theta = b_0 + b_1 s$), where the weights are inversely proportional to the variance of the effect size. The greater the value of the regression coefficient b_1, the greater the evidence for small study effects. Because each of these approaches looks for an association between treatment effect (e.g. log odds ratio) and its standard error in each study, they can be seen as statistical analogues of funnel plots of treatment effect against standard error. Both methods have been implemented in the statistical package Stata (see Chapter 18).

Sterne et al.[44] used simulation studies to investigate the sensitivity of the two methods (i.e. their ability to detect small study effects). The sensitivity of the methods was low in meta-analyses based on less than 20 trials, or in the absence of substantial bias. The regression method appeared more sensitive than the rank correlation method.

It has been claimed that the methods may give evidence of bias when bias is not in fact present (false-positive test results).[45] Sterne et al. found that the methods gave false-positive rates which were too high when there were large treatment effects, or few events per trial, or all trials were of similar sizes.[44] They concluded that the weighted regression method is appropriate and reasonably powerful in the situations where meta-analysis generally makes sense – in estimating moderate treatment effects, based on a reasonable number of trials – but that it should only be used if there is clear variation in trial sizes, with one or more trials of medium or large size.

Meta-regression

An obvious extension to the methods described above is to consider a measure of study size (for example the standard error of the effect estimate) as one of a number of different possible explanations for between-study heterogeneity in a multivariable 'meta-regression' model (see also Chapters 8 to 10 for a discussion of the use of regression models in meta-analysis).

For example, the effects of study size, adequacy of randomisation and type of blinding might be examined simultaneously. Thompson and Sharp[46] recently reviewed different methods for meta-regression. These have been implemented in Stata (see Chapter 18).

Three notes of caution are necessary. Users of standard regression models know that it is unwise to include large numbers of covariates, particularly if the sample size is small. In meta-regression the number of data points corresponds to the number of studies, which is usually less than 50 and often less than 10.[44] Thus tests for association between treatment effect and large numbers of study characteristics may lead to "overfitting" and spurious claims of association. Secondly, all associations observed in such analyses are observational, and may therefore be confounded by other unknown or unmeasured factors. Thirdly, regression analyses using averages of patient characteristics from each trial (such as the mean age of all the patients) can give a misleading impression of the relation for individual patients. As discussed in Chapter 9, there is potential for the so-called ecological fallacy,[47] whereby the relation with treatment benefit may be different across trials as compared to within trials.

Meta-regression could be used to examine associations between clinical outcomes and markers of adherence to treatment or of the biological effects of treatment, weighting appropriately for study size. As discussed above, the intercept (coefficient of the constant term) should be zero if there is no biological effect so a non-zero intercept may be evidence of bias, or of a treatment effect which is not mediated via the marker. Unless the error in estimating the effect of treatment on the marker is small, this error must be incorporated in models of the association between the treatment effect and the change in the surrogate marker. Daniels and Hughes[48] discuss this issue and propose a Bayesian estimation procedure. This method has been applied in a study of CD4 cell count as a surrogate endpoint in HIV clinical trials.[49]

The case study illustrates the use of some of the methods described in this chapter, using the example of a widely cited meta-analysis of placebo-controlled trials of homoeopathy.

Case study: is the effect of homoeopathy due to the placebo effect?

The placebo effect is a popular explanation for the apparent efficacy of homoeopathic remedies.[50,51,52] Linde et al. addressed this question in a fascinating systematic review and meta-analysis of placebo-controlled trials of homoeopathy, in which all trials, independent of clinical condition and outcomes, were included.[34] The authors performed an extensive literature search, without language restrictions, covering a wide range of bibliographic databases and complementary medicine registries. Linde et al. included 89 published and unpublished reports of randomised placebo-controlled trials. Quality assessment covered the dimensions of internal validity that are

known to be associated with treatment effects[9,10] (see Chapter 5): concealment of the allocation of homoeopathic remedies or placebo, blinding of
outcome assessment and handling of withdrawals and dropouts.

The funnel plot of the 89 homoeopathy trials is clearly asymmetrical
(Figure 11.5(a)) and both the rank correlation and the weighted regression

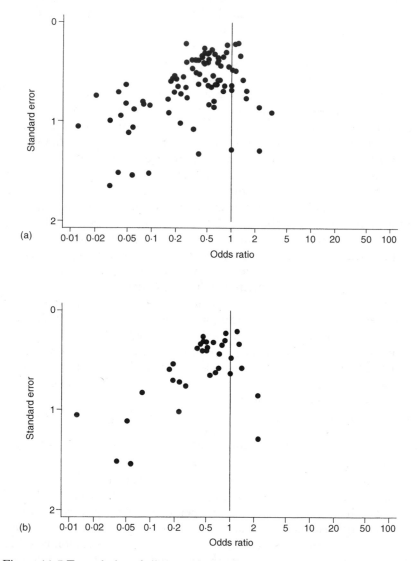

Figure 11.5 Funnel plot of all 89 randomised controlled trials comparing homoeopathic medicine with placebo identified by Linde *et al.*[34] (a) and 34 trials of high
methodological quality (b).

test indicated clear asymmetry (P<0·0001). This asymmetry remained (Figure 11.5(b)) when the plot was restricted to 34 double-blind trials with adequate concealment of treatment allocation (P = 0·014 with rank correlation and <0·001 with regression method). The authors used a selection model (assuming that the likelihood that a study was reported depended on the one-tailed P value)[32,33] to correct for publication bias, and found that the odds ratio was increased from 0·41 (95% confidence interval 0·34 to 0·49) to 0·56 (0·32 to 0·97) after correcting for bias. Similar results are obtained with the fill and trim method (Figure 11.6). To make the funnel plot symmetric, 16 studies are added. The adjusted odds ratio (including the filled studies) is 0·52 (0·43 to 0·63).

Linde *et al.* therefore concluded that the clinical effects of homoeopathy are unlikely to be due to placebo.[34] However the method they used does not allow simultaneously for other sources of bias, and thus assumes that publication bias is the sole cause of funnel plot asymmetry. Table 11.2 shows the results from meta-regression analyses of associations between trial characteristics and the estimated effect of homoeopathy. Results are presented as ratios of odds ratios (ORs) comparing the results from trials with to trials without the characteristic. Thus ratios below 1 correspond to a smaller treatment odds ratio for trials with the characteristic, and hence a larger apparent benefit of homoeopathic treatment. For example, in univariable analysis the odds ratio was reduced by factor 0·24 (ratio of ORs

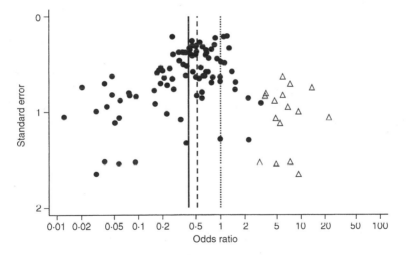

Figure 11.6 Application of the "trim and fill" method to the funnel plot of 89 trials comparing homoeopathic medicine with placebo. The solid circles represent the 89 trials, while the open triangles are the "filled" studies. The solid line is the original (random-effects) estimate of the pooled odds ratio, the dashed line is the adjusted estimate (including the filled studies) and the dotted line is the null value (1).

Table 11.2 Meta-regression analysis of 89 homoeopathy trials.

Study characteristic	Univariable analysis		Controlling for all variables	
	Ratio of odds ratios* (95% CI)	P	Ratio of odds ratios* (95% CI)	P
Unit increase in standard error of log OR	0·18 (0·10 to 0·34)	<0·001	0·20 (0·11 to 0·37)	<0·001
Language (Non-English vs. English)	0·73 (0·51 to 1·06)	0·097	0·73 (0·55 to 0·98)	0·038
Study quality				
Allocation concealment (not adequate vs. adequate)	0·70 (0·49 to 1·01)	0·054	0·98 (0·73 to 1·30)	0·87
Blinding (not double-blind vs. double-blind)	0·24 (0·12 to 0·46)	<0·001	0·35 (0·20 to 0·60)	<0·001
Handling of withdrawals (not adequate vs. adequate)	1·32 (0·87 to 1·99)	0·19	1·10 (0·80 to 1·51)	0·56
Publication type (not MEDLINE-indexed vs. MEDLINE-indexed)	0·61 (0·42 to 0·90)	0·013	0·91 (0·67 to 1·25)	0·57

*Odds ratio with characteristic divided by odds ratio without characteristic. Ratios below 1 correspond to a smaller treatment odds ratio for trials with the characteristic, and hence a larger apparent benefit of homoeopathic treatment.

0·24, 95% confidence interval 0·12 to 0·46) if outcome assessment was not blinded. Inadequate concealment of allocation, and publication in a non-MEDLINE-indexed journal were also associated with greater estimated benefits. Univariable analyses provided strong evidence of small study effects: trials with larger standard errors had substantially greater estimated benefits of homoeopathic treatment. When the effect of each variable was controlled for all others there remained strong associations with standard error (ratio of ORs 0·20, 95% confidence interval 0·11 to 0·37), and inadequate blinding of outcome assessment (ratio of ORs 0·35, 95% confidence interval 0·20 to 0·60).

Meta-regression analysis and funnel plots indicate that the treatment effects seen are strongly associated with both methodological quality and study size. The two largest (i.e. with the smallest standard error) trials of homoeopathy which were double blind and had adequate concealment of randomisation (on 300 and 1270 patients) show no effect. This is consistent with the intercept from the regression of effect size on standard error, which can be interpreted as the estimated effect in large trials (OR = 1·02, 95% confidence interval 0·71 to 1·46). The evidence is thus compatible with the hypothesis that the clinical effects of homoeopathy are completely due to placebo. This example illustrates that publication bias is only one of the reasons why the results from small studies may be misleading. However, we emphasise that our results cannot *prove* that the apparent benefits of homoeopathy are due to bias.

Conclusions

Prevention is better than cure. In conducting a systematic review and meta-analysis, investigators should make strenuous efforts to ensure that they find all published studies, and to search for unpublished work, for example in trial registries or conference abstracts (see Chapter 4). The quality of component studies should also be carefully assessed (Chapter 5). Summary recommendations on examining for and dealing with bias in meta-analysis are shown in Box 11.2. Selection models for the process of publication bias are likely to be of most use in sensitivity analyses in which the robustness of a meta-analysis to possible publication bias is assessed. Funnel plots should be used in most meta-analyses, to provide a visual assessment of whether treatment effect estimates are associated with study

Box 11.1 Summary recommendations on investigating and dealing with publication and other biases in a meta-analysis

Examining for bias

- Check for funnel plot asymmetry using graphical and statistical methods.
- Consider meta-regression to look for associations between key measures of trial quality and treatment effect size.
- Consider meta-regression to examine other possible explanations for heterogeneity.
- If available, examine associations between treatment effect size and changes in biological markers or patients' adherence to treatment.

Dealing with bias

- If there is evidence of bias, report this with the same prominence as any combined estimate of treatment effect.
- Consider sensitivity analyses to establish whether the estimated treatment effect is robust to reasonable assumptions about the effect of bias.
- Consider excluding studies of lower quality.
- If sensitivity analyses show that a review's conclusions could be seriously affected by bias, then consider recommending that the evidence to date be disregarded.

size. Statistical methods which examine the evidence for funnel plot asymmetry are now available, and meta-regression methods may be used to examine competing explanations for heterogeneity in treatment effects between studies. The power of all of these methods is limited, however, particularly for meta-analyses based on a small number of small studies, and the results from such meta-analyses should therefore always be treated with caution.

Statistically combining data from new trials with a body of flawed evidence will not remove bias. However there is currently no consensus on how to guide clinical practice or future research when a systematic review suggests that the evidence to date is unreliable for one or more of the reasons discussed in this chapter. If there is clear evidence of bias, and if sensitivity analyses show that this could seriously affect a review's conclusions, then reviewers should not shrink from recommending that some or all of the evidence to date be disregarded. Future systematic reviews could then be based on new, high-quality evidence. Important improvements such as better conduct and reporting of trials, prospective registration, easier access to data from published and unpublished studies and comprehensive literature searching are being made to the process of assessing the effect of medical interventions. It is to be hoped that these will mean that bias will be a diminishing problem in future systematic reviews and meta-analyses.

Acknowledgements

We are grateful to Klaus Linde and Julian Midgley who provided unpublished data from their meta-analyses.

1 Easterbrook PJ, Berlin JA, Gopalan R, Matthews DR. Publication bias in clinical research. *Lancet* 1991;**337**:867–72.
2 Dickersin K, Min YI, Meinert CL. Factors influencing publication of research results: follow-up of applications submitted to two institutional review boards. *JAMA* 1992;**263**:374–8.
3 Stern JM, Simes RJ. Publication bias: evidence of delayed publication in a cohort study of clinical research projects. *BMJ* 1997;**315**:640–5.
4 Egger M, Zellweger-Zähner T, Schneider M, Junker C, Lengeler C, Antes G. Language bias in randomised controlled trials published in English and German. *Lancet* 1997;**350**:326–9.
5 Gøtzsche PC. Reference bias in reports of drug trials. *BMJ* 1987;**295**:654–6.
6 Ravnskov U. Cholesterol lowering trials in coronary heart disease: frequency of citation and outcome. *BMJ* 1992;**305**:15–19.
7 Tramèr MR, Reynolds DJ, Moore RA, McQuay HJ. Impact of covert duplicate publication on meta-analysis: a case study. *BMJ* 1997;**315**:635–40.
8 Gøtzsche PC. Multiple publication of reports of drug trials. *Eur J Clin Pharmacol* 1989;**36**:429–32.
9 Schulz KF, Chalmers I, Hayes RJ, Altman DG. Empirical evidence of bias. Dimensions of methodological quality associated with estimates of treatment effects in controlled trials. *JAMA* 1995;**273**:408–12.

10 Moher D, Pham B, Jones A, et al. Does quality of reports of randomised trials affect estimates of intervention efficacy reported in meta-analyses? *Lancet* 1998;**352**:609–13.

11 Light RJ, Pillemer DB. *Summing up: the science of reviewing research.* Cambridge: Harvard University Press, 1984.

12 Galbraith RF. A note on graphical presentation of estimated odds ratios from several clinical trials. *Stat Med* 1988;**7**:889–94.

13 Egger M, Davey Smith G, Schneider M, Minder C. Bias in meta-analysis detected by a simple, graphical test. *BMJ* 1997;**315**:629–34.

14 Begg CB, Mazumdar M. Operating characteristics of a rank correlation test for publication bias. *Biometrics* 1994;**50**:1088–101.

15 Begg CB, Berlin JA. Publication bias: a problem in interpreting medical data. *J R Statist Soc A* 1988;**151**:419–63.

16 Villar J, Piaggio G, Carroli G, Donner A. Factors affecting the comparability of meta-analyses and the largest trials results in perinatology. *J Clin Epidemiol* 1997;**50**:997–1002.

17 Davey Smith G, Egger M. Who benefits from medical interventions? Treating low risk patients can be a high risk strategy. *BMJ* 1994;**308**:72–4.

18 Glasziou PP, Irwig LM. An evidence based approach to individualising treatment. *BMJ* 1995;**311**:1356–9.

19 Davey Smith G, Song F, Sheldon TA. Cholesterol lowering and mortality: the importance of considering initial level of risk. *BMJ* 1993;**306**:1367–73.

20 Baxter GF, Sumeray MS, Walker JM. Infarct size and magnesium: insights into LIMIT-2 and ISIS-4 from experimental studies. *Lancet* 1996;**348**:1424–6.

21 ISIS-4 (Fourth International Study of Infact Survival) Collaborative Group. ISIS-4: a randomised factorial trial assessing early oral captopril, oral mononitrate, and intravenous magnesium sulphate in 58 050 patients with suspected acute myocardial infarction. *Lancet* 1995;**345**:669–85.

22 Collins R, Peto R. Magnesium in acute myocardial infarction. *Lancet* 1997;**349**:282

23 Stuck AE, Siu AL, Wieland GD, Adams J, Rubenstein LZ. Comprehensive geriatric assessment: a meta-analysis of controlled trials. *Lancet* 1993;**342**:1032–6.

24 Thompson SG. Controversies in meta-analysis: the case of the trials of serum cholesterol reduction. *Stat Methods Med Res* 1993;**2**:173–92.

25 Holme I. Cholesterol reduction and its impact on coronary artery disease and total mortality. *Am J Cardiol* 1995;**76**:10C–17C.

26 Midgley JP, Matthew AG, Greenwood CMT, Logan AG. Effect of reduced dietary sodium on blood pressure. A meta-analysis of randomized controlled trials. *JAMA* 1996;**275**:1590–7.

27 Prentice RL. Surrogate endpoints in clinical trials: definition and operational criteria. *Stat Med* 1989; **8**:431–40.

28 Fleming TR, Demets DL. Surrogate end points in clinical trials: are we being misled? *Ann Intern Med* 1996;**125**:605–13.

29 Rosenthal R. The "file drawer" problem and tolerance for null results. *Psychol Bull* 1979;**86**:638–41.

30 Iyengar S, Greenhouse JB. Selection problems and the file drawer problem. *Stat Sci* 1988;109–35.

31 Dear KBG, Begg CB. An approach to assessing publication bias prior to performing a meta-analysis. *Stat Sci* 1992;**7**:237–45.

32 Hedges LV. Modeling publication selection effects in meta-analysis. *Stat Sci* 1992;**7**:246–55.

33 Vevea JL, Hedges LV. A general linear model for estimating effect size in the presence of publication bias. *Psychometrika* 1995;**60**:419–35.

34 Linde K, Clausius N, Ramirez G, et al. Are the clinical effects of homeopathy placebo effects? A meta-analysis of placebo-controlled trials. *Lancet* 1997;**350**:834–43.

35 Givens GH, Smith DD, Tweedie RL. Publication bias in meta-analysis: a Bayesian data-augmentation approach to account for issues exemplified in the passive smoking debate. *Stat Sci* 1997;**12**:221–50.

36 Taylor SJ, Tweedie RL. Practical estimates of the effect of publication bias in meta-analysis. *Austral Epidemiol* 1998;**5**:14–17.

207

37 Duval SJ, Tweedie RL. Trim and fill: a simple funnel plot based method of testing and adjusting for publication bias in meta-analysis. *Biometrics* 2000;**56**:455–63.
38 Duval SJ, Tweedie RL. A non-parametric "trim and fill" method of assessing publication bias in meta-analysis. *J Am Stat Assoc* 2000;**95**:89–98.
39 Sutton AJ, Duval SJ, Tweedie RL, *et al*. Empirical assessment of effect of publication bias on meta-analyses. *BMJ* 2000;**320**:1574–7.
40 Sterne JAC, Egger M. High false positive rate for trim and fill method (electronic letter). http://www.bmj.com/cgi/eletters/320/7249/1574
41 Begg CB. Publication bias in meta-analysis. *Stat Sci* 1997;**12**:241–4.
42 Copas J. What works?: selectivity models and meta-analysis. *J R Statist Soc A* 1999;**162**:95–109.
43 Copas JB, Shi JQ. Reanalysis of epidemiological evidence on lung cancer and passive smoking. *BMJ* 2000;**320**:417–18.
44 Sterne JAC, Gavaghan D, Egger M. Publication and related bias in meta-analysis: power of statistical tests and prevalence in the literature. *J Clin Epidemiol* 2000;**53**:1119–29.
45 Irwig L, Macaskill P, Berry G, Glasziou P. Graphical test is itself biased. *BMJ* 1998;**316**:470–1.
46 Thompson SG, Sharp SJ. Explaining heterogeneity in meta-analysis: a comparison of methods. *Stat Med* 1999;**18**:2693–708.
47 Morgenstern H. Uses of ecologic analysis in epidemiologic research. *Am J Public Health* 1982;**72**:1336–44.
48 Daniels MJ, Hughes MD. Meta-analysis for the evaluation of potential surrogate markers. *Stat Med* 1997;**16**:1965–82.
49 Hughes MD, Daniels MJ, Fischl MA, Kim S, Schooley RT. CD4 cell count as a surrogate endpoint in HIV clinical trials: a meta-analysis of studies of the AIDS Clinical Trials Group. *AIDS* 1998;**12**:1823–32.
50 Maddox J, Randi J, Stewart WW. "High-dilution" experiments a delusion. *Nature* 1988;**334**:287–91.
51 Gøtzsche PC. Trials of homeopathy. *Lancet* 1993;**341**:1533.
52 Vandenbroucke JP. Homoeopathy trials: going nowhere. *Lancet* 1997;**350**:824.

Part III: Systematic reviews of observational studies

12 Systematic reviews of observational studies

MATTHIAS EGGER, GEORGE DAVEY SMITH,
MARTIN SCHNEIDER

Summary points

- Systematic reviews and meta-analyses of observational studies are as common as reviews of randomised controlled trials.
- In contrast to high-quality randomised trials, confounding and selection bias often distort the findings of observational studies. Bigger is not necessarily better: smaller studies can devote more attention to characterising confounding factors than larger studies.
- There is a danger that meta-analyses of observational data produce very precise but spurious results. The statistical combination of data should therefore not be a prominent component of systematic reviews of observational studies.
- More is gained by carefully examining possible sources of heterogeneity between the results from observational studies. Individual participant data may often be required for this purpose.

The previous chapters focused on the potentials, principles and pitfalls of systematic reviews and meta-analysis of randomised controlled trials. Systematic reviews of observational, non-randomised data are, however, also common. An early example of an observational meta-analysis can be found in the 1964 Surgeon General's report on Smoking and Health which calculated summary estimates of cancer risk for smokers from seven cohort studies.[1] In a MEDLINE search using keyword "meta-analysis" we identified 755 articles (excluding letters, editorials or commentaries) that were published in 1999. We randomly selected 100 of these articles and examined them further. Fifty-nine reported on actual meta-analyses, and 41 were methodological papers, traditional reviews or reports of other types of studies (Table 12.1). Among the meta-analyses, about 40% were based

211

Table 12.1 Characteristics of 100 articles sampled at random from articles published in 1999 and identified in MEDLINE using "meta-analysis" as keyword.

Type of article	Articles (n)
Meta-analysis of:	
Controlled trials	34
Observational studies*	25
Methodological article	15
Traditional review	15
Other	11

* Including eight meta-analyses of observational studies of aetiological associations, six of therapeutic or preventive interventions and four of prognostic factors.

on observational studies, mainly cohort and case–control studies of aetiological associations or medical interventions. In this chapter we will examine systematic reviews and meta-analyses of such studies, with an emphasis on observational studies from aetiological epidemiology and research into the effectiveness of medical interventions. Systematic reviews of prognostic studies and evaluations of diagnostic studies will be discussed in Chapters 13 and 14.

Why do we need systematic reviews of observational studies?

The randomised controlled trial is the principal research design in the evaluation of medical interventions. Aetiological hypotheses, however, cannot generally be tested in randomised experiments. For example, does breathing other people's tobacco smoke promote the development of lung cancer, drinking coffee cause coronary heart disease, and eating a diet rich in unsaturated fat induce breast cancer? Studies of such 'menaces of daily life'[2] employ observational designs, or examine the presumed biological mechanisms in the laboratory. In these situations the risks involved are generally small, but once a large proportion of the population is exposed, the potential public health impact of these associations, if they are causal, can be striking.

Analyses of observational data also have a role in medical effectiveness research.[3] The evidence that is available from clinical trials will rarely answer all the important questions. Most trials are conducted to establish efficacy and safety of a single agent in a specific clinical situation. Due to the limited size of such trials,[4–6] less common adverse effects of drugs may only be detected in case–control studies, or in analyses of databases from postmarketing surveillance schemes. Also, because follow-up is generally limited, adverse effects occurring later will not be identified. If established

212

interventions are associated with adverse effects many years after their introduction, there will be ethical, political and legal obstacles to the conduct of a new trial. Recent examples for such situations include the controversy surrounding intramuscular administration of vitamin K to newborns and the risk of childhood cancer[7] and oral contraceptive use and breast cancer.[8]

The patients that are enrolled in randomised trials often differ from the average patient seen in clinical practice. Women, the elderly and minority ethnic groups are often excluded from randomised trials.[9,10] Similarly, the university hospitals typically participating in clinical trials differ from the settings where most patients are treated. In the absence of randomised trial evidence from these settings and patient groups, the results from observational database analyses may appear more relevant and more readily applicable to clinical practice.[11] Finally, both patient and therapist preferences may preclude a randomised controlled experiment. In the field of complementary medicine, for example, consider a therapy which involves ingesting your own urine.[12] Because of strong preferences determined by prior belief and taste, it would probably be impossible to recruit sufficient patients into a controlled trial.

As discussed in Chapter 1 it is always appropriate and desirable to review a body of data systematically, independent of the design and type of studies reviewed. Statistically combining results from separate studies in meta-analysis may, however, sometimes be inappropriate. Meta-analysis may be particularly attractive to reviewers in aetiological epidemiology and observational effectiveness research, promising a precise and definite answer when the magnitude of the underlying risks are small, or when the results from individual studies disagree. The possibility of producing a spuriously precise, but misleading overall estimate of an association or treatment effect is a problem in meta-analysis in general but this danger is particularly great when combining observational studies.

Confounding and bias

Meta-analysis of randomised trials is based on the assumption that each trial provides an unbiased estimate of the effect of an experimental treatment, with the variability of the results between the studies being attributed to random variation. The overall effect calculated from a group of sensibly combined and representative randomised trials will provide an essentially unbiased estimate of the treatment effect, with an increase in the precision of this estimate. A fundamentally different situation arises in the case of observational studies. Such studies yield estimates of association that may deviate from true underlying relationships beyond the play of chance. This may be due to the effects of confounding factors, biases, or both. Those exposed to the factor under investigation may differ in a number of other aspects that are relevant to the risk of developing the disease in question. Consider, for example, smoking as a risk factor for suicide.

Does smoking cause suicide?

A large number of cohort studies have shown a positive association between smoking and suicide, with a dose–response relationship being evident between the amount smoked and the probability of committing suicide.[13-18] Figure 12.1 illustrates this for four prospective studies of middle-aged men, including the massive cohort of men screened for the Multiple Risk Factor Intervention Trial (MRFIT).[19] Based on over 390 000 men and almost five million years of follow-up, a meta-analysis of these cohorts produces very precise and statistically significant estimates of the increase in suicide risk that is associated with smoking different daily amounts of cigarettes: relative rate for 1–14 cigarettes 1·43 (95% confidence interval 1·06 to 1·93), for 15–24 cigarettes 1·88 (1·53 to 2·32), 25 or more cigarettes 2·18 (1·82 to 2·61).

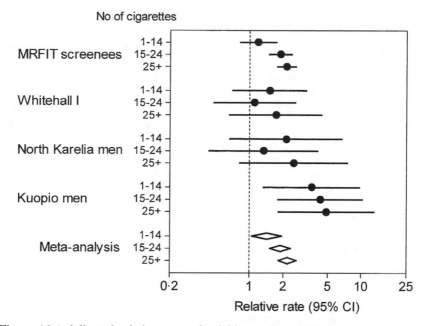

Figure 12.1 Adjusted relative rates of suicide among middle-aged male smokers compared to non-smokers. Results from four cohort studies adjusted for age, and income, ethnicity, cardiovascular disease, diabetes (Multiple Risk Factor Intervention Trial; MRFIT), employment grade (Whitehall I), alcohol use, serum cholesterol, systolic blood pressure, education (North Karelia and Kuopio). Meta-analysis by fixed effects model. CI: confidence interval.

Based on established criteria,[20] many would consider the association to be causal – if only it were more plausible. It is improbable that smoking is causally related to suicide.[13] Rather, it is the social and mental states predisposing to suicide that are also associated with the habit of smoking. Factors that are related to both the exposure and the disease under study, confounding factors, may thus distort results. If the factor is known and has been measured, the usual approach is to adjust for its influence in the analysis. For example, any study assessing the influence of coffee consumption on the risk of myocardial infarction should make statistical adjustments for smoking, since smoking is generally associated with drinking larger amounts of coffee and smoking is a cause of coronary heart disease.[21] However, even if adjustments for confounding factors have been made in the analysis, *residual confounding* remains a potentially serious problem in observational research. Residual confounding arises whenever a confounding factor cannot be measured with sufficient precision – a situation which often occurs in epidemiological studies.[22,23] Confounding is the most important threat to the validity of results from cohort studies whereas many more difficulties, in particular selection biases, arise in case-control studies.[24]

Plausible but spurious findings

Implausible results, such as in the case of smoking and suicide, rarely protect us from reaching misleading conclusions. It is generally easy to produce plausible explanations for the findings from observational research. For example, one group of researchers which investigated co-factors in heterosexual HIV transmission in a cohort study of sex workers found a strong association between the use of oral contraceptives and HIV infection which was independent of other factors.[25] The authors hypothesised that, among other mechanisms, the risk of transmission could be increased with oral contraceptives due to "effects on the genital mucosa, such as increasing the area of ectopy and the potential for mucosal disruption during intercourse." In a cross-sectional study another group produced diametrically opposed findings, indicating that the use of oral contraceptives actually protects against the virus.[26] This was considered to be equally plausible, "since progesterone-containing oral contraceptives thicken cervical mucus, which might be expected to hamper the entry of HIV into the uterine cavity." It is likely that confounding and bias had a role in producing these contradictory findings. Epidemiological studies produce a large number of seemingly plausible associations. Some of these findings will be spurious but all are eagerly reported in the media. Figure 12.2 shows how one member of the public, the cartoonist Jim Borgman, reflects on this situation.

215

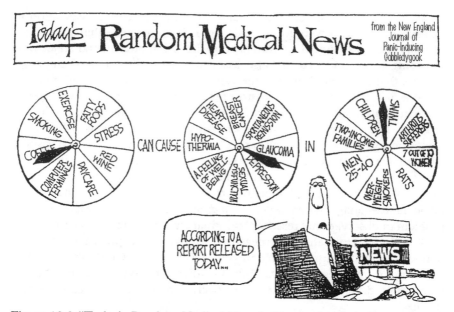

Figure 12.2 "Today's Random Medical News": Observational studies produce a large number of seemingly plausible associations. Some of these findings will be spurious due to bias and confounding but they are nevertheless eagerly reported in the media. Cartoon by Jim Borgman (copyright: Hearst Corporation. Reprinted with special permission of King Features Syndicate).

The fallacy of bigger being better

In meta-analysis the weight given to each study generally reflects the statistical power of the study: the larger the study, the greater the weight (see Chapters 2 and 15). In the case of well-conducted randomised controlled trials, when the main problem is lack of precision in effect estimates, giving the greatest weight to studies that provide the most information is appropriate. In the field of observational meta-analysis, however, the main problem is not lack of precision but that some studies produce findings that are seriously biased or confounded. The statistical power of a study is not the best indicator of which study is likely to have the least biased or confounded results. Indeed, the opposite may be the case. Other things being equal, smaller studies can devote more attention to characterising both the exposure of interest and confounding factors than larger studies. Collecting more detailed data on a smaller number of participants is, in many cases, a better strategy for obtaining an accurate result from a study than is collecting cruder data on a larger number of participants.[27] The most informative studies are those which give the answer nearest to the correct one; in observational studies this is unlikely to be the case for large, but poorly conducted studies.

For example, in a meta-analysis of observational studies of the association of *Helicobacter pylori* infection and coronary heart disease a large case-control study of 1122 survivors of acute myocardial infarction and 1122 controls with no history of coronary heart disease would receive much weight.[28] Cases were participants in the UK arm of the third International Study of Infarct Survival (ISIS-3),[29] a trial of thrombolytic therapy in acute myocardial infarction. Controls were selected from the siblings, children and spouses of cases. The final response rate in controls was less than 20% and around 60% for the cases, which leaves ample room for bias. It is well known that people from less favourable social circumstances are more likely to be non-responders in such studies.[30,31] This would lead to a greater proportion of socio-economically disadvantaged people among the cases. Since *H. pylori* infection is strongly influenced by adverse social circumstances in childhood[32,33] the more affluent control group would be expected to have lower infection rates than the case group, even if *H. pylori* is not causally associated with coronary heart disease. Such selection bias would be expected to produce a strong but spurious association between *H. pylori* infection and coronary heart disease risk. Indeed, the study yielded an odds ratio of 2·28 which was statistically significantly different from no effect (P < 0·0001) and adjustment for a limited array of confounders left a residual odds ratio of 1·75 (P < 0·0001). Several well-conducted prospective studies have been carried out in which response rates were high, *H. pylori* infection status was determined before onset of coronary heart disease and there was greater ability to control for confounding.[34,35] In these studies there is no good evidence that *H. pylori* infection contributes to coronary risk. It is thus likely that despite its large size the result of this case–control study was strongly confounded and biased.

Rare insight? The protective effect of beta-carotene that wasn't

Observational studies have consistently shown that people eating more fruits and vegetables, which are rich in beta-carotene, and people having higher serum beta-carotene concentrations have lower rates of cardiovascular disease and cancer.[36] Beta-carotene has antioxidant properties and could thus plausibly be expected to prevent carcinogenesis and atherogenesis by reducing oxidative damage to DNA and lipoproteins. Unlike many other associations found in observational studies, this hypothesis could be, and was, tested in experimental studies. The findings of four large trials have recently been published.[37–40] The results were disappointing and for the two trials conducted in men at high risk, smokers and workers exposed to asbestos, even disturbing.[37,38]

We performed a meta-analysis of the findings for cardiovascular

217

mortality, comparing the results from the six observational studies recently reviewed by Jha *et al.*[36] with those from the four randomised trials. In observational studies we compared groups with high and low beta-carotene intake or serum beta-carotene level, and in trials participants randomised to beta-carotene supplements were compared with participants randomised to placebo. Using a fixed effects model, meta-analysis of the cohort studies shows a significantly lower risk of cardiovascular death (relative risk reduction 31%, 95% confidence interval 41 to 20%, $P < 0.0001$) (Figure 12.3). The results from the randomised trials, however, indicate a moderate adverse effect of beta-carotene supplementation (relative increase in the risk of cardiovascular death 12%, 4 to 22%, $P = 0.005$). Discrepant results between epidemiological studies and trials of the effects of beta-carotene have also been observed for cancer,[41,42] age-related maculopathy[43-45] and cataract.[46,47] Similar discrepancies are evident for other antioxidants, including vitamin E and vitamin C.[48-50]

The situation with antioxidants is not unique. Meta-analyses of the observational evidence of the association between oestrogen-replacement therapy and coronary heart disease concluded that postmenopausal

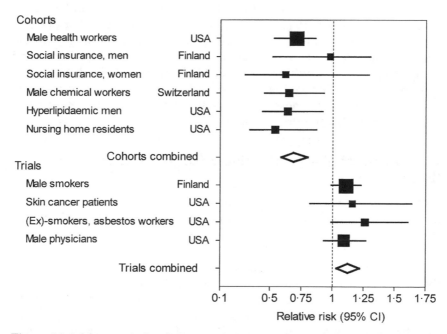

Figure 12.3 Meta-analysis of the association between beta-carotene intake and cardiovascular mortality: Results from observational studies[36] indicate considerable benefit whereas the findings from randomised controlled trials show an increase in the risk of death.[37-40] CI: confidence interval.

218

oestrogen use reduced the risk of coronary heart disease by 35 to 45% and that this effect was unlikely to be explained by confounding or bias.[51,52] One review argued that the protective effect of oestrogen was even stronger in women with established coronary heart disease than in healthy women.[52] Women who use hormone-replacement therapy may, however, be a selected group of relatively healthy women who comply with treatment. Such selection bias ("compliance bias",[53] "prevention bias"[54]) could explain the apparent beneficial effect that was observed in observational studies. This is supported by the observation that women using hormone-replacement therapy are also less likely to develop diseases that are unlikely to be influenced by hormone-replacement therapy.[55] More recently, the large Heart and Estrogen/progestin Replacement Study (HERS) in women with established coronary heart disease[56] and a meta-analysis of smaller trials in postmenopausal women[57] showed that hormone-replacement therapy does not reduce the risk of coronary events.

There are, of course, examples of observational studies that produced results similar to those from randomised controlled trials.[58 60] However, the fact that in observational studies the intervention was deliberately chosen and not randomly allocated means that selection bias and confounding will often distort results.[61] Bias and confounding is particularly likely for preventive interventions, which are more likely to be chosen and adhered to by people with healthier lifestyles, and for treatments that physicians tend to selectively prescribe to some groups of patients,[62] for example the very sick or relatively healthy, but the direction and degree of bias is difficult to predict in individual cases.[63] This means that in meta-analyses of observational studies, the analyst may often unknowingly and naïvely be producing tight confidence intervals around biased results.

Exploring sources of heterogeneity

Some observers suggest that meta-analysis of observational studies should be abandoned altogether.[64] We disagree, but think that the statistical combination of studies should not, in general, be a prominent component of reviews of observational studies. The thorough consideration of possible sources of heterogeneity between observational study results will provide more insights than the mechanistic calculation of an overall measure of effect, which may often be biased. We re-analysed a number of examples from the literature to illustrate this point. Consider diet and breast cancer: the hypothesis from ecological analyses[65] that higher intake of saturated fat could increase the risk of breast cancer generated much observational research, often with contradictory results. A comprehensive meta-analysis[66] showed an association for case–control but not for cohort studies (odds ratio 1·36 for case–control studies versus rate ratio 0·95 for cohort studies comparing highest with lowest categories of saturated fat intake, P = 0·0002 for difference) (Figure 12.4). This discrepancy was also shown in two separate large collaborative pooled analyses of cohort and case–control studies.[67,68] The most likely explanation for this situation is that biases in the recall of dietary items, and in the selection of study participants, have produced a spurious association in the case–control comparisons.[68]

That differential recall of past exposures may introduce bias is also evident from a meta-analysis of case–control studies of intermittent sunlight exposure and melanoma[69] (Figure 12.4). When combining studies in which some degree of blinding to the study hypothesis was achieved, only a small and statistically non-significant effect (odds ratio 1·17, 95% confidence interval 0·98 to 1·39) was evident. Conversely, in studies without blinding, the effect was considerably greater and statistically significant (odds ratio 1·84, 1·52 to 2·25). The difference between these two estimates is unlikely to be a product of chance (P = 0·0004 in our calculation).

The importance of the methods used for exposure assessment is further illustrated by a meta-analysis of cross-sectional data of dietary calcium intake and blood pressure from 23 different studies.[70] As shown in Figure 12.5(a), the regression slope describing the change in systolic blood pressure (in mmHg) per 100 mg of calcium intake was reported to be strongly influenced by the approach employed for assessment of the amount of calcium consumed. The association was small with diet histories (slope –0·01) and 24-hour recall (slope –0·06) but large and statistically highly significant when food frequency questionnaires, which assess habitual diet and long-term calcium intake, were used (slope –0·15). The authors argued that "it is conceivable that any 'true' effect of chronic dietary calcium intake on blood pressure or on the development of hypertension could be estimated better by past exposure since it allows for a latency period between exposure and outcome".[70] However, it was subsequently pointed out[71] that errors had occurred when extracting the data from the original publications. This meant that the weight given to one study[72] was about 60 times greater than it should have been and this study erroneously dominated the meta-analysis of diet history trials. Correcting the meta-analysis for this error and several other mistakes leads to a completely different picture (12.5(b)). There is no suggestion that the explanation put forward by the authors for the different findings from studies using different dietary methodologies holds true. This is another demonstration that plausible reasons explaining differences found between groups of trials can easily be generated.[73] It also illustrates the fact that the extraction of data from published articles which present data in different, complex formats is prone to error. Such errors can be avoided in collaborative analyses where investigators make their primary data available.[74]

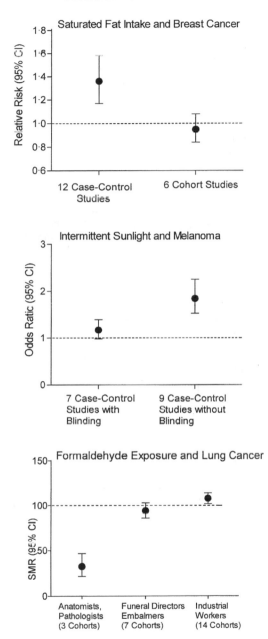

Figure 12.4 Examples of heterogeneity in published observational meta-analyses: saturated fat intake and cancer,[66] intermittent sunlight and melanoma,[69] and formaldehyde exposure and lung cancer.[75] SMR: standardised mortality ratio; CI: confidence interval.

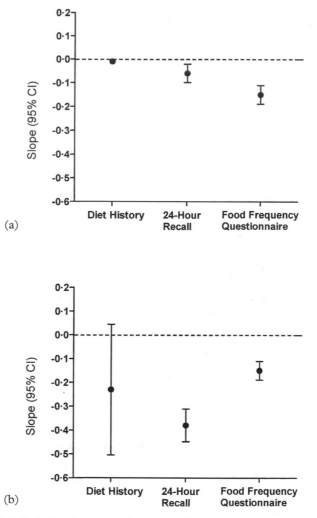

Figure 12.5 Relation between dietary calcium and systolic blood pressure by method of dietary assessment. Initial analysis, which was affected by data extraction errors (a),[70] and corrected analysis (b).[71] CI: confidence interval.

Analyses based on individual participant data (see also Chapter 6) also allow a more thorough investigation of confounding factors, bias and heterogeneity.

An important criterion supporting causality of associations is the demonstration of a dose–response relationship. In occupational epidemiology, the quest to demonstrate such an association can lead to very different groups of employees being compared. In a meta-analysis examining formaldehyde

222

exposure and cancer, funeral directors and embalmers (high exposure) were compared with anatomists and pathologists (intermediate to high exposure) and industrial workers (low to high exposure, depending on job assignment).[75] As shown in Figure 12.4, there is a striking deficit of lung cancer deaths among anatomists and pathologists (standardised mortality ratio [SMR] 33, 95% confidence interval 22 to 47) which is most likely to be due to a lower prevalence of smoking among this group. In this situation few would argue that formaldehyde protects against lung cancer. In other instances such selection bias may be less obvious, however.

In these examples heterogeneity was explored in the framework of sensitivity analysis[76] (see Chapter 2) to test the stability of findings across different study designs, different approaches to exposure ascertainment and to selection of study participants. Such sensitivity analyses should alert investigators to inconsistencies and prevent misleading conclusions. Although heterogeneity was noticed, explored and sometimes extensively discussed, the way the situation was interpreted differed considerably. In the analysis examining studies of dietary fat and breast cancer risk, the authors went on to combine case–control and cohort studies and concluded that "higher intake of dietary fat is associated with an increased risk of breast cancer".[66] The meta-analysis of sunlight exposure and melanoma risk was exceptional in its thorough examination of possible reasons for heterogeneity and the calculation of a combined estimate was deemed appropriate in one subgroup of population-based studies only.[69] Conversely, uninformative and potentially misleading combined estimates were calculated both in the dietary calcium and blood pressure example[70] and the meta-analysis of occupational formaldehyde exposure.[75] These case studies indicate that the temptation to combine the results of studies is hard to resist.

Conclusion

The suggestion that formal meta-analysis of observational studies can be misleading and that insufficient attention is often given to heterogeneity does not mean that a return to the previous practice of highly subjective narrative reviews is called for. Many of the principles of systematic reviews remain: a study protocol should be written in advance, complete literature searches should be carried out, and studies selected in a reproducible and objective fashion. Individual participant data will often be required to allow differences and similarities of the results found in different settings to be inspected thoroughly, hypotheses to be formulated and the need for future studies, including randomised controlled trials, to be defined.

Acknowledgements

We are grateful to Iain Chalmers for helpful comments on an earlier draft of this chapter. We thank Jim Neaton (MRFIT Research Group), Juha Pekkanen and Erkki Vartiainen (North Karelia and Kuopio Cohorts) and Martin Shipley (Whitehall Study) for providing additional data on suicides. This chapter draws on material published earlier in the *BMJ*.[77]

1 Surgeon General. *Smoking and Health*. Washington: US Government Printing Office, 1964.
2 Feinstein AR. Scientific standards in epidemiological studies of the menace of daily life. *Science* 1988;**242**:1257–63.
3 Black N. Why we need observational studies to evaluate the effectiveness of health care. *BMJ* 1996;**312**:1215–18.
4 Freiman JA, Chalmers TC, Smith H, Kuebler RR. The importance of beta, the type II error, and sample size in the design and interpretation of the randomized controlled trial. In Bailar JC, Mosteller F, eds. *Medical uses of statistics*, pp. 357–73. Boston, MA: NEJM Books, 1992.
5 Moher D, Dulberg CS, Wells GA. Statistical power, sample size, and their reporting in randomized controlled trials. *JAMA* 1994;**272**:122–4.
6 Mulward S,.Gøtzsche PC. Sample size of randomized double-blind trials 1976–1991. *Dan Med Bull* 1996;**43**:96–8.
7 Brousson MA, Klein MC. Controversies surrounding the administration of vitamin K to newborns: a review. *Can Med Ass J* 1996;**154**:307–15.
8 Collaborative Group on Hormonal Factors in Breast Cancer. Breast cancer and hormonal contraceptives: collaborative reanalysis of individual data on 53 297 women with breast cancer and 100 239 women without breast cancer from 54 epidemiological studies. *Lancet* 1996;**347**:1713–27.
9 Gurwitz JH, Col NF, Avorn J. The exclusion of the elderly and women from clinical trials in acute myocardial infarction. *JAMA* 1992;**268**:1417–22.
10 Levey BA. Bridging the gender gap in research. *Clin Pharmacol Therapeut* 1991;**50**:641–6.
11 Hlatky MA. Using databases to evaluate therapy. *Stat Med* 1991;**10**:647–52.
12 Wilson CWM. The protective effect of auto-immune buccal urine therapy (AIBUT) against the Raynaud phenomenon. *Med Hypotheses* 1984;**13**:99–107.
13 Davey Smith G, Phillips AN, Neaton JD. Smoking as "independent" risk factor for suicide: illustration of an artifact from observational epidemiology. *Lancet* 1992;**340**:709–11.
14 Doll R, Peto R, Wheatley K, Gray R, Sutherland I. Mortality in relation to smoking: 40 years' observation on male British doctors. *BMJ* 1994;**309**:901–11.
15 Doll R, Gray R, Hafner B, Peto R. Mortality in relation to smoking: 22 years' observations on female British doctors. *BMJ* 1980;**280**:967–71.
16 Tverdal A, Thelle D, Stensvold I, Leren P, Bjartveit K. Mortality in relation to smoking history: 13 years follow-up of 68 000 Norwegian men and women 35–49 years. *J Clin Epidemiol* 1993;**46**:475–87.
17 Vartiainen E, Puska P, Pekkanen J, Tuomilehto J, Lannquist J, Ehnholm C. Serum cholesterol concentrations and mortality from accidents, suicide, and other violent causes. *BMJ* 1994;**309**:445–7.
18 Hemenway D, Solnick SJ, Colditz GA. Smoking and suicide among nurses. *Am J Public Health* 1993;**83**:249–51.
19 Multiple Risk Factor Intervention Trial Research Group. Multiple Risk Factor Intervention Trial. Risk factor changes and mortality results. *JAMA* 1982;**248**:1465–77.
20 Bradford Hill A. The environment and disease: association or causation? *Proc R Soc Med* 1965;**58**:295–300.
21 Leviton A, Pagano M, Allred EN, El Lozy M. Why those who drink the most coffee appear to be at increased risk of disease: a modest proposal. *Ecol Food Nutr* 1994;**31**:285–93.

22 Phillips AN, Davey Smith G. How independent are "independent" effects? Relative risk estimation when correlated exposures are measured imprecisely. *J Clin Epidemiol* 1991;**44**:1223–31.
23 Davey Smith G, Phillips AN. Confounding in epidemiological studies: why "independent" effects may not be all they seem. *BMJ* 1992;**305**:757–9.
24 Sackett DL. Bias in analytical research. *J Chronic Dis* 1979;**32**:51–63.
25 Plummer FA, Simonsen JN, Cameron D, *et al*. Cofactors in male-female sexual transmission of human immunodeficiency virus type 1. *J Infect Dis* 1991;**233**:233–9.
26 Lazzarin A, Saracco A, Musicco M, Nicolosi A. Man-to-woman sexual transmission of the human immunodeficiency virus. *Arch Intern Med* 1991;**151**:2411–16.
27 Phillips AN, Davey Smith G. The design of prospective epidemiological studies: more subjects or better measurements? *J Clin Epidemiol* 1993;**46**:1203–11.
28 Danesh J, Youngman L, Clark S, Parish S, Peto R, Collins R. *Helicobacter pylori* infection and early onset myocardial infarction: case-control and sibling pairs study. *BMJ* 1999;**319**:1157–62.
29 ISIS-3 Collaborative Group. ISIS-3: a randomised comparison of streptokinase vs tissue plasminogen activator vs anistreplase and of aspirin plus heparin vs aspirin alone among 41 299 cases of suspected acute myocardial infarction. *Lancet* 1992;**339**:753–70.
30 Sheikh K, Mattingly S. Investigating non-response bias in mail surveys. *J Epidemiol Community Health* 1981;**35**:293–6.
31 Hill A, Roberts J, Ewings P, Gunnell D. Non-response bias in a lifestyle survey. *J Public Health Med* 1997;**19**:203–7.
32 Boffetta P. Infection with *Helicobacter pylori* and parasites, social class and cancer. *IARC Sci Publ* 1997;325–9.
33 Sitas F, Forman D, Yarnell JW, *et al*. *Helicobacter pylori* infection rates in relation to age and social class in a population of Welsh men. *Gut* 1991;**32**:25–8.
34 Danesh J. Coronary heart disease, *Helicobacter pylori*, dental disease, *Chlamydia pneumoniae*, and cytomegalovirus: meta-analyses of prospective studies. *Am Heart J* 1999;**138**:S434–S437.
35 Whincup P, Danesh J, Walker M, *et al*. Prospective study of potentially virulent strains of *Helicobacter pylori* and coronary heart disease in middle-aged men. *Circulation* 2000;**101**:1647–52.
36 Jha P, Flather M, Lonn E, Farkouh M, Yusuf S. The antioxidant vitamins and cardiovascular disease. *Ann Intern Med* 1995;**123**:860–72.
37 The Alpha-Tocopherol BCCPSG. The effect of vitamin E and beta carotene on the incidence of lung cancer and other cancers in male smokers. *N Engl J Med* 1994;**330**:1029–35.
38 Omenn GS, Goodman GE, Thornquist MD, *et al*. Effects of a combination of beta carotene and vitamin A on lung cancer and cardiovascular disease. *N Engl J Med* 1996;**334**:1150–5.
39 Hennekens CH, Buring JE, Manson JE, *et al*. Lack of effect of long-term supplementation with beta carotene on the incidence of malignant neoplasms and cardiovascular disease. *N Engl J Med* 1996;**334**:1145–9.
40 Greenberg ER, Baron JA, Karagas MR, *et al*. Mortality associated with low plasma concentration of beta carotene and the effect of oral supplementation. *JAMA* 1996;**275**:699–703.
41 Peto R, Doll R, Buckley JD, Sporn MB. Can dietary beta-carotene materially reduce human cancer rates? *Nature* 1981;**290**:201–8.
42 Smigel K. Beta-carotene fails to prevent cancer in two major studies; CARET intervention stopped. *J Natl Cancer Inst* 1995;**88**:145.
43 Goldberg J, Flowerdew G, Smith E, Brody JA, Tso MO. Factors associated with age-related macular degeneration. An analysis of data from the first National Health and Nutrition Examination Survey. *Am J Epidemiol* 1988;**128**:700–10.
44 West S, Vitale S, Hallfrisch J, *et al*. Are antioxidants or supplements protective for age-related macular degeneration? *Arch Ophthalmol* 1994;**112**:222–7.
45 Teikari JM, Laatikainen L, Virtamo J, *et al*. Six-year supplementation with alpha-tocopherol and beta-carotene and age-related maculopathy. *Acta Ophthalmol Scand* 1998;**76**:224–9.

225

46 Leske MC, Chylack LT, Jr, Wu SY. The Lens Opacities Case–Control Study. Risk factors for cataract. *Arch Ophthalmol* 1991;**109**:244–51.

47 Teikari JM, Virtamo J, Rautalahti M, Palmgren J, Liesto K, Heinonen OP. Long-term supplementation with alpha-tocopherol and beta-carotene and age-related cataract. *Acta Ophthalmol Scand* 1997;**75**:634–40.

48 Lonn EM, Yusuf S. Is there a role for antioxidant vitamins in the prevention of cardio-vascular diseases? An update on epidemiological and clinical trials data. *Can J Cardiol* 1997;**13**:957–65.

49 Yusuf S, Dagenais G, Pogue J, Bosch J, Sleight P. Vitamin E supplementation and cardio-vascular events in high-risk patients. The Heart Outcomes Prevention Evaluation Study Investigators. *N Engl J Med* 2000;**342**:154–60.

50 Ness A, Egger M, Davey Smith G. Role of antioxidant vitamins in prevention of cardio-vascular diseases. Meta-analysis seems to exclude benefit of vitamin C supplementation. *BMJ* 1999;**319**:577.

51 Stampfer MJ, Colditz GA. Estrogen replacement therapy and coronary heart disease: a quantitative assessment of the epidemiologic evidence. *Prevent Med* 1991;**20**:47–63.

52 Grady D, Rubin SM, Petitti DB, *et al.* Hormone therapy to prevent disease and prolong life in postmenopausal women. *Ann Intern Med* 1992;**117**:1016–37.

53 Petitti DB. Coronary heart disease and estrogen replacement therapy. Can compliance bias explain the results of observational studies? *Ann Epidemiol* 1994;**4**:115–18.

54 Barrett-Connor E. Postmenopausal estrogen and prevention bias. *Ann Intern Med* 1991;**115**:455–6.

55 Posthuma WF, Westendorp RG, Vandenbroucke JP. Cardioprotective effect of hormone replacement therapy in postmenopausal women: is the evidence biased? *BMJ* 1994;**308**:1268–9.

56 Hulley S, Grady D, Bush T, *et al.* Randomized trial of estrogen plus progestin for secondary prevention of coronary heart disease in postmenopausal women. Heart and Estrogen/progestin Replacement Study (HERS) Research Group. *JAMA* 1998;**280**:605–13.

57 Hemminki E, McPherson K. Impact of postmenopausal hormone therapy on cardio-vascular events and cancer: pooled data from clinical trials. *BMJ* 1997;**315**:149–53.

58 McKee M, Britton A, Black N, McPherson K. Interpreting the evidence: choosing between randomised and non-randomised studies. *BMJ* 1999;**319**:312–15.

59 Benson K, Hartz AJ. A comparison of observational studies and randomized, controlled trials. *N Engl J Med* 2000;**342**:1878–86.

60 Concato J, Shah N, Horwitz RI. Randomized, controlled trials, observational studies, and the hierarchy of research designs. *N Engl J Med* 2000;**342**:1887–92.

61 Pocock SJ, Elbourne DR. Randomized trials or observational tribulations? *N Engl J Med* 2000;**342**:1907–9.

62 Green SB, Byar DP. Using observational data from registries to compare treatments: the fallacy of omnimetrics. *Stat Med* 1984;**3**:361–70.

63 Kunz R, Oxman AD. The unpredictability paradox: review of empirical comparisons of randomised and non-randomised clinical trials. *BMJ* 1998;**317**:1185–90.

64 Shapiro S. Meta-analysis/Shmeta-analysis. *Am J Epidemiol* 1994;**140**:771–8.

65 Armstrong B, Doll R. Environmental factors and cancer incidence and mortality in different countries with special reference to dietary practices. *Int J Cancer* 1975;**15**:617–31.

66 Boyd NF, Martin LJ, Noffel M, Lockwood GA, Trichler DL. A meta-analysis of studies of dietary fat and breast cancer. *Br J Cancer* 1993;**68**:627–36.

67 Howe GR, Hirohata T, Hislop TG, *et al.* Dietary factors and risk of breast cancer: combined analysis of 12 case–control studies. *J Natl Cancer Inst* 1990;**82**:561–9.

68 Hunter DJ, Spiegelman D, Adami H-O, *et al.* Cohort studies of fat intake and the risk of breast cancer – a pooled analysis. *N Engl J Med* 1996;**334**:356–61.

69 Nelemans PJ, Rampen FHJ, Ruiter DJ, Verbeek ALM. An addition to the controversy on sunlight exposure and melanoma risk: a meta-analytical approach. *J Clin Epidemiol* 1995;**48**:1331–42.

70 Cappuccio FP, Elliott P, Allender PS, Pryer J, Follman DA, Cutler JA. Epidemiologic

association between dietary calcium intake and blood pressure: a meta-analysis of published data. *Am J Epidemiol* 1995;**142**:935–45.

71 Birkett NJ. Comments on a Meta-analysis of the Relation between Dietary Calcium Intake and Blood Pressure. *Am J Epidemiol* 1999;**148**:223–8.

72 Kromhout D, Bosschieter EB, Coulander CD. Potassium, calcium, alcohol intake and blood pressure: the Zutphen Study. *Am J Clin Nutr* 1985;**41**:1299–304.

73 Smith GD, Egger M. Meta-analyses of observational data should be done with due care. *BMJ* 1999;**318**:56.

74 Beral V. "The practice of meta-analysis": Discussion. Meta-analysis of observational studies: A case study of work in progress. *J Clin Epidemiol* 1995;**48**:165–6.

75 Blair A, Saracci R, Stewart PA, Hayes RB, Shy C. Epidemiologic evidence on the relationship between formaldehyde exposure and cancer. *Scand J Work Environ Health* 1990;**16**:381–93.

76 Egger M, Davey Smith G, Phillips AN. Meta-analysis: principles and procedures. *BMJ* 1997;**315**:1533–7.

77 Egger M, Schneider M, Davey Smith G. Spurious precision? Meta-analysis of observational studies. *BMJ* 1998;**316**:140–5.

13 Systematic reviews of evaluations of prognostic variables

DOUGLAS G ALTMAN

Summary points

- Systematic reviews are applicable to all types of research design. Studies of prognostic variables are an important additional area where appropriate methodology should be applied.
- Difficulties in searching the literature for prognostic studies mean that there is a higher risk of missing studies than for randomised trials.
- Prognostic variables should be evaluated in a representative sample of patients assembled at a common point in the course of their disease. Ideally they should all have received the same medical treatment or have been in a double-blind randomised study.
- Evaluation of study quality is essential. When examined critically, a high proportion of prognostic studies are found to be methodologically poor, in particular in relation to the analysis of continuous prognostic variables and the adjustment for other factors.
- Meta-analysis based on published data is often hampered by difficulties in data extraction and variation in study and patient characteristics.
- The poor quality of the published literature is a strong argument in favour of systematic reviews but simultaneously also an argument against formal meta-analysis. The main outcome from a systematic review may well be the demonstration that there is little good quality published information.
- Meta-analysis of prognostic studies using individual patient data may overcome many of these difficulties. Access to individual patient data is therefore highly desirable, to allow comparable analyses across studies.

Systematic reviews are equally valuable for all types of research, and studies of prognosis are an important area to which the methodology should be extended. Prognostic studies include clinical studies of variables predictive of future events as well as epidemiological studies of aetiological or risk factors. As multiple similar studies accumulate, it becomes increasingly important to identify and evaluate all of the relevant studies to develop a more reliable overall assessment. As I will show, for prognostic studies this is not straightforward.

As noted by Mackenzie in 1921, "To answer [patients'] questions requires a knowledge of prognosis . . . Moreover, common sense tells us that the public is perfectly justified in expecting from the doctor a knowledge so manifestly essential to medicine".[1] Windeler[2] noted the close link between prognosis and therapy. He observed that summaries of prognosis are not meaningful unless associated with a particular therapeutic strategy and suggested that the greatest importance of prognostic studies is to aid in treatment decisions. Windeler[2] also observed that a prognostic study is similar to a diagnostic study but with the added dimension of time. The clinical importance of information on prognostic factors is summarised in Table 13.1.[3]

Table 13.1 Purpose of prognostic factor studies.

- Improve understanding of the disease process.
- Improve the design and analysis of clinical trials (for example, risk stratification).
- Assist in comparing outcome between treatment groups in non-randomised studies, by allowing adjustment for case mix.
- Define risk groups based on prognosis.
- Predict disease outcome more accurately or parsimoniously.
- Guide clinical decision making, including treatment selection, and patient counselling.

The emphasis in this chapter is primarily on clinical studies to examine the variation in prognosis in relation to a single putative prognostic variable of interest (also called a prognostic marker or factor). Many of the issues discussed are also relevant to epidemiological studies of aetiological or risk factor studies (as discussed in Chapter 12), especially cohort studies. I will also consider some issues relating to systematic reviews of studies of multiple prognostic variables.

Systematic review of prognostic studies

Prognostic studies take various forms. Some studies investigate the prognostic value of a particular variable, while others investigate many variables simultaneously in order either to evaluate which are prognostic or to develop a "prognostic model" for making prognoses for individual patients. In practice, it is not always easy to discern the aims of a particular study. Also, some studies are carried out to try to identify variables that predict response to treatment; in oncology these are called "predictive factors". I will not consider such studies here, although several of the issues discussed will also be relevant to studies of predictive factors.

Some features of prognostic studies lead to particular difficulties for the systematic reviewer. First, in most clinical prognostic studies the outcome of primary interest is the time to an event, often death. Meta-analysis of such studies is rather more difficult than for binary data or continuous measurements. Second, as already indicated, in many contexts the prognostic variable of interest is often one of several prognostic variables. When examining a variable of interest researchers should consider other prognostic variables with which it might be correlated. Third, many prognostic factors are continuous variables, for which researchers use a wide variety of methods of analysis.

Identifying relevant publications

It is probably more difficult to identify all prognostic studies by literature searching than for randomised trials, which itself is problematic (Chapter 4). There is as yet no widely acknowledged optimal strategy for searching the literature for such studies. However, McKibbon et al.[4] have developed search strategies for prognostic studies (see Box 13.1).

It is probable, and is supported by anecdote, that there is considerable publication bias (see Chapter 3), such that studies showing a strong (often statistically significant) prognostic ability are more likely to

---

Box 13.1 Effective MEDLINE searching strategies for studies of prognosis[4]

Best single term:
    explode cohort studies (MeSH).

The best complex search strategy with the highest sensitivity is:
    incidence (MeSH)
    OR explode mortality (MeSH)
    OR follow-up studies (MeSH)
    OR mortality (subheading)
    OR prognos* (text word)
    OR predict* (text word)
    OR course (text word)

MeSH: Medical subject heading

---

be published. This would be in keeping with the finding that epidemiological studies are more prone to publication bias than randomised trials.[5] Indeed, publication bias may be worse as many prognostic studies are based on retrospective analysis of clinical databases. These "studies" thus do not really exist until and unless published.

In addition, it is likely that some researchers selectively report those findings which are more impressive (usually those which are statistically significant) from a series of exploratory analyses of many variables.

Data extraction

A particular problem is that some authors fail to present a numerical summary of the prognostic strength of a variable, such as a hazard ratio, especially in cases where the analysis showed that the effect of the variable was not statistically significant. Even when numerical results are given, they may vary in format – for example, survival proportions may be given for different time points. Also, odds ratios or hazard ratios from grouped or ungrouped analyses are not comparable. Systematic reviewers often find that a quantitative synthesis (meta-analysis) is not possible because the published papers do not all include adequate or compatible information.

Assessing methodological quality – design

There are no widely agreed quality criteria for assessing prognostic studies. As yet there is very little empirical evidence to support the importance of particular study features affecting the reliability of study findings, including the avoidance of bias. Nevertheless, theoretical considerations and common sense point to several methodological aspects that are likely to be important. It is likely that several methodological issues are similar to those relevant to studies of diagnosis (see Chapter 14).

As a consequence, systematic reviewers tend either to ignore the issue or to devise their own criteria. Unfortunately the number of different criteria and scales is likely to continue to increase and cause confusion, as has happened for randomised trials (Chapter 5), systematic reviews (Chapter 7), and diagnostic tests (Chapter 14). As in those contexts, the various scales that have been proposed vary considerably, both in their content and complexity.

Generic criteria

Table 13.2 shows a list of methodological features that are likely to be important for internal validity. This list draws in particular on previous suggestions.[6-10] The items in Table 13.2 are not phrased as questions but rather as domains of likely importance. Most authors have

Table 13.2 A framework for assessing the internal validity of articles dealing with prognosis.

Study feature	Qualities sought
Sample of patients	Inclusion criteria defined Sample selection explained Adequate description of diagnostic criteria Clinical and demographic characteristics fully described Representative Assembled at a common (usually early) point in the course of their disease Complete
Follow up of patients	Sufficiently long
Outcome	Objective Unbiased (for example, assessment blinded to prognostic information) Fully defined Appropriate Known for all or a high proportion of patients
Prognostic variable	Fully defined, including details of method of measurement if relevant Precisely measured Available for all or a high proportion of patients
Analysis	Continuous predictor variable analysed appropriately Statistical adjustment for all important prognostic factors
Treatment subsequent to inclusion in cohort	Fully described Treatment standardised or randomised

presented their checklists as questions. For example, Laupacis et al.[8] included the question "Was there a representative and well-defined sample of patients at a similar point in the course of the disease?," which includes three elements from Table 13.2. Their checklist is widely quoted, for example in a guide for clinicians,[11] but it omits several of the items in Table 13.2.

There seems to be wide agreement that a reliable prognostic study requires a well-defined cohort of patients at the same stage of their disease. Some authors suggest that the sample should be an "inception" cohort of patients very early in the course of the disease (perhaps at diagnosis).[6] This is just one example of a more general requirement that the cohort can be clearly described, which is necessary for the study to have external validity. While homogeneity is often desirable, heterogeneous cohorts can be stratified in the analysis. Not all prognostic studies relate to patients with overt disease. It would be very reasonable to study prognostic factors in a cohort of asymptomatic persons infected with the human immunodeficiency virus (HIV)[12] or risk factors for myocardial infarction in a cohort of men aged 50–55 most of whom will have atherosclerotic plaques in their coronary arteries. One important difference between clinical and epidemiological studies is that the latter are often not cohort studies. Both case–control and cross-sectional studies may be used to examine risk factors, but these designs are much weaker. Case–control designs have been shown to yield optimistic results for evaluations of diagnostic tests,[13] a result which is likely to be relevant to prognostic studies. In cross-sectional studies it may be very difficult to determine whether the exposure or outcome came first, for example in studies study examining the association between oral contraceptive use and HIV infection.

Most authors of checklists have not considered the issue of subsequent treatment. If the treatment received varies in relation to prognostic variables then the study cannot deliver an unbiased and meaningful assessment of prognostic ability unless the different treatments are equally effective (in which case why vary the treatment?). Such variation in treatment may be quite common once there is some evidence that a variable is prognostic. Ideally, therefore, prognostic variables should be evaluated in a cohort of patients treated the same way, or in a randomised trial.[9,14]

The important methodological dimensions will vary to some extent according to circumstances. For example, in some prognostic studies the reliability of the measurements may be of particular importance. Many biochemical markers can be measured by a variety of methods (such as assays), and studies comparing these often show that the agreement is not especially good. It is desirable, therefore, that the method of measurement is stated and that the same method was used throughout a study; this information may not be given explicitly.

Study-specific criteria

The inclusion of context-specific as well as generic aspects of methodological quality may sometimes be desirable. For example, Marx and Marx[10] included two questions on the nature of the endpoints, reflecting particular problems encountered in their review of prognosis of idiopathic membranous nephropathy, where many studies used ill-defined surrogate endpoints.

As well as internal validity some checklists consider aspects of external validity and clinical usefulness of studies. Notably, Laupacis et al.[8] included five questions relating to the clinical usefulness of a study.

Further, some checklists very reasonably include items relating to the clinical area of the review. For example, in their review of the association between maternal HIV infection and perinatal outcome, Brocklehurst and French[15] considered whether there was an adequate description of the maternal stage of disease.

One difficulty with quality assessment is that answering the questions posed, such as those in Table 13.2, often requires judgement. An

233

example is the question quoted above from Laupacis *et al.*[8] relating to the derivation of the sample. Thus even if consensus could be reached on the important dimensions of quality, they would probably still be replete with judgmental terms such as "adequate", "appropriate", "representative", and "similar".

Assessing methodological quality – analysis

The criteria in Table 13.2 include two items relating to difficult aspects of data analysis – adjustment for other variables and the analysis of continuous prognostic variables. In this section I consider in some detail these important issues, which have a major influence on whether any meta-analysis might be possible.

Adjustment for covariates

It is important to adjust for other prognostic variables to get a valid picture of the relative prognosis for different values of the primary prognostic variable. This procedure is often referred to as "control of confounding". It is necessary because patients with different values of the covariate of primary interest are likely to differ with respect to other prognostic variables. Also, in contexts where much is known about prognosis, such as breast cancer, it is important to know whether the variable of primary interest (such as a new tumour marker) offers prognostic value over and above that which can be achieved with previously identified prognostic variables. It follows that prognostic studies generally require some sort of multiple regression analysis, although stratification may be useful in simpler situations. For outcomes which are binary or time to a specific event, logistic or Cox proportional hazards regression models respectively are appropriate for examining the influence of several prognostic factors simultaneously.

Many studies seek parsimonious prediction models by retaining only the most important prognostic factors, most commonly by using multiple regression analysis with stepwise variable selection. Unfortunately, this method is quite likely to be misleading.[14] Recognised or "standard" prognostic factors should not be subjected to the selection process. Even though such variables may not reach specified levels of significance in a particular study, they should be included in the models generated in order to compare results to other reported studies.[3] Comparison of models with and without the variable of interest provides an estimate of its independent effect and a test of statistical significance of whether it contains additional prognostic information.

Two problems for the systematic reviewer are that different researchers use different statistical approaches to adjustment, and that they adjust for different selections of variables. One way round the latter problem is to use unadjusted analyses. While this approach is common in systematic reviews of randomised controlled trials, in prognostic studies it replaces one problem with a worse one; it is rare that unadjusted analyses will be unbiased.

Handling continuous predictor variables

Many prognostic variables are continuous measurements, including many tumour markers and levels of environmental exposure. If such a variable were prognostic, the risk of an event would usually be expected to increase or decrease systematically as the level increases. Nonetheless, many researchers prefer to categorise patients into high- and low-risk groups based on a threshold or cutpoint. This type of analysis discards potentially important quantitative information and considerably reduces the power to detect a real association with outcome.[16,17] If a cutpoint is used, it should not be determined by a data-dependent process. Reasonable approaches include using a cutpoint reported in another study, one based on the reference interval in healthy individuals, or the median or other pre-specified centile from the present study.

Some investigators compute the statistical significance level for all possible cutpoints and then select the cutpoint giving the smallest P value. There are several serious problems associated with this so-called "optimal" cutpoint approach.[18,19] In particular, the P values and regression coefficients resulting from these analyses are biased, and in general the prognostic value of the variable of interest will be over-estimated. The bias cannot be adjusted for in any simple manner, and it is carried across into subsequent multiple regression analyses. Misleading results from individual studies are bad enough, but when such studies are included in a meta-analysis they may well distort the results (as in the case study presented below).

Keeping variables continuous in the analysis has the considerable advantages of retaining all the information and avoiding arbitrary cut-points. It may also greatly simplify any subsequent meta-analysis. Many researchers, however, are unwilling to assume that the relationship of marker with outcome is log-linear, i.e. that the risk (expressed as the log odds ratio or log hazard ratio) either increases or decreases linearly as the variable increases, and investigations of non-linear (curved) relation-ships are uncommon. The assumption of linearity may well be more reasonable than the assumptions that go with dichotomising, namely constant risk either side of the cutpoint.

Using a small number of groups, say four, offers a good compromise between dichotomising and treating the data as continuous, which requires assumptions about the shape of the relation with the probability of the event. This approach is common in epidemiology. However, it may lead to problems for the systematic reviewer, because it is rare that different studies use the same groupings. For example, Buettner et al.[20] summarised 14 studies that had examined the prognostic importance of tumour thickness in primary cutaneous melanoma. As shown in Table 13.3, the number of cutpoints varied between two and six. Despite their clear similarities, no two studies had used the same cutpoints. Further, several studies had used the "optimised" approach that, as noted above, is inherently overoptimistic.

Table 13.3 Tumour thickness in primary cutaneous melanoma.[20] Cutpoints are shown in clusters around 0.75, 1, 1.5, 2, 3, 4, and > 5 mm.

Study	Patients (n)	Groups (n)	Cut-off point (mm)							Method
1	2012	3		1		2				Optimised
2	581	3			1·5		3			Unclear
3	339	4	0·75		1·5			4		Optimised
4	598	4	0·85		1·7		3·6			Optimised
5	739	4		1		2		4		Unclear
6	971	4	0·75		1·7		3·6			Optimised
7	648	4	0·75		1·7		3·65			Optimised
8	98	5	0·75		1·5	2·25	3			Optimised
9	699	5		1		2	3	4		Linear
10	585	5	0·75		1·5		3		5	Unclear
11	1082	5	0·75		1·7		3	4		Optimised
12	769	6		1		2	3	4	5	Unclear
13	8500	6	0·75		1·5	2·5		4	8	Optimised
14	2012	7	0·75		1·5	2·25	3	4·5	6	Unclear

Meta-analysis of prognostic factor studies

It can be seen that prognostic studies raise several particular difficulties for the systematic reviewer. These are summarised in Box 13.2. Most have been discussed above. The last two items relate to inadequate reporting of results in the primary studies, discussed below.

There are clearly major difficulties in trying to get a quantitative synthesis of the prognostic literature. In this section I consider when it might be reasonable to proceed to formal meta-analysis, and how this might be achieved.

Whether to carry out a meta-analysis

Two of the main concerns regarding prognostic studies are the quality of the primary studies – both methodological quality and quality of reporting – and the possibility of publication bias. While quality is not considered in some systematic reviews, others have adopted strict inclusion criteria based on methodological quality. For example, in their systematic review of psychosocial factors in the aetiology and prognosis

Box 13.2 Problems with systematic reviews of prognostic studies from publications

- Difficulty of identifying all studies
- Negative (non-significant) results may not be reported (publication bias)
- Inadequate reporting of methods
- Variation in study design
- Most studies are retrospective
- Variation in inclusion criteria
- Lack of recognised criteria for quality assessment
- Different assays/measurement techniques
- Variation in methods of analysis
- Differing methods of handling of continuous variables (some data-dependent)
- Different statistical methods of adjustment
- Adjustment for different sets of variables
- Inadequate reporting of quantitative information on outcome
- Variation in presentation of results (for example, survival at different time points)

of coronary heart disease, Hemingway and Marmot[21] included only prospective cohort studies with at least 500 (aetiology) or 100 participants (prognosis). They included only those psychosocial factors used in two or more studies. Nonetheless, because of the risk of publication bias and the lack of standardised measurement methods, they did not attempt a statistical synthesis.

More commonly, authors have concluded that a set of studies was either too diverse or too poor, or both, to allow a meaningful meta-analysis. Box 13.3 shows details of a systematic review of prognosis in elbow disorders which reached such a conclusion. Likewise, in a systematic review of studies of the possible relation between hormonal contraception and risk of HIV transmission, Stephenson[22] concluded that a meta-analysis was unwise. By contrast, Wang et al.[23] performed such a meta-analysis on a similar set of studies, arguing that this enabled the quantitative investigation of the impact of various study features. Because of the likelihood of serious methodological difficulties, some authors have suggested that in general it is unwise to carry out a sensible meta-analysis without access to individual patient data.[3,24]

This gloomy picture does not apply always, however. In the next section I consider in outline how a meta-analysis might proceed, on the assumption that a subset of studies has been identified which are deemed similar enough and of acceptable quality.

Box 13.3 Prognosis in elbow disorders

Hudak et al.[9] carried out a systematic review of the evidence regarding prognostic factors that affect elbow pain duration and outcomes. Selected papers were subjected to a detailed quality assessment using a scheme adapted from other publications. Each paper was assessed on six dimensions: case definition, patient selection, follow up (completeness and length), outcome, information about prognostic factors, and analysis. Each dimension was scored from 0 to 2 or 3, and a minimum score for "strong evidence" specified. Their pre-specified minimum requirements for studies providing strong evidence were as follows (with the number of studies meeting the criteria shown in brackets):

- provided an operational definition of cases [15/40];
- included an inception cohort (defined in relation to onset of symptoms) or a survival cohort that included a subset of patients in whom duration of symptoms was less than four months [5/40];
- demonstrated follow up of >80% of cases for at least one year [8/40];
- used a blinded and potentially replicable outcome measure appropriate to the research question [20/40];
- used adequate measurement and reporting of potential prognostic factors [36/40];
- provided crude proportions for at least one of response, recovery, and recurrence [34/40].

Papers were identified from a comprehensive literature search of multiple databases. The authors included the search strategy they used.

Of the 40 eligible studies assessed using the above criteria, none provided "strong evidence" and just four provided "moderate evidence", none of which followed patients for more than one year. The authors note that several studies with excellent follow up were not based on inception cohorts. Only three of the 40 studies had used a statistical method to derive results adjusted for other factors.

Among the four providing "moderate-level" evidence there was variation in study design (one cases series, three randomised trials), patient selection, interventions, and length of follow up. As a consequence, meta-analysis was not attempted. The authors made several suggestions for the methodological requirements for future studies.

Methods of meta-analysis of prognostic factor studies

Even if it is felt that a set of published studies is of good enough quality to attempt a formal meta-analysis, there are many potential barriers to success. In essence, we wish to compare the outcome for groups with different values of the prognostic variable. The method of analysis suitable for pooling values across several studies will depend on whether the prognostic variable is binary, categorical, or continuous. In principle, it should be relatively easy to combine data from studies which have produced compatible estimates of effect, with standard errors. I will consider only binary or continuous variables, and will not consider the more complex case of categorical outcomes.

Outcome is occurrence of event, regardless of time

In many studies the time to an event is ignored and the question is simply whether the factor of interest predicts the outcome. For a binary outcome, standard methods for comparative studies, notably Mantel–Haenszel or inverse variance methods, can be used to pool the data when the prognostic variable is binary using risk ratio, odds ratio or risk difference (Chapter 15). Such data arise especially from case–control studies (for which only the odds ratio would be appropriate). For an unadjusted analysis of a single continuous prognostic variable there is no simple approach, but the data can be analysed using logistic regression.

As already noted, however, in general it is necessary to allow for other potentially confounding variables in such a meta-analysis. Here too, for both binary and continuous prognostic variables, logistic regression is used to derive an odds ratio after adjustment for other prognostic or potentially confounding variable. Logistic regression yields an estimated log odds ratio with its standard error, from which the odds ratio and confidence interval are obtained. For a binary prognostic variable the odds ratio gives the ratio of the odds of the event in those with and without that feature. For continuous predictors, it relates to the increase in odds associated with an increase of one unit in the value of the variable. Estimated log odds ratios from several studies can be combined using the inverse variance method (Chapter 15).

Even when a study considers the time to the event of interest, attention may focus on an arbitrary but much-used time point, such as death within five years after a myocardial infarction. Although explicit "survival" times are often ignored in such studies, if any patients are lost to follow up before the specified time point (as is usual) it is preferable to use methods intended for time-to-event data, such as the log rank test. Meta-analysis would then be based on the methods described in the following section. However, it is possible to use the Mantel–Haenszel method by suitably modifying the sample size to allow for loss to follow up, as was done by Bruinvels *et al.*[25] to combine data from several studies. Unusually, these authors used the risk difference as effect measure, on the grounds that the odds ratio is intuitively hard to interpret (see Chapter 16). (Their meta-analysis was of non-randomised intervention studies rather than prognostic studies, although the statistical principles are the same.)

Some prognostic studies relate to time-specific events, most notably studies in pregnancy or surgery. In such cases one can also treat the problem using the framework of a diagnostic study (Chapter 14). For example, in their systematic review of eight studies of intrapartum umbilical artery Doppler velocimetry as a predictor of adverse perinatal outcome, Farrell et al.[26] used positive and negative likelihood ratios (see Chapter 14).

Outcome is time to event

When the time to event is explicitly considered for each individual in a study, the data are analysed using "survival analysis" methods – most often the log rank test for simple comparisons or Cox regression for analyses of multiple predictor variables or where one or more variables is continuous. By analogy with logistic regression discussed above, these analyses yield hazard ratios, which are similar to relative risks. Log rank statistics and log hazard ratios can be combined using the Peto method or the inverse variance method respectively (see Chapter 15). Although in principle it would also be possible sometimes to combine estimated Kaplan–Meier survival probabilities at a single time point, it is unlikely that adequately detailed data will be presented.

Practical difficulties are likely to make meta-analysis much more difficult than the preceding explanation suggests. Most obviously, the hazard ratio is not always explicitly presented for each study. Parmar et al.[27] described a number of methods of deriving estimates of the necessary statistics in a variety of situations. For example, an estimate can be derived from the P value of the log-rank test. Of note, they also explain how to estimate the standard errors of these estimates.

Several authors have proposed more complex methods for combining data from studies of survival.[28,29] All can be applied in this context if it is possible to extract suitable data, but some require even more data than the basic items just discussed. As is true more generally, the use of sophisticated statistical techniques may be inappropriate when several much more basic weaknesses exist. Indeed, some reviewers (for example, Fox et al.[30]) have had to summarise the findings of the primary studies as P values as it is very difficult to extract useful and usable quantitative information from many papers. For some studies the direction of the association between the prognostic factor and outcome may even not be clear.

General issues

The preceding comments implicitly assume that the prognostic variable was handled in a like manner in all studies. In practice this will often not be the case. In the simplest case, researchers may all have dichotomised but using different cutpoints. A meta-analysis is possible comparing "high" and "low" values, using whatever definition was used in the primary studies, but interpretation is not simple. Patients with the same values would be "high" in some studies and "low" in others. It is important to recognise that, in a given study, moving the cutpoint to a higher value increases the mean in both the high and low groups. This phenomenon is known as "stage migration" as discussed, for example, by Feinstein et al.[31] At the very least this is a source of heterogeneity, and its effect is amenable to study. As noted above, the analysis will be biased if any studies used a cutpoint derived by the minimum P value method.

When authors have presented results for more than two categories it may be impossible to combine estimates. In some situations it is possible to convert results from a group of studies with diverse categorical presentation to the same format. Chêne and Thompson[32] presented a method that can be used when results relate to groups defined by different quantiles of the observed distribution of data values, and can combine these with estimates from ungrouped analyses. In practice, it is likely that studies have used a mixture of categorical and continuous representations of the prognostic variable which cannot be combined in any simple manner.

Some of these difficulties are illustrated in the following case study.

Case study: Cathepsin D and disease-free survival in node-negative breast cancer

Ferrandina et al.[33] described a meta-analysis of 11 studies which examined the relation between cathepsin D (a proteolytic enzyme) and disease-free survival (time to relapse) in node-negative breast cancer. Their inclusion criteria included the presentation of outcome separately for groups with "high" and "low" cathepsin D values. Studies were included if they had used a cytosol assay with a cutpoint in the range 20–78 pmol/mg or a semiquantitative method based on histochemical assay. It is not clear why this range was chosen. It seems that no studies were excluded because they treated cathepsin D values as a continuous variable. Some studies were excluded because they did not present results separately for patients with node-negative breast cancer and others because they reported overall survival rather than disease-free survival. These exclusions are carefully documented in an appendix. The authors apparently did not evaluate methodological quality and included all studies that had relevant data. The studies are summarised in Table 13.4.

The authors had used a variety of cutpoints in the range 20–78

Table 13.4 Some characteristics of 11 studies included in the meta-analysis of Ferrandina et al.[33]

First author	Sample size	Cutoff (pmol/mg)	Percentage positive	Assay	P
Thorpe	119	78	22%	ELISA	0·06
Kute	138	39	28%	RIA	0·0001
Tandon	199	75	32%	WB	0·0001
Janicke	97	50	34%	ELSA	0·08
Isola	262	*	36%	IHC	0·0001
Kandalafi	135	*	38%	IHC	0·07
Pujol	64	20	40%	ELISA	0·07
Spyratos	68	45	43%	ELISA	0·001
Namer	246	35	46%	ELSA	NS
Ravdin	927	54	50%	WB, IHC	NS
Seshadri	354	25	67%	ELSA	NS
Thorpe	71	24	70%	ELISA	0·04

*Positivity defined from immunohistochemical assay.
NS: not significant (P > 0·05).

pmol/mg derived by various methods. As a consequence, the proportion of patients classified as "high" varied markedly across studies. Ferrandina et al.[33] also noted that inter-study heterogeneity in the relative risk was "remarkably high", which was probably partly due to the use of the minimum P value method in some studies. The use of optimal cutpoints will also have led to an exaggeration of the prognostic importance of cathepsin D in some studies. It is regrettable, therefore, that they did not specify which studies used this approach, and did not present results in relation to the method of deriving the cutpoint.

P values from individual studies are shown. In addition, values extracted from survival curves were used to produce estimates of the log-rank odds ratio for different time intervals from the start of follow up.[29,34] In this case the authors produced estimates for each 12-month period up to 84 months. The estimated pooled odds ratios were remarkably consistent across these periods, varying only between 0·53 and 0·62. As noted, however, these values are biased to an unknown extent by inclusion of an unspecified number of studies which had used a data-derived cutpoint. The authors noted that the results were similar when they excluded those studies which had not used a cytosol assay. There was some indication that the findings were not as strong in those studies using an immunohistochemical method.

Overall the conclusion that cathepsin D does have some prognostic value is probably fair, but the quantitative results are unreliable, which puts into question the considerable effort in obtaining them.

Studies of many prognostic factors

The above discussion has concentrated on the case where there is a single prognostic or risk factor of prior interest. Some systematic reviews consider a set of research studies where the aim was to investigate many factors simultaneously, to identify important risk factors. The primary studies here are likely to be even more variable than those examining a specific factor, and there is considerable risk of false-positive findings in individual studies. Systematic review of these exploratory studies is certainly desirable, but it is unlikely that there will often be scope for sensible meta-analysis.

Problems of such studies include the examination of different factors, reporting of only the statistically significant factors, possibly without declaring which had been examined, and a mixture of adjusted and unadjusted estimates (with the latter adjusted for a variety of other variables). Pooling of quantitative estimates will be problematic. Ankum et al.[35] produced pooled estimates of odds ratios associated with various risk factors for ectopic pregnancy. Studies varied in their design and identified different risk factors. Results for individual factors were based on between one and ten studies. They did not comment on the methods used in the primary studies to develop estimates of risk.

Randolph et al.[36] presented a checklist of ten questions to ask regarding a study reporting a clinical prediction tool.

Discussion

While it is clearly desirable that the principles of the systematic review should be extended to studies of prognosis, it is abundantly clear that this is by no means straightforward. The prognostic literature features studies of poor quality and variable methodology, and the difficulties are exacerbated by poor reporting of methodology. The poor quality of the published literature is actually a strong argument in favour of systematic reviews but simultaneously also an argument against formal meta-analysis. To this end, it is valuable if a systematic review includes details of the methodology of each study and its principal numerical results.

As discussed above, there are particular issues for prognostic studies that make meta-analysis based on published information difficult or impossible. One is the way continuous prognostic variables have been analysed, which usually varies among studies. Another is the adjustment for other prognostic variables, which is not always done and when done is likely to be poorly reported[37] and the adjustment made for different variables. While meta-analyses may sometimes be useful, especially when the study characteristics do not vary too much and only the best studies are included, the findings will rarely be convincing. The main outcome from such systematic reviews may well be the realisation that

243

there is very little good quality information in the literature. Even an apparently clear result may best be seen as providing the justification for a well-designed prospective study.[38] For these and other reasons, some authors have suggested that meta-analysis of the published literature will rarely be justified for prognostic studies.[3,24]

By contrast, meta-analysis based on individual patient data (Chapter 6) is highly desirable. Among several advantages of individual patient data, it is possible to analyse all the data in a consistent manner. Such meta-analysis of the raw data from all (or almost all) relevant studies is a worthy goal and there have been some notable examples, especially in a more epidemiological setting.[39] Apart from the considerable resources needed to carry out such a review (Chapter 6), in most cases it is likely that many of the data sets will be unobtainable. However, a careful collaborative re-analysis of the raw data from several good studies may well be more valuable than a more superficial review which mixes good and poor studies. Two examples of such collaborative meta-analyses of raw data are a study of the relation between alcohol consumption and development of breast cancer[40] and a study of the relation between vegetarian diet and mortality.[41] The same approach has also been adopted in some reviews of multiple prognostic variables.[42,43] Clearly, the suitability of this less than systematic approach will depend upon the representativeness of the studies being analysed, which may be hard to establish. Studies for which individual patient data are available may be unrepresentative of all studies. It may be possible, however, to combine individual patient data with summary statistics from studies for which the raw data were not available.[44]

It is particularly important to recognise that individual studies that are open to bias may distort the results of a subsequent meta-analysis. Evaluation of study quality is thus essential, although it is not always done (see case study above). When examined critically, a high proportion of prognostic studies are found to be methodologically poor.[6,45] Prognostic studies are generally too small, and too poorly designed and analysed to provide reliable evidence. Fox et al.[30] noted that their review "highlights the need for journal editors to have a minimal set of criteria for accepting papers on prognostic factors". Similar sentiments were expressed by Ferrandina et al.[33] in their review (described above). Some suggested guidelines have appeared,[3,10] but there is little evidence that methodological guidelines are observed by authors or editors, and they would be unlikely to influence research in other medical specialties. Progress may depend upon developing a consensus regarding the main methodological requirements for reliable studies of prognostic factors, as has happened for randomised trials.[46]

As a consequence of the poor quality of research, prognostic markers may remain under investigation for many years after initial studies without any resolution of the uncertainty. Multiple separate and unco-ordinated studies may actually delay the process of defining the role of prognostic markers. Cooperation from the outset between different research groups could lead to clear results emerging more rapidly than is commonly the case.

In relation to the ten methodological standards they suggested, Marx and Marx[10] noted that "rather than create a rigid scoring system for quality, our aim was to describe general methodologic problems that investigators could note and try to avoid in future research". Systematic reviews can thus draw attention to the paucity of good quality evidence and, we may hope, help to improve the quality of future research.

1 Mackenzie J. A defence of the thesis that "the opportunities of the general practitioner are essential for the investigation of disease and the progress of medicine". *BMJ* 1921;1:797–804.
2 Windeler J. Prognosis – what does the clinician associate with this notion? *Stat Med* 2000;19:425–30.
3 Altman DG, Lyman GH. Methodological challenges in the evaluation of prognostic factors in breast cancer. *Breast Cancer Res Treat* 1998;52:289–303.
4 McKibbon K, Eady A, Marks S. *Evidence-based principles and practice*. PDQ Series. Hamilton, Canada: Dekker, 1999.
5 Easterbrook PJ, Berlin J, Gopalan R, Matthews DR. Publication bias in clinical research. *Lancet* 1991;337:867–72.
6 Kernan WN, Feinstein AR, Brass LM. A methodological appraisal of research on prognosis after transient ischemic attacks. *Stroke* 1991;22:1108–16.
7 Levine MN, Browman GP, Gent M, Roberts R, Goodyear M. When is a prognostic factor useful?: A guide for the perplexed. *J Clin Oncol* 1991;9:348–56.
8 Laupacis A, Wells G, Richardson S, Tugwell P. Users' guides to the medical literature – V. How to use an article about prognosis. *JAMA* 1994;272:234–7.
9 Hudak PL, Cole DC, Haines T. Understanding prognosis to improve rehabilitation: the example of lateral elbow pain. *Arch Phys Med Rehabil* 1996;77:586–93.
10 Marx BE, Marx M. Prognosis of idiopathic membranous nephropathy: a methodologic meta-analysis. *Kidney Int* 1997;51:873–9.
11 Straus SE, McAlister FA. A clinician's guide to journal articles about prognosis. *ACP J Club* 1999;May–June:A13–A15.
12 Low N, Egger M. Can we predict the prognosis of HIV infection? How to use the findings of a prospective study. *Sex Transm Inf* 1998;74:149–54.
13 Lijmer JG, Mol BW, Heisterkamp S, *et al.* Empirical evidence of design-related bias in studies of diagnostic tests. *JAMA* 1999;282:1061–6.
14 Simon R, Altman DG. Statistical aspects of prognostic factor studies in oncology. *Br J Cancer* 1994;69:979–85.
15 Brocklehurst P, French R. The association between maternal HIV infection and peri-natal outcome: a systematic review of the literature and meta-analysis. *Br J Obstet Gynaecol* 1998;105:836–48.
16 Cohen J. The cost of dichotomization. *Appl Psychol Meas* 1983;7:249–53.
17 Morgan TM, Elashoff RM. Effect of categorizing a continuous covariate on the com-parison of survival time. *J Am Stat Assoc* 1986;81:917–21.
18 Altman DG, Lausen B, Sauerbrei W, Schumacher M. Dangers of using "optimal" cut-points in the evaluation of prognostic factors. *J Natl Cancer Inst* 1994;86:829–35.
19 Altman DG. Suboptimal analysis using "optimal" cutpoints. *Br J Cancer* 1998;78:556–7.

20 Buettner P, Garbe C, Guggenmoos-Holzmann I. Problems in defining cutoff points of continuous prognostic factors: example of tumor thickness in primary cutaneous melanoma. *J Clin Epidemiol* 1997;**50**:1201–10.

21 Hemingway H, Marmot M. Psychosocial factors in aetiology and prognosis of coronary heart disease: systematic review of prospective cohort studies. *BMJ* 1999;**318**:1460–7.

22 Stephenson JM. Systematic review of hormonal contraception and risk of HIV transmission: when to resist meta-analysis. *AIDS* 1998;**12**:545–53.

23 Wang CC, Kreiss JK, Reilly M. Risk of HIV infection in oral contraceptive pill users: a meta-analysis. *J Acquir Immune Defic Syndr* 1999;**21**:51–8.

24 Blettner M, Sauerbrei W, Schlehofer B, Scheuchenpflug T, Friedenreich C. Traditional reviews, meta-analyses and pooled analyses in epidemiology. *Int J Epidemiol* 1999;**28**:1–9.

25 Bruinvels DJ, Stiggelbout AM, Kievit J, van Houwelingen HC, Habbema JD, van de Velde CJ. Follow-up of patients with colorectal cancer. A meta-analysis. *Ann Surg* 1994;**219**:174–82.

26 Farrell T, Chien PFW, Gordon A. Intrapartum umbilical artery Doppler velocimetry as a predictor of adverse perinatal outcome: a systematic review. *Br J Obstet Gynaecol* 1999;**106**:783–92.

27 Parmar M, Torri V, Stewart L. Extracting summary statistics to perform meta-analyses of the published literature for survival endpoints. *Stat Med* 1998;**17**:2815–34.

28 Hunink MGM, Wong JB. Meta-analysis of failure-time data with adjustment for covariates. *Med Decis Making* 1994;**14**:59–70.

29 Dear KBG. Iterative generalised least squares for meta-analysis of survival data at multiple times. *Biometrics* 1994;**50**:989–1002.

30 Fox SB, Smith K, Hollyer J, Greenall M, Hastrich D, Harris AL. The epidermal growth factor receptor as a prognostic marker: results of 370 patients and review of 3009 patients. *Breast Cancer Res Treat* 1994;**29**:41–9.

31 Feinstein AR, Sosin DM, Wells CK. The Will Rogers phenomenon. Stage migration and new diagnostic techniques as a source of misleading statistics for survival in cancer. *N Engl J Med* 1985;**312**:1604–8.

32 Chêne G, Thompson SG. Methods for summarizing the risk associations of quantitative variables in epidemiological studies in a consistent form. *Am J Epidemiol* 1996;**144**:610–21.

33 Ferrandina G, Scambia G, Bardelli F, Benedetti Panici P, Mancuso S, Messori A. Relationship between cathepsin-D content and disease-free survival in node-negative breast cancer patients: a meta-analysis. *Br J Cancer* 1997;**76**:661–6.

34 Fine HA, Dear KBG, Loeffler JS, Black PM, Canellos GP. Meta-analysis of radiation therapy with and without adjuvant chemotherapy for malignant gliomas in adults. *Cancer* 1993;**71**:2585–92.

35 Ankum WM, Mol BW, Van der Veen F, Bossuyt PM. Risk factors for ectopic pregnancy: a meta-analysis. *Fertil Steril* 1996;**65**:1093–9.

36 Randolph AG, Guyatt GH, Calvin JE, Doig G, Richardson WS. for the Evidence Based Medicine in Critical Care Group. Understanding articles describing clinical prediction tools. *Crit Care Med* 1998;**26**:1603–12.

37 Müllner M, Matthews H, Altman DG. Reporting on statistical methods to adjust for confounding: a cross sectional survey (submitted, 2000).

38 Ray JG. Meta-analysis of hyperhomocysteinemia as a risk factor for venous thromboembolic disease. *Arch Intern Med* 1998;**158**:2101–6.

39 Collaborative Group on Hormonal Factors in Breast Cancer. Breast cancer and hormonal contraceptives: collaborative reanalysis of individual data of 53 297 women with breast cancer and 100 239 women without breast cancer from 54 epidemiological studies. *Lancet* 1996;**347**:1713–27.

40 Key TJ, Fraser GE, Thorogood M, *et al*. Mortality in vegetarians and nonvegetarians: detailed findings from a collaborative analysis of five prospective studies. *Am J Clin Nutr* 1999;**70**(3 suppl):516S–524S.

41 Smith-Warner SA, Spiegelman D, Yaun S-S, *et al*. Alcohol and breast cancer in women. A pooled analysis of cohort studies. *JAMA* 1998;**279**:535–40.

42 Rawson NSB, Peto J. An overview of prognostic factors in small cell lung cancer. *Br J Cancer* 1990;**61**:597–604.
43 The International Non-Hodgkin's Lymphoma Prognostic Factors Project. A predictive model for aggressive lymphoma. *N Engl J Med* 1993;**329**:987–94.
44 Steyerberg EW, Eijkemans MJC, van Houwelingen JC, Lee KL, Habbema JDF. Prognostic models based on literature and individual patient data in logistic regression analysis. *Stat Med* 2000;**19**:141–60.
45 Borghouts JAJ, Koes BW, Bouter LM. The clinical course and prognostic factors of non-specific neck pain: a systematic review. *Pain* 1998;**77**:1–13.
46 Begg C, Cho M, Eastwood S, *et al.* Improving the quality of reporting of randomized controlled trials: the CONSORT Statement. *JAMA* 1996;**276**:637–9.

14 Systematic reviews of evaluations of diagnostic and screening tests

JONATHAN J DEEKS

Summary points

- The main differences between systematic reviews of studies of diagnostic accuracy and systematic reviews of randomised controlled trials arise in the identification of studies, assessments of the potential for bias and the methods used to statistically combine their results.
- Electronic literature searches for reviews of diagnostic accuracy can be difficult due to a lack of suitable design-related indexing terms.
- Empirical research suggests that the most important aspects of study quality include the selection of a clinically relevant cohort, the consistent use of a single good reference standard, and the masking of experimental and reference test results. Incomplete reporting is also associated with bias.
- The choice of a statistical method for pooling study results depends on the sources of heterogeneity, especially variation in diagnostic thresholds (whether through explicit numerical differences in cutpoints, or natural variation between locations and operators).
- Sensitivities, specificities and likelihood ratios may be combined directly if the results are reasonably homogeneous. When a threshold effect exists, the study results may best be summarised as a summary receiver operating characteristic (ROC) curve. Such a curve can prove difficult to interpret and apply in practice. When study results are strongly heterogeneous it may be most appropriate not to attempt statistical pooling.
- The full evaluation of the performance of a diagnostic test involves studying test reliability, diagnostic accuracy, diagnostic and therapeutic impact, and the net effect of the test on patient outcomes. Separate systematic reviews can be performed for each of these

aspects of test evaluation depending on the availability of suitable studies.

Tests are routinely used in medicine to screen for, diagnose, grade and monitor the progression of disease. Diagnostic information is obtained from a multitude of sources, including imaging and biochemical technologies, pathological and psychological investigations, and signs and symptoms elicited during history-taking and clinical examinations.[1] Each item of information obtained from these sources can be regarded as a result of a separate diagnostic or screening "test", whether it is obtained for the purpose of identifying diseases in sick people, or for detecting early disease in asymptomatic individuals. Systematic reviews of assessments of the reliability, accuracy and impact of these "tests" are essential to guide optimal test selection and the appropriate interpretation of test results.

To make sense of a diagnostic investigation a clinician needs to be able to make an inference regarding the probability that a patient has the disease in question according to the result obtained from the test. Tests rarely make a diagnosis 100% certain, but they may provide enough information to rule-in or rule-out a diagnosis in a pragmatic manner.[2,3] That is, they may make a diagnosis certain enough for the expected benefits of treating the patient to outweigh the expected consequences of not treating them. This chapter focuses on systematic reviews of studies of diagnostic accuracy which describe the probabilistic relationships between positive and negative test results and the presence or absence of disease, and therefore indicate how well a test can separate diseased from non-diseased patients.

Rationale for undertaking systematic reviews of studies of test accuracy

Systematic reviews of tests are undertaken for the same reasons as systematic reviews of therapeutic interventions: to produce estimates of performance based on all available evidence, to evaluate the quality of published studies, and to account for variation in findings between studies.[4–7] Reviews of studies of diagnostic accuracy, in common with systematic reviews of randomised controlled trials, involve key stages of question definition, literature searching (see Chapter 4), evaluation of studies for eligibility and quality (see Chapter 5), data extraction and data synthesis (see Chapter 9 and Chapter 15). However, the details within many of the stages differ. In particular, the design of test accuracy evaluations differs from the design of studies that evaluate the effectiveness of treatments, which means that different criteria are needed when assessing study quality and the potential for bias. Additionally, each study reports a pair of related summary statistics (for example, sensitivity and specificity) rather than a single statistic, requiring alternative statistical methods for pooling study results.

Systematic reviews of randomised controlled trials are often justified on the grounds that they increase statistical power: by assimilating participants recruited to a series of trials they increase our ability to detect small but clinically important differences in outcomes between treated and control groups. Statistical power is rarely discussed in studies of diagnostic accuracy as they do not compare two groups, and they do not formally test hypotheses. However, increasing sample size by pooling the results of several studies does improve the precision of estimates of diagnostic performance. Whilst it has not been formally documented that individual studies of test performance are on average too small, informal reviews of the literature usually reveal that individual studies often estimate test sensitivity in particular, on the basis of a very small sample of cases, especially when the disease is rare. Pooling results across studies provides an opportunity to improve the precision of these estimates, and to investigate the consistency of test performance and compare results between studies of different designs and from different settings.

In this chapter I provide an overview of the most established methods and current issues in undertaking systematic reviews of diagnostic tests. Whilst the science of systematically reviewing studies of test accuracy is developing fast, the methods are less established than those for reviewing randomised controlled trials. I will highlight some deficiencies of current methodologies and knowledge that limit their usefulness and application.

Features of studies of test accuracy

Studies of test performance (or accuracy) compare test results between separate groups of patients with and without the target disease, each of whom undergoes the experimental test as well as a second "gold standard" reference test. The relationship between the test results and disease status is described using probabilistic measures, such as sensitivity, specificity and likelihood ratios. It is important that the results of the reference test are very close to the truth, or else the performance of the experimental test will be poorly estimated.[8] To achieve this, reference tests sometimes involve combining several pieces of information, undertaking invasive procedures, or following the patient for lengthy periods of time.

Summary measures of diagnostic accuracy

Sensitivity, specificity and likelihood ratios

Both the reference and experimental diagnostic tests may naturally report the result as a binary classification (disease present / disease absent). This allows the results to be presented in a 2×2 table, with individuals classified as true positives (TP) and true negatives (TP) (correct test results), or false positives (FP) and false negatives (FN) (incorrect test results). The standard summaries of sensitivity, specificity and likelihood ratios are calculated from the numbers of individuals classified as TP, TN, FP and FN, as shown in Box 14.1. Note that all these calculations are undertaken on the columns, and give the same results if the numbers of participants with the disease and the numbers without the disease within the study sample change. These values are therefore not *directly* affected by changes in the prevalence of the disease in the study sample.

In some circumstances the test under assessment will yield results as a set of ordered categories, perhaps derived from a continuous measurement. For example, the results of magnetic resonance imaging scans for detecting the presence of some anatomical feature may be reported as definitely positive, probably positive, unclear, probably negative or definitely negative. Sensitivity and specificity apply naturally only in situations where there are two categories of results, but can be calculated in these situations by select-ing a diagnostic threshold to define positive and negative test outcomes.[9] The results can then be presented in a 2×2 table combining categories above and below the threshold (for example, combining definitely and probably positive compared to combining unclear or definitely or probably negative). Different thresholds will produce different sensitivities and specificities. When several thresholds have been considered for a single set of data the diagnostic characteristics of the test can be illustrated graphically using a graph known as a receiver operating characteristic (ROC) plot of the true positive rate (sensitivity) against the false positive rate (1 – specificity). This plot is explained in detail in Box 14.2.

A likelihood ratio describes how many times a person with disease is more likely to receive a particular test result than a person without disease. Binary tests have two likelihood ratios: a positive likelihood ratio (LR +ve) (usually a number greater than one) and a negative likelihood ratio (LR –ve) (usually a number between zero and one).

A guide to using likelihood ratios in clinical practice suggests that positive likelihood ratios greater than 10 or negative likelihood ratios less than 0·1 can provide convincing diagnostic evidence, whilst those above 5 and below 0·2 give strong diagnostic evidence, although this depends on the pre-test probability and the context to which they are applied.[10]

Box 14.1 Calculation of sensitivity, specificity and likelihood ratios

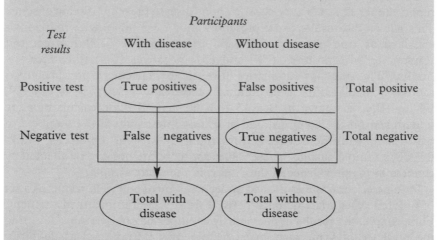

The sensitivity is the proportion of those with disease who have positive test results:

Sensitivity = number of true positives/total with disease

The specificity is the proportion of those without disease who have negative test results:

Specificity = number of true negatives/total without disease

The positive likelihood ratio is the ratio of the true positive rate to the false positive rate:

LR +ve = (number of true positives/total with disease)/
(number of false positives/total without disease)
LR +ve = sensitivity/(1 − specificity)

The negative likelihood ratio is the ratio of the false negative rate to the true negative rate:

LR −ve = (number of false negatives/total with disease)/
(number of true negatives/total without disease)
LR −ve = (1 − sensitivity)/specificity

Likelihood ratios can be applied in clinical practice to update an individual's estimated chances of disease according to their test result using Bayes' theorem[11]: the post-test odds that a patient has the disease are estimated by multiplying the pre-test odds by the likelihood ratio. Simple nomograms are available[1,3,12] for this calculation which avoid the need to convert probabilities to odds and *vice versa* (see Chapter 16 for a detailed explanation of the differences between odds and probabilities). Likelihood ratios are also a preferable measure of diagnostic performance when test results are reported in more than two categories, as they can be calculated separately for each category, making best use of all available diagnostic information.

Box 14.2 Receiver operating characteristic (ROC) curves

ROC curves are used to depict the patterns of sensitivities and specificities observed when the threshold at which results are classified as positive or negative changes. Figure 14.1 shows a ROC curve from a study of the detection of endometrial cancer by ultrasound measurement of endometrial thickness.[13] Women with endometrial cancer are likely to have increased endometrial thicknesses: very few women who do not have cancer will have thicknesses exceeding a high threshold whereas very few women with endometrial cancer will have thicknesses below a low threshold. This pattern of results is seen in the figure, with the 5 mm threshold demonstrating high sensitivity (0·98) and poor specificity (0·59), whilst the 25 mm threshold demonstrates poor sensitivity (0·24) but high specificity (0·98).

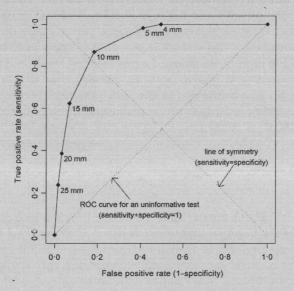

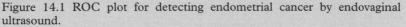

Figure 14.1 ROC plot for detecting endometrial cancer by endovaginal ultrasound.

The overall diagnostic performance of a test can be judged by the position of the ROC line. Poor tests have ROC lines close to the rising diagonal, whilst the ROC lines for perfect tests would rise steeply and pass close to the top left-hand corner, where both the sensitivity and specificity are 1. Later in the chapter I will consider the issue of whether ROC curves are symmetrical – this curve demonstrates reasonable reflective symmetry around the indicated line, but it is not perfectly symmetrical. This means that the overall diagnostic performance (the diagnostic odds ratio, see main text) varies somewhat according to the cutpoint chosen for endometrial thickness.

The diagnostic odds ratio

Summaries of diagnostic accuracy describe either how well the test works in those with the disease and those without (sensitivity and specificity), or the discriminatory properties of the positive and negative test results (positive and negative likelihood ratios). The ROC plot clearly demonstrated the trade-off for tests between high sensitivity and high specificity: a similar tension also exists between positive and negative likelihood ratios. These trade-offs are inconvenient when we consider how to combine the results, as the measurements within each pair are interdependent, and therefore cannot be considered separately. However, sensitivities and specificities, and positive and negative likelihood ratios, can be combined into the same single summary of diagnostic performance, known as the diagnostic odds ratio. This statistic is not easy to apply in clinical practice (it describes the ratio of the odds of a positive test result in a patient with disease compared to a patient without disease), but it is a convenient measure to use when combining studies in a systematic review as it is often reasonably constant regardless of the diagnostic threshold. The diagnostic odds ratio (DOR) is defined as:

$$DOR = \frac{TP \times TN}{FP \times FN},$$

where TP, TN, FP, FN are the numbers of true positive, true negative, false positive and false negative diagnoses, as denoted in the 2×2 table in Box 14.1. It is necessary to add a small quantity (typically 0·5) to the all four counts if any of them are zero before computing this statistic to avoid computational problems (see Chapter 15). Some authors advise doing this routinely to all studies.[5]

The diagnostic odds ratio can also be computed from the sensitivity and specificity or from the likelihood ratios as:

254

$$DOR = \frac{\left(\dfrac{sensitivity}{1 - sensitivity}\right)}{\left(\dfrac{1 - specificity}{specificity}\right)} = \frac{LR + ve}{LR - ve}$$

where $LR +ve$ is the likelihood ratio for a positive result, and $LR -ve$ is the likelihood ratio for a negative result. Examples of diagnostic odds ratios for different sensitivities, specificities, and positive and negative likelihood ratios are given in Table 14.1.

Note that when a test provides no diagnostic evidence (sensitivity + specificity = 1) the diagnostic odds ratio is 1, which corresponds to the rising diagonal in Figure 14.1. Considering diagnostic odds ratios that correspond to Jaeschke's guides[10] for convincing and strong diagnostic evidence gives a gauge to values of the DOR which could be usefully high. A DOR of 25 could for example, correspond to a positive likelihood ratio of 5 and negative likelihood ratio of 0·2, whilst a DOR of 100 may correspond to a positive likelihood ratio of 10 and a negative likelihood ratio of 0·1, if both criteria are met in the same test. For the data in Figure 14.1, the DORs for the cutpoints of 25 mm, 20 mm, 15 mm and 10 mm are 19, 19, 22, and 29 respectively, around Jaeschke's values for strong diagnostic evidence.

Table 14.1 Examples of diagnostic odds ratios.

Sensitivity	Specificity	LR +ve	LR −ve	Diagnostic OR
0·50	0·50	1·0	1·00	1·0
0·60	0·60	1·5	0·67	2·3
0·70	0·70	2·3	0·43	5·4
0·80	0·80	4·0	0·25	16·0
0·90	0·90	9·0	0·11	81·0
0·95	0·95	19·0	0·05	361·0
0·99	0·99	99·0	0·01	9801·0
0·90	0·60	2·3	0·17	13·5
0·90	0·70	3·0	0·14	21·0
0·90	0·80	4·5	0·13	36·0
0·95	0·60	2·4	0·08	28·5
0·95	0·70	3·2	0·07	44·3
0·95	0·80	4·8	0·06	76·0
0·95	0·90	9·5	0·06	171·0
0·99	0·60	2·5	0·02	148·5
0·99	0·70	3·3	0·01	231·0
0·99	0·80	5·0	0·01	396·0
0·99	0·90	9·9	0·01	891·0
0·99	0·95	19·8	0·01	1881·0

It is important to note that whilst the diagnostic odds ratio summarises the results into a single number, crucial information contained in sensitivity and specificity or in likelihood ratios is discarded. Notably, it cannot distinguish between tests with high sensitivity and low specificity and tests with low sensitivity and high specificity. For example, the DOR for a test with a sensitivity of 0·90 and specificity of 0·60 is exactly the same as the DOR for a test with sensitivity 0·60 and specificity 0·90.

Predictive values

A fourth set of measures of diagnostic performance, predictive values, describe the probabilities that positive or negative test results are correct, and are calculated as indicated in Box 14.3. Note that in contrast to the calculations in Box 14.1, the calculations of predictive values are undertaken on the rows of the 2×2 table, and therefore do depend on the prevalence of the disease in the study sample. The more common a disease is, the more likely it is that a positive result is right and a negative result is wrong. Whilst clinicians often consider predictive values to be the most useful measures of diagnostic performance when interpreting the test results of a single patient, they are rarely used in systematic reviews. Disease prevalence is rarely constant across studies included in a systematic review, so there is often an unacceptably high level of heterogeneity among positive and negative predictive values, making them unsuitable choices of effect measures. There is an analogy here with the estimation of risk differences in systematic reviews of RCTs (Chapter 16), which are the easiest summary statistics to understand and apply, but are rarely the summary of choice for a meta-analysis as they are commonly heterogeneous across trials.

However, predictive values can be estimated indirectly from the results of systematic reviews. The predictive values of a test can be thought of as post-test probabilities, and hence estimated from summary likelihood ratios by application of Bayes' Theorem[11] as described previously. In this situation the pre-test probability is estimated by the population prevalence: application of the positive likelihood ratio yields the positive predictive value. The negative predictive value can be calculated by application of the negative likelihood ratio, and subtracting the resulting post-test probability from one.

Systematic reviews of studies of diagnostic accuracy

There are three major ways in which systematically reviewing studies of diagnostic accuracy differs from reviewing therapeutic interventions: the

Box 14.3 Calculation of positive and negative predictive values

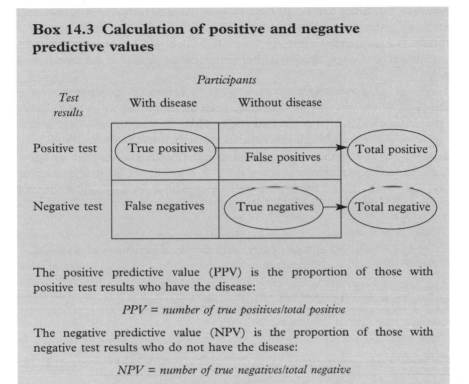

The positive predictive value (PPV) is the proportion of those with positive test results who have the disease:

PPV = number of true positives/total positive

The negative predictive value (NPV) is the proportion of those with negative test results who do not have the disease:

NPV = number of true negatives/total negative

choice of search terms for electronic literature searches, the criteria for the assessment of study quality, and the methods for the statistical combination of results.

Literature searching

The identification of studies for a systematic review typically involves undertaking both electronic and manual searches. The manual searches may include hand-searching key or or unindexed journals, reviewing reference lists and bibliographies, and contacting experts (see Chapter 5). This process is no different for systematic reviews of diagnostic accuracy than for reviews of randomised controlled trials.

However, electronic database searches for studies of diagnostic accuracy can be more difficult and less productive than those for randomised trials. Occasionally a simple search using just the test name will prove to be sensitive, but many diagnostic technologies (such as ultrasound, x rays, and serology tests) are used across a variety of fields in medicine, so that a mixture of appropriate and inappropriate studies will be retrieved, and the search will not be specific. Including terms for the disease in the search may help.

Names of diagnostic tests may also be routinely mentioned in the abstracts of studies of other designs, such as in the descriptions of entry criteria for randomised controlled trials. This can lead to searches retrieving large numbers of irrelevant studies. Research has been undertaken to develop methodological search filters to identify the studies that are most likely to consider diagnostic accuracy.[14,15] A summary of the indexing terms and text-words that have been found to be useful for locating studies of diagnostic accuracy is given in Table 14.2.

Table 14.2 Useful MEDLINE search terms for detecting studies of diagnostic accuracy.[14,15]

Useful subject headings (MeSH terms)
Explode "SENSITIVITY-AND-SPECIFICITY"/ all subheadings
Explode "MASS-SCREENING"
"PREDICTIVE-VALUE-OF-TESTS"
"ROC-CURVE"

Textwords

Specificit*	Sensitivit*
False negative*	Predictive value*
Accuracy	Likelihood ratio*
Screening	

Sub-headings
Sub-headings are used with other subject headings to limit the type of articles retrieved. The sub-heading /*diagnostic use* can be added to names of agents, investigations, etc. to restrict the findings to those mentioning using the agent or investigation for diagnostic purposes. Similarly the subheading /*diagnosis* can be added to names of diseases to identify articles on those diseases associated with diagnosis, likewise the subheading /*pathology*. However the rigor with which subheadings are applied in the indexing of medical journals is unclear.

The indexing term "sensitivity-and-specificity" appears to be the most appropriate for these studies, but it is inconsistently used and insensitive. The alternative MeSH term "diagnosis" includes a whole tree of additional terms and consequently has low specificity. The term "diagnosis" can more usefully be used as a subheading added to a disease term to limit a search to articles concerning the diagnosis of the particular disease. The increased use of words like "sensitivity", "specificity", "predictive value" and "likelihood ratio" in reporting results also make them useful candidates for textwords to include in a methodological filter.

Assessment of study quality

Selection of study sample

The ideal study sample for inclusion in a review is a consecutive (or randomly selected) series of patients recruited from a relevant clinical population. Selection bias may be introduced by selecting patients for inclusion in a non-random manner. This can present as a form of spectrum bias (see below) that arises whenever the study population is not representative of the spectrum of diseases within which the test will be applied in practice.[16]

In practice it is often easier to recruit patients with out or without disease as separate groups, as in a case-control study. This can lead to bias, however, as detection rates vary according to the severity of disease, and the chances of receiving a falsely positive diagnosis will vary between patients according to the the alternative diseases that they do have. Choosing cases that have already been identified as having the disease will introduce bias into the estimates of test sensitivity, choosing controls that are completely healthy will introduce bias into the estimates of test specificity. For example, Table 14.3 shows for hypothetical data sensitivities for three stages of disease ("early", "intermediate", "advanced") and in Table 14.4 specificities for two alternative diseases within the differential diagnosis (alternative "X" and alternative "Y") as well as for healthy subjects. A case-control design may sample cases solely from those with "intermediate" and "advanced" disease. This gives very high estimates of sensitivity: much higher than those observed in the general practice and hospital samples that contain a more typical mixture of patients. Similarly, use of a group of healthy controls gives artificially high estimates of specificity, higher than those which will be encountered in practice where some of the patients on whom the test will be used are not healthy but actually have other routinely encountered diseases.

Table 14.3 Effect of spectrum bias on sensitivity.

Disease grade	Sensitivity	Spectrum of disease		
		Cases in case–control study (n = 100)	General practice (n = 100)	Hospital (n = 100)
Early	0·50	0	80	20
Intermediate	0·75	20	15	30
Advanced	1·00	80	5	50
Observed sensitivity		0·95	0·56	0·83

259

Table 14.4 Effect of spectrum bias on specificity.

Disease	Specificity	Spectrum of alternative diagnoses		
		Controls in case–control study (n = 100)	General practice (n = 100)	Hospital (n = 100)
Alternative "X"	0·30	0	30	75
Alternative "Y"	0·95	0	65	25
Healthy adults	0·99	100	5	0
Observed specificity		0·99	0·76	0·46

As well as being selected in the correct manner, it is also important that the study samples are selected from similar healthcare settings. This is more a matter of the applicability of a study rather than study quality. Importantly, it is possible that the spectrum of disease and alternative diagnoses varies between different points in the health care referral process, such as between primary and secondary care. To illustrate this point, consider the hypothetical data in Table 14.3 and Table 14.4 again. The general practice sample relates to a point early in the referral process where the majority of diseased patients have early disease, or an alternative condition "Y". The hospital sample is more typical of a secondary care stage of the referral process where there are many more patients with advanced disease, and fewer with the alternative condition "Y" (who may have been treated in primary care or referred elsewhere). As the sensitivity and specificity are not constant across the spectrum of disease or across the alternative conditions, the observed values of test sensitivity and specificity in the two samples differ. This variation has nothing directly to do with disease prevalence within the study group: although it is likely that the prevalence of the disease will also differ between points in a referral process, the observed sensitivity and specificity will only change if the proportionate mix of the spectrum of diseased and non-diseased patients varies as well. Variation in prevalence may be a hint of the presence of spectrum bias, but it is not its cause.

Ascertainment of reference diagnosis

The selection of a good reference standard is crucial. Typically the reference standard is considered a "gold standard", and the comparison is one-sided: if there are any disagreements between the reference standard and the experimental test it is always assumed that the experimental test is incorrect.

It is important that the two tests are based on independent measurements. In some circumstances the reference diagnosis may be made on the basis of a battery of clinical tests and other available clinical evidence. If this is the case, the battery of results should not include the experimental test result, or else diagnostic accuracy will most likely be overestimated. Such an effect is known as *incorporation bias*.[16]

Verification bias is a problem when the decision to undertake the reference investigation is influenced by the result of the experimental test or other factors which indicate that the disease is unlikely,[17] as clinicians are often hesitant in using an invasive test in these circumstances. There are two levels of incomplete verification: *partial verification* where not all participants undergo the reference investigation, and *differential verification* where different reference tests are used according to the results of the experimental test. Partial verification bias usually leads to the numbers of true negative and false negative participants being reduced, so that sensitivity is biased upwards and specificity biased downwards. In contrast, differential verification bias may lead to both estimates being biased upwards.

Blinding

Blinding involves each test being undertaken and interpreted without knowledge of the result of the other. This is especially important for tests that involve subjective judgements, such as those that rely on human perceptions in interpreting images and sounds.

Other aspects of design

Another important aspect of quality is whether both diagnostic tests were undertaken before any treatment was started. Where this does not occur a *treatment paradox* can be introduced: patients who are diagnosed with the disease at the first test can be treated and cured before the second test, and misclassified as false positives or false negatives depending on which test was used first.[18]

Inclusion of the test results of all participants in the analysis is important. Many tests report some results as being in a *grey-zone*, or occasionally as *test failures*. Although including these outcomes in an analysis is not always straightforward, ignoring them will present a test more favourably than is justified.

Aspects of the quality of reporting

Ideally a study report should include clear descriptions of the reference and experimental tests, with definitions of positive and negative outcomes for both, and descriptions of demographic characteristics, co-morbidities, the source and referral history of the patients.

261

Empirical evidence of bias

Lijmer *et al.* have recently undertaken an empirical study to evaluate which of these particular aspects of design and execution are of most importance.[19] They analysed the results of 218 test evaluations from 18 separate meta-analyses to determine which features of studies of diagnostic accuracy alter the observed diagnostic performance. A full summary of their results is given in Table 14.5. The relative diagnostic odds ratios describe how many times greater the diagnostic odds ratio was for studies with the characteristic: relative diagnostic odds ratios greater than one therefore indicate increases in observed diagnostic accuracy.

Table 14.5 Impact of aspects of study quality on diagnostic odds ratios.[19]

Feature	Relative diagnostic odds ratios (95% CI)
Case–control design rather than clinical cohort	3·0 (2·0 to 4·5)
Different reference tests according to test result	2·2 (1·5 to 3·3)
Partial verification of cases	1·0 (0·8 to 1·3)
Assessors not blinded	1·3 (1·0 to 1·9)
Cases were non-consecutive	0·9 (0·7 to 1·1)
Retrospective study design	1·0 (0·7 to 1·4)
No description of the test	1·7 (1·1 to 2·5)
No description of the population	1·4 (1·1 to 1·7)
No description of the reference test	0·7 (0·6 to 0·9)

Their study provided evidence that case-control study designs over-estimated diagnostic accuracy and that this was the greatest potential source of bias, although very few of the studies included in their analysis were of this design. Studies using differential reference standards were also found to overestimate diagnostic performance compared to those using the same reference standard for both, whilst partial verification did not introduce a consistent effect. Unblinded studies were on average more likely to overestimate diagnostic accuracy.

Lijmer *et al.* also noted that the omission of reporting specific details of a study was associated with systematic differences in results.

Incorporation of quality assessments in a systematic review

Several authors have developed checklists for assessing the quality of a diagnostic accuracy evaluation[6,7,20-22] although not all of these have been designed specifically for use in a systematic review. However, these check-lists were developed prior to Lijmer's empirical evaluation of aspects of quality, and may require updating and consolidating.

To be reliable, a systematic review should aim to include only studies of the highest scientific quality, as assessed according to the criteria listed above. Systematic reviews should aim either to exclude studies which do not meet these criteria and are susceptible to bias, or alternatively to include studies with a mixture of quality characteristics and explore the differences.[5,7] Whichever approach is adopted, it is essential that the quality of the studies included in the review is assessed and reported, so that appropriately cautious inferences can be drawn.

Meta-analysis of studies of diagnostic accuracy

As with systematic reviews of RCTs it is not essential that every systematic review of studies of diagnostic accuracy includes a meta-analysis. Meta-analysis should only be considered when the studies have recruited from clinically similar populations, used comparable experimental and reference tests, and are unlikely to be biased. Even when these criteria are met there may still be such gross heterogeneity between the results of the studies that it is inappropriate to summarise the performance of a test as a single number.

Meta-analysis is a two-stage process, involving the derivation of a single summary statistic for each study, and then computation of a weighted average of the summary statistics across the studies (see Chapter 15). Three general approaches commonly used to pool results of studies of diagnostic accuracy that are described below. The selection of a method depends on the choice of a summary statistic, and potential causes of heterogeneity.

Sources of heterogeneity: importance of the diagnostic threshold

The choice of statistical method for combining study results depends on the pattern of heterogeneity observed between the results of the studies. The degree of variability between study results should first be considered graphically by plotting the sensitivity and specificity from each study on a ROC plot. Some divergence of the study results is to be expected by chance, but variation in other factors, such as patient selection and features of study design may increase the observed variability or heterogeneity,[23] as they do for randomised controlled trials (see Chapter 9).

There is also one important extra source of variation to consider in meta-analyses of diagnostic accuracy: variation introduced by changes in diagnostic threshold. The studies included in a systematic review may have used different thresholds to define positive and negative test results. Some may have done this explicitly, for example by varying numerical cut-points used to classify a biochemical measurement as positive or negative. For others there may be naturally occurring variations in diagnostic thresholds between observers or between laboratories. The choice of a threshold may

also have been determined according to the prevalence of the disease –
when the disease is rare a low threshold may have been used to avoid large
numbers of false positive diagnoses being made. Unlike random variability
and other sources of heterogeneity, varying the diagnostic threshold
between studies introduces a particular pattern into the ROC plot of study
results. If such variation is present, the points will demonstrate curvature
that parallels the underlying ROC curve for that test, such as is illustrated
in Figure 14.1. The approach to combining studies in these situations
involves deriving the best-fitting ROC curve rather than summarising the
results as a single point. As explained below, there is a simple method to do
this that assumes that the ROC curve is symmetrical around the "sensitivity
= specificity" line, and another method for more complex situations where
the curve is asymmetrical. Examples of symmetrical and asymmetrical
ROC curves are given later in the chapter in Figures 14.6(b) and 14.6(d)
respectively.

> **Case study: Ruling out endometrial cancer with transvaginal ultrasound**
>
> Endovaginal ultrasound (EVUS) is a non-invasive diagnostic test
> which can be used to investigate causes of postmenopausal vaginal
> bleeding, one of which is endometrial cancer. Smith-Bindman *et al.*
> published a systematic review of 35 studies evaluating the diagnostic
> accuracy of EVUS for endometrial cancer and other endometrial
> disorders.[24] All studies included in the review were of prospective
> cohort designs, and used the results of endometrial biopsy, dilation
> and curettage, or hysterectomy as a reference standard. Most of the
> studies presented sensitivities and specificities at several EVUS thick-
> nesses (the ROC curve in Figure 14.1 is in fact from one of these
> studies): the authors of the review present separate analyses for each
> EVUS thickness. Using this case study I will illustrate the various
> methods of meta-analysis as they are described below, using the
> subset of 20 studies from this review that consider the diagnostic
> performance of ultrasound measurements of less than 5 mm in ruling
> out a diagnosis of endometrial cancer.

Pooling sensitivities and specificities

The simplest method of combining studies of diagnostic accuracy is to
compute weighted averages of the sensitivities, specificities or likelihood

ratios. This method can should only be applied in the absence of variability of the diagnostic threshold. The possibility of a threshold effect can be investigated before this method is used, both graphically by plotting the study results on an ROC plot, and statistically, by undertaking tests of the heterogeneity of sensitivities and specificities and investigating whether there is a relationship between them.[25] The homogeneity of the sensitivities and specificities from the studies can be tested using standard chi-squared tests as both measures are simple proportions. Calculation of the correlation coefficient between sensitivities and specificities will test whether they are related, as would be the case if there was variation in the diagnostic threshold. If an association between the sensitivities and specificities is detected, use of weighted averages will lead to underestimation of diagnostic performance, as the point corresponding to the average of the sensitivities and the average of the specificities always falls below the ROC curve.[26] As an illustration of the error which could arise if a trade-off relationship is ignored, consider averaging the six numbered points in Figure 14.1. This gives a sensitivity of 0·67 and a specificity of 0·78, which falls below the curve and is therefore a poor summary. Note that when the studies in the systematic reviews have small sample sizes, tests for heterogeneity and correlation have low statistical power, and therefore a threshold related effect may exist but remain undetected by the statistical tests.[26]

Computation of an average sensitivity and specificity is straightforward. Considering the sensitivity and specificity in each study i to be denoted as a proportion p_i,

$$p_i = \frac{y_i}{n_i}; \; sensitivity_i = \frac{true\ positives_i}{all\ with\ disease_i}; \; specificity_i = \frac{true\ negatives_i}{all\ without\ disease_i}.$$

Using an approximation to the inverse variance approach (effectively weighting each study according to its sample size) (see Chapter 15), the estimate of the overall proportion is

$$p = \frac{\sum y_i}{\sum n_i}$$

where $\sum y_i$ is the sum of all true positives (for sensitivity) or true negatives (for specificity), and $\sum n_i$ is the sum of diseased (for sensitivity) or not diseased (for specificity). The large sample approximation for the standard error of this estimate is:

$$SE(p) = \sqrt{\frac{p(1-p)}{\sum n_i}}.$$

More complex statistical methods, such as bootstrapping, can be used to compute confidence intervals when samples are small, or when the sensitivity or specificity is close to 1.[27,28]

Case study (continued): Pooling sensitivities and specificities

Sensitivities and specificities for the 20 studies are presented in Figure 14.2. From the graph it appears that the sensitivities are relatively homogenous (nearly all of the confidence intervals overlap) whereas it is clearly evident that the specificities are grossly heterogeneous.

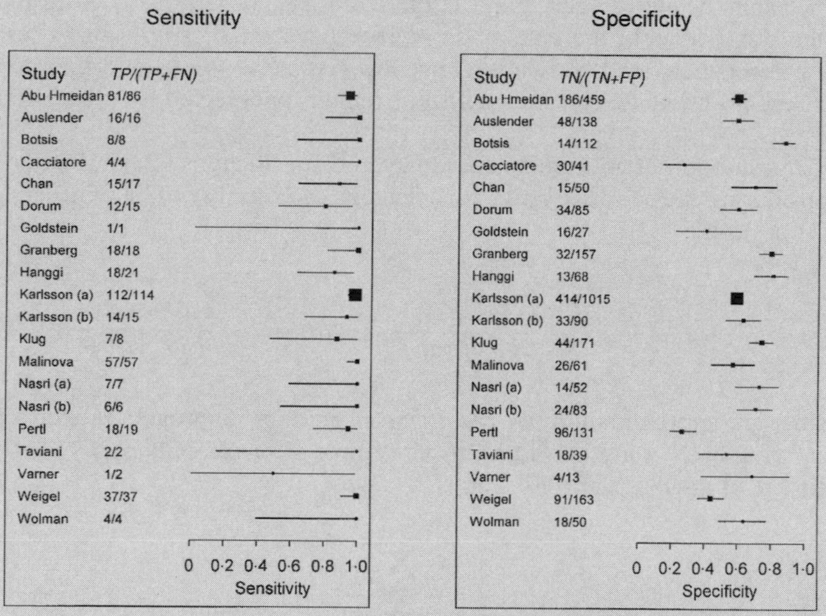

Figure 14.2 Estimates from 20 studies of the sensitivity and specificity of a 5 mm cutpoint for detecting endometrial cancer by endovaginal ultrasound.

The simplest analysis pools the estimates of sensitivity and specificity separately across the studies, but is only appropriate if there is no variation in diagnostic threshold. Even though all these studies claimed to use a cutpoint of endometrial thicknesses of 5 mm, it is still possible for unobserved variation in diagnostic threshold to occur through differences in machine calibration and measurement technique. We can crudely test for a threshold effect by computing the correlation between sensitivities and specificities across the 20 studies. Where sensitivities and specificities are not normally distributed a non-parametric correlation is preferable: for these data Spearman's rho is estimated to be 0·14, which is not statistically significant (P=0·6).

Sensitivity

Using the formulae given above, estimates of the pooled sensitivity and its standard error are:

$$p = \frac{\sum y_i}{\sum n_i} = \frac{438}{457} = 0\cdot958;$$

$$SE(p) = \sqrt{\frac{p(1-p)}{\sum n_i}} = \sqrt{\frac{0\cdot958 \times 0\cdot042}{457}} = 0\cdot009,$$

yielding an overall sensitivity (95% CI) of 0·958 (0·928 to 0·977).

Using a chi-squared test to check homogeneity of sensitivities across the studies is difficult as the assumption of minimum expected frequencies for a chi-squared test is not met (many of studies have expected values of less that 5 for the number of false negatives) and computation of Fisher's exact test on a 2×20 table is not computationally trivial. An alternative likelihood ratio test gives a chi-squared value of 31·2 on 19 degrees of freedom (P=0·04). Whilst this is formally statistically significant, the degree of heterogeneity between the results is small, with only one of the twenty studies (Dorum) not including the overall value within its confidence interval. The horizontal line on the ROC plot in Figure 14.3 corresponds to this summary estimate and lies reasonably close to the majority of the studies. The overall estimate for sensitivity of 0·958 therefore seems to be a reasonable summary, and we can conclude that the test has suitably high sensitivity for use in detecting endometrial cancer.

Specificity

Following the same calculations as for the sensitivities the overall estimate of mean specificity (95% CI) is 0·608 (0·590 to 0·626). However, a chi-squared test confirms the statistical significance of the heterogeneity observed in Figure 14.2 (χ^2=201, df=19, P<0·001). The extra uncertainty arising through the between study variation can be incorporated by use of a logistic model with adjustment to account for overdispersion.[29] This produces a confidence interval of (0·549 to 0·664), more than 3 times as wide as the original estimate. The large between study heterogeneity is clearly evident in Figure 14.3, with the results of many of the studies lying some distance from the summary specificity. In such a situation it is probably inappropriate to consider pooling specificities at all, and it may be best to note the heterogeneity by describing the range [0·267 to 0·875] between which the specificities were seen to vary.

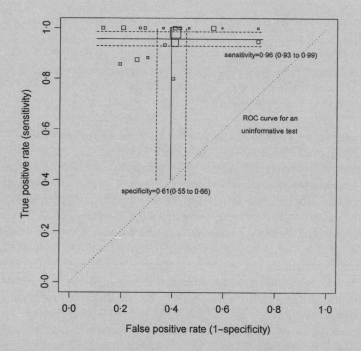

Figure 14.3 Summary sensitivity and specificity (with 95% CI) for a 5 mm cutpoint.

Pooling likelihood ratios

Likelihood ratios are ratios of probabilities, and in a meta-analysis can be treated as risk ratios (albeit calculated between the columns of a 2×2 table and not the rows as for RCTs).[30] A weighted average of the likelihood ratios can be computed using the standard Mantel-Haenszel or inverse variance methods of meta-analysis of risk ratios outlined in Chapter 15. The heterogeneity of likelihood ratios can also be tested by standard heterogeneity tests after combining the statistics in a meta-analysis.

Case study (continued): Pooling likelihood ratios

Likelihood ratios can be estimated either from the summary estimates of sensitivity and specificity:

$$LR + ve = \frac{sensitivity}{1 - specificity} = \frac{0 \cdot 958}{1 - 0 \cdot 608} = 2 \cdot 44;$$

$$LR - ve = \frac{1 - sensitivity}{specificity} = \frac{1 - 0 \cdot 958}{0 \cdot 608} = 0 \cdot 07,$$

or by pooling likelihood ratios calculated for each study using risk ratio methods of meta-analysis (see Chapter 15). The pooling method is preferable as it allows the investigation of heterogeneity in likelihood ratios between the studies and does not use the unreliable estimate of specificity computed above.

Combining positive likelihood ratios using the Mantel-Haenszel method yields an overall estimate (95% CI) of 2·38 (2·26 to 2·51). However, as with the specificities, there is significant heterogeneity in positive likelihood ratios between studies (Cochran's Q=187, df=19, P<0.001), and the estimate of 2·38 is outside the 95% confidence intervals of 8 of the 20 studies. The between study variation can be incorporated using a DerSimonian and Laird random effects model (positive LR (95% CI): 2·54 (2·16 to 2·98)) but again it is debatable whether combining such heterogeneous results is sensible. In Figure 14.4 it is quite clear that the summary positive likelihood ratio lies some distance from many of the study values. However, regardless of whether a formal pooled estimate of the likelihood ratio is presented, it is evident from the values of the positive likelihood ratios across the studies (they are all well below 10) that a positive test result cannot provide convincing evidence of the presence of endometrial cancer.

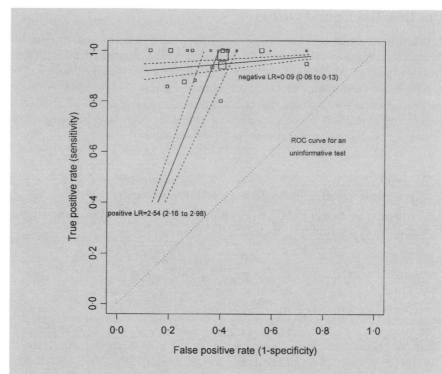

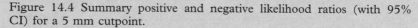

Figure 14.4 Summary positive and negative likelihood ratios (with 95% CI) for a 5 mm cutpoint.

The negative likelihood ratios show no evidence of significant heterogeneity (Cochran's $Q=27\cdot9$, $df=19$, $P=0\cdot09$), the Mantel-Haenszel pooled estimate (95% CI) being $0\cdot09$ ($0\cdot06$ to $0\cdot13$), and the summary line on the ROC plot in Figure 14.4 lying close to most of the study results. This finding is very useful as it shows that an EVUS measurement of less than 5 mm can provide reasonably convincing evidence that rule outs endometrial cancer. The probability of endometrial cancer in a woman with a EVUS less than 5 mm depends on the local prevalence of endometrial cancer among women presenting with postmenopausal vaginal bleeding. Taking the average prevalence across the 20 studies of 13% and applying Bayes' theorem[1,3,11] we can estimate that only $1\cdot3\%$ of women with an EVUS measurement <5 mm will have endometrial cancer as follows:

$$\text{pre-test odds} = \frac{prevalence}{1 - prevalence} = \frac{0\cdot13}{0\cdot87} = 0\cdot15$$

$$\text{post-test odds} = \text{pre-test odds} \times \text{negative likelihood ratio} = 0\cdot15 \times 0\cdot09 = 0\cdot014$$

$$\text{post-test probability} = \frac{post\text{-}test\ odds}{1 + post\text{-}test\ odds} = \frac{0\cdot014}{0 + 1.014} = 0\cdot013$$

For the particular clinical example, pooling of likelihood ratios probably provides the most crucial clinical summary information from these studies

Combining symmetric ROC curves: pooling diagnostic odds ratios

If there is any evidence that the diagnostic threshold varies between the studies, the best summary of the results of the studies will be an ROC curve rather than a single point. The full method for deciding on the best fitting summary ROC is explained below, but first it is worth noting that a simple method for estimating a summary ROC curve exists when it can be assumed that the curve is symmetrical around the "sensitivity = specificity" line.

Diagnostic tests where the diagnostic odds ratio is constant regardless of the diagnostic threshold have symmetrical ROC curves. In these situations it is possible to use standard meta-analysis methods for combining odds ratios (see Chapter 15) to estimate the common diagnostic odds ratio, and hence to determine the best-fitting ROC curve.[26,31,32] Once the summary odds ratio, *DOR*, has been calculated the equation of the corresponding ROC curve is given by:

$$sensitivity = \frac{1}{1 + \dfrac{1}{DOR \times \left(\dfrac{1 - specificity}{specificity}\right)}}.$$

Methods of testing whether the data can be summarised using a symmetrical ROC curve are described below.

271

Case study (continued): Pooling diagnostic odds ratios

A model which assumes constant diagnostic odds ratios regardless of diagnostic threshold corresponds to a summary ROC curve that is symmetrical about a descending diagonal line where sensitivity equals specificity. As the sensitivities of all 20 studies are higher than the specificities, the results of all 20 studies lie above this diagonal line in the ROC plot. A symmetrical summary ROC line is tenable in this situation.

Computing a summary diagnostic odds ratio using the Mantel-Haenszel method for pooling odds ratios (see Chapter 15) yields an estimate (95% CI) of 28·0 (18·2 to 43·2). There was no evidence of gross heterogeneity (Cochran's Q=22·0, df=19, P=0·3), so this diagnostic odds ratio appears to be a reasonably consistent summary measure of diagnostic performance across the studies. The diagnostic odds ratio can be interpreted in terms of sensitivities and specificities by consulting the figures in Table 14.1 (which suggests that a DOR of 28·5 would occur if sensitivity=0·95 and specificity=0·60) or by plotting the summary ROC curve, as is done in Figure 14.5.

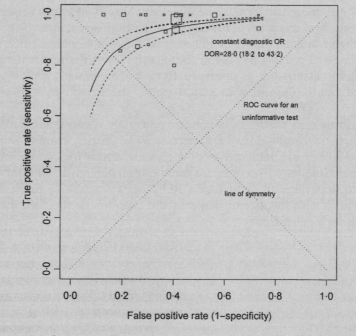

Figure 14.5 Summary diagnostic odds ratio (with 95% CI) for a 5 mm cutpoint.

> However, there is no unique joint summary estimate of sensitivity and specificity: it is only possible to obtain a summary estimate of one value conditional on the value of the other.

Littenberg and Moses methods for estimation of summary ROC curves

Asymmetrical ROC curves occur when the diagnostic odds ratio changes with diagnostic threshold. Littenberg and Moses proposed a method for fitting a whole family of summary ROC curves which allow for variation in DOR with threshold.[31,33] The method considers the relationship between the DOR and a summary measure of diagnostic threshold, given by the product of the odds of true positive and the odds of false positive results. As a diagnostic threshold decreases, the numbers of positive diagnoses (both correct and incorrect) increases, and the measure of threshold increases.

In the equations and figures which follow the logarithm of the diagnostic odds ratio is denoted by D, and the logarithm of the measure of threshold by S. D and S can be calculated (from the true positive rate (TPR) and false positive rate (FPR)) using any of the following equations:

$$S = \ln \left(\frac{TPR}{(1-TPR)} \times \frac{FPR}{(1-FPR)} \right) = \text{logit } (TPR) + \text{logit } (FPR)$$

$$D = \ln (DOR) = \ln \left(\frac{TPR}{(1-TPR)} \times \frac{(1-FPR)}{FPR} \right) = \ln \left(\frac{LR + ve}{LR - ve} \right) = \text{logit } (TPR) - \text{logit } (FPR)$$

(where the *logit* indicates the *log of the odds*, as used in logistic regression).

Littenberg and Moses' method first considers a plot of the log of the diagnostic odds ratio (D) against the measure of threshold (S) calculated for each of the studies. They then propose computing the best fitting straight line through the points on the graph. If the equation of the fitted line is given by:

$$D = a + bS$$

testing the significance of the estimate of the slope parameter b tests whether there is significant variation in diagnostic performance with threshold. If the line can be assumed horizontal (as illustrated in Figure 14.6(a)), the diagnostic odds ratio does not change with threshold, and the

273

method yields symmetrical ROC curves (as shown in Figure 14.6(b)), similar to those obtained from directly pooling odds ratios as explained above. However, if there is a significant trend in the diagnostic odds ratio with diagnostic threshold (as is the case in Figure 14.6(c)) then ROC curves are asymmetrical (as shown in Figure 14.6(d)), the summary ROC curve being calculated as:

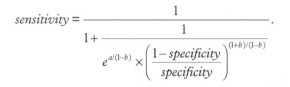

$$ sensitivity = \cfrac{1}{1 + \cfrac{1}{e^{a/(1-b)} \times \left(\cfrac{1 - specificity}{specificity} \right)^{(1+b)/(1-b)}}}. $$

(a) D vs S plot for constant odds ratios   (b) Summary ROC curve for constant odds ratios

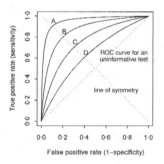

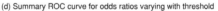

(c) D vs S plot for odds ratios varying with threshold   (d) Summary ROC curve for odds ratios varying with threshold

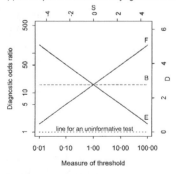

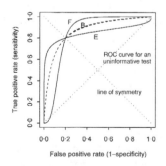

Figure 14.6 Littenberg–Moses plots and corresponding ROC curves with constant DOR (a) and (b), and DOR varying with diagnostic threshold (c) and (d).

274

Estimates of the parameters a and b can be obtained from either ordinary least squares regression (which weights each study equally), weighted least squares regression (where the weights can be taken as the inverse variance weights of the diagnostic log odds ratio, or simply the sample size) or robust methods of regression (which are not so strongly influenced by outliers).[26]

Expositions of this method most commonly formulate it in terms of the *logits* of the true positive and false positive rates.[4,5,31,33] As shown in the equations above the log of the diagnostic odds ratio is in fact the difference of these logits, whilst the log of the measure of diagnostic threshold is the sum of these logits. Hence the choice of notation: D for the difference, and S for the sum.

Case study (continued): Calculating a summary ROC curve

An alternative summary ROC curve allowing for variation in diagnostic odds ratio with diagnostic threshold can be estimated by the method of Moses and Littenberg.[31] First, the log of the diagnostic odds ratio, D, and the measure of diagnostic threshold, S, are computed for each study. Regression of the log diagnostic odds ratio (D) on the measure of diagnostic threshold (S), weighting by study size, produces estimates of the parameters a and b from the regression equation, $D = a + bS$. The parameter estimates are as follows:

Parameter	Estimate	SE	95% CI	P value
a	2·701	0·524	(1·600 to 3·801)	<0·001
b	0·359	0·174	(−0·006 to 0·724)	0·054

These results suggest that there is weak evidence (P=0·054) that the diagnostic odds ratio changes with threshold. To illustrate the impact of this, compare the ROC curve corresponding to this regression equation given in Figure 14.7, with the symmetric curve of Figure 14.5. The values of sensitivity and specificity are similar in the middle of the range of values of the observed studies, but differ at higher and lower specificities. Again the method does not provide a unique joint summary estimate of sensitivity and specificity suitable for use in clinical practice.

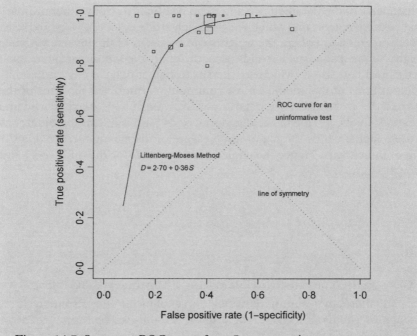

Figure 14.7 Summary ROC curve for a 5 mm cutpoint.

Investigation of sources of heterogeneity

Differences between studies in patient groups, test execution and study design can introduce variability in diagnostic odds ratios.[23] Both methods of pooling odds ratios can be extended to investigate the possible importance of these features. If it can be assumed that the summary ROC curves are symmetrical, the impact of other factors can be investigated using standard methods of meta-regression for odds ratios (see Chapter 9). Alternatively, the Littenberg–Moses regression method can be extended by adding a covariate to the regression equation for each potential effect modifier.[23,31] The exponential of each of these terms estimates multiplicative increases in diagnostic odds ratios for each factor. Lijmer *et al.* used this approach to investigate the effects of aspects of study quality on diagnostic odds ratios as reported in Table 14.5.[19]

Pooling ROC curves

All the methods described above consider the situation where each study provides estimates of sensitivity and specificity at one diagnostic threshold.

276

Case study (continued): Investigating sources of heterogeneity

Several of the studies include women who were receiving hormone replacement therapy (HRT). The Littenberg–Moses summary ROC curve method can investigate whether the diagnostic accuracy of EVUS is similar in studies that did or did not include women receiving HRT. A hypothesis of equal diagnostic odds ratios can be tested formally by adding a term to the weighted regression indicating which studies included women receiving HRT:

$$D = a + bS + cHRT,$$

where HRT is 1 for the studies including women receiving HRT and 0 otherwise. The estimates of the parameters a, b and c are now:

Parameter	Estimate	SE	95% CI	P value
a	2·684	0·697	(1·213 to 4·156)	0·001
b	0·362	0·198	(−0·056 to 0·781)	0·085
c	0·017	0·476	(−0·989 to 1·021)	0·971

There is no evidence that the diagnostic odds ratio is any different in the subset of studies which included women receiving HRT (P=0·97).

Occasionally, individual studies will publish ROC curves, or data from which they can be constructed. To undertake a meta-analysis of such data using the methods outlined above it is possible (a) to pool data separately for each cutpoint or (b) to fit a summary ROC curve through all the published data points (allowing multiple points per study). Neither of these approaches seems entirely satisfactory as they both involve multiple analyses of the same data.

One alternative is to compute *area under the curve* (AUC) statistics from the ROC plot[34] which summarise the diagnostic power as a single number which can be pooled across studies.[35] Perfect tests will have an AUC close to 1 and poor tests have AUCs closer to 0·5. However ROC curves of different shapes can have the same AUC, so it is not possible to interpret a summary AUC in terms of a set of unique combinations of sensitivity and specificity.

A second alternative is to compute the equations of the ROC curves for each of the studies[36] which yields estimates of intercept and slope parameters similar to those described for the Littenberg and Moses method. These parameters can be pooled to give an "average" ROC curve, but this

277

method is unsatisfactory as it ignores the correlation between the intercept and slope parameters for each study.[37]

In addition, neither of these alternative approaches can be used in the common situation where several of the studies report ROC curves whilst others report test performance at only one cutpoint.

Discussion

There are many factors that currently limit the usefulness of systematic reviews of diagnostic test accuracy. Several of these have already been mentioned, such as the lack of a method for pooling ROC curves, whilst others have been demonstrated in the case study, such as problems introduced by heterogeneity and difficulties in the interpretation of a summary ROC curve.

Whilst a health care practitioner desires valid summary estimates of the sensitivity and specificity (or positive and negative likelihood ratios) for a given value of a diagnostic test, the presence of gross between-study-heterogeneity (as was observed for specificity and the positive likelihood ratio in the case study) can often prohibit their estimation. The use of summary statistics which are more consistent across studies, such as the diagnostic odds ratio or a summary ROC curve, does allow the computation of a valid summary estimate of diagnostic performance, but produces statistics which cannot be applied directly to clinical practice. To interpret both diagnostic odds ratios and summary ROC curves it is necessary to have some knowledge of either the sensitivity or specificity of the test in the population to which it will be applied: unfortunately neither of these figures is estimable without undertaking yet another study of diagnostic accuracy.

In fact, the need to summarise information with a summary ROC technique due to variability and interdependence between the observed sensitivities and specificities can be considered to indicate a problem with the application of a diagnostic technology. This is especially the case when an ROC-like relationship is observed for a test that purports not to have explicit variation in cut-points (such as many imaging technologies), or where such variation is observed at a common cut-point. In these cases the ROC-like relationship indicates that test performance differs between the studies, and most likely will differ between test operators. Whilst the summary ROC method allows for this variation, it does not attempt to characterise or explain it, so that the meta-analysis fails to provide information that will assist an operator in using the technology in the most accurate manner.

It should also be noted that an apparent threshold effect can arise through variation in other factors which simultaneously increase (or decrease) both true positive and false positive diagnosis rates. For example, reconsider the data in Tables 14.3 and 14.4 illustrating the hypothetical effect of a change in the spectrum of disease and alternative diagnoses on sensitivity and specificity. The change from the general practice sample to the hospital sample is marked by increases in the true positive rate (sensitivity) and the false positive rate (1-specificity), whilst the diagnostic odds ratio remains relatively constant (around 4). Analysis of these studies using summary ROC methods will misappropriate the effect of varying spectrum as a threshold effect. It is unclear the extent to which variations in spectrum masquerade as apparent threshold effects in practice, rather than as differences in diagnostic odds ratios as detected by Lijmer and colleagues.[19]

Bearing all these points in mind, the promotion of summary ROC methods as the default method for pooling diagnostic study data[4-6] can be justly criticised. Empirical research is required to assess whether the simpler methods for pooling sensitivities, specificities and likelihood ratios are likely to be seriously misleading in practice, and whether apparent threshold effects are really due to variations in diagnostic threshold rather than alternative sources of heterogeneity. Given the clinical utility and promotion of likelihood ratios[1,3] for the practice of clinical medicine, the ability to derive validly these simpler summaries of diagnostic accuracy rather than diagnostic odds ratios and summary ROC curves is highly desirable.

In addition, meta-analyses of diagnostic test accuracy are hindered by a lack of appreciation and knowledge of the important aspects of study design, poor standards of reporting, and publication bias. None of these problems are unique to studies of diagnostic accuracy, but there is concern that they may be more problematic than for RCTs.[4,5] Lijmer and colleagues have made headway into understanding the importance of particular features of study design,[19] which may in turn lead to evidence based reporting guidelines similar to those for randomised controlled trials (Chapter 5) and systematic reviews (Chapter 7).

The problems of publication bias are more difficult: there are no studies in the literature which estimate rates of publication bias for diagnostic accuracy studies, and such investigations are difficult to undertake, as studies cannot easily be identified before they are undertaken. Also, there is no equivalent of the funnel plot (Chapter 11) to investigate whether or not the studies identified are a biased sample. Some authors have suggested that publication bias may in fact be a greater problem for studies of diagnostic accuracy than for randomised controlled trials.[4,5]

The evaluation of the diagnostic accuracy of a test is also only one component of assessing whether it is of clinical value.[38,39] Therapeutic interventions can only be recommended for use in health care only if they are shown on average to be of benefit to patients: the same criterion applies for the use of a diagnostic test, and even the most accurate of tests can be clinically useless and do more harm than good. Studies of diagnostic accuracy cannot prove that a diagnostic investigation is effective, but can discern whether the performance of a test is satisfactory for it to have the potential to be effective.

A reviewer should consider whether undertaking a systematic review of studies of diagnostic accuracy is likely to provide the most useful evidence of the value of a diagnostic intervention. Studies of patient outcomes, or the impact of using a test of therapeutic and diagnostic decisions, may provide more convincing evidence of the incremental benefit of using a new diagnostic test. But such studies are not available for many tests, especially for new technologies and components of the clinical examination. Conversely, practical issues (such as the absence of good independent reference standards for some diseases) occasionally mean that reliable studies of diagnostic accuracy cannot be undertaken, and studies of test reliability, management decisions and patient outcomes will provide the only evidence of the value of a diagnostic test.

Whilst the basic methodology for undertaking rigorous systematic reviews of studies of diagnostic accuracy exists, the greatest barrier to its practical application is the absence of appropriately designed, conducted and reported primary studies[5]. Whilst in some fields useful estimates of diagnostic performance can be obtained, in many the role of systematic reviews is limited to highlighting deficiencies in the primary studies.

Acknowledgements

I am grateful to Jeroen Lijmer and Walter Deville for providing access to pre-publication copies of their manuscripts, and to Rebecca Smith-Bindman for giving access to the data upon which the case study is based. Thanks also to Patrick Bossuyt, Daniel Pewsner and Rebecca Smith-Bindman for reviewing draft versions of the chapter and for making useful comments.

1 Sackett DL, Haynes RB, Guyatt GH, Tugwell P. *Clinical epidemiology: a basic science for clinical medicine*, 2nd edn. Boston: Little, Brown, 1991.
2 Pauker SG, Kassirer JP. The threshold approach to clinical decision making. *N Engl J Med* 1980;**302**:1109–17.
3 Sackett DL, Richardson WS, Rosenberg W, Haynes RB. *Evidence-based medicine: how to practice and teach EBM*. New York: Churchill Livingstone, 1997.
4 Irwig L, Tosteson AN, Gatsonis CA, *et al* Guidelines for meta-analyses evaluating diagnostic tests. *Ann Intern Med* 1994;**120**:667–76.
5 Irwig L, Macaskill P, Glasziou P, Fahey M. Meta-analytical methods for diagnostic test accuracy. *J Clin Epidemiol* 1995;**48**:119–30.
6 *Cochrane methods group on systematic review of screening and diagnostic tests*. Recommended methods, updated 6 June 1996. Available at <http://som.flinders.edu.au/cochrane/>
7 Vamvakas EC. Meta-analyses of studies of diagnostic accuracy of laboratory tests: a review of concepts and methods. *Arch Pathol Lab Med* 1998;**122**:675–86.

8 Valenstein PN. Evaluating diagnostic tests with imperfect standards. *Am J Clin Pathol* 1990;**93**:252–8.
9 Feinstein AR. The inadequacy of binary models for the clinical reality of three-zone diagnostic decisions. *J Clin Epidemiol* 1990;**43**:109–13.
10 Jaeschke R, Guyatt GH, Sackett DL for the Evidence-based Medicine Working Group. Users' guides to the medical literature. VI. How to use an article about a diagnostic test. B: What are the results and will they help me in caring for my patients? *JAMA* 1994;**271**:703–7.
11 Ingelfinger JA, Mosteller F, Thibodeau LA, Ware JH. *Biostatistics in clinical medicine*, 3rd edn. New York: McGraw-Hill, 1994;26–50.
12 Fagan TJ. Nomogram for Bayes' theorem. *N Engl J Med* 1975;**293**:257.
13 Deeks JJ, Morris JM. Evaluating diagnostic tests. *Ballière's Clin Obstet Gynaecol* 1996;**10**:613–30.
14 Haynes RB, Wilczynski N, McKibbon KA, Walker CJ, Sinclair JC. Developing optimal search strategies for detecting clinically sound studies in MEDLINE. *J Am Med Inform Assoc* 1994;**1**:447–58.
15 Devillé WLJM, Bezemer PD, Bouter LM. Publication on diagnostic test evaluation in family medicine journals: an optimal search strategy. *J Clin Epidemiol* 2000;**53**:65–9.
16 Ransohoff DF, Feinstein AR. Problems of spectrum and bias in evaluating the efficacy of diagnostic tests. *N Engl J Med* 1978;**299**:926–30.
17 Choi BCK. Sensitivity and specificity of a single diagnostic test in the presence of work-up bias. *J Clin Epidemiol* 1992;**45**:581–6.
18 Deeks JJ. Pressure sore prevention: using and evaluating risk assessment tools. *Br J Nursing* 1996;**5**:313–20.
19 Lijmer JG, Mol BW, Heisterkamp S, *et al.* Empirical evidence of design-related bias in studies of diagnostic tests. *JAMA* 1999;**282**:1061–6.
20 Jaeschke R, Guyatt GH, Sackett DL for the Evidence-based Medicine Working Group. Users' guides to the medical literature. VI. How to use an article about a diagnostic test. A: Are the results of the study valid? *JAMA* 1994;**271**:289–91.
21 Mulrow CD, Linn WD, Gaul MK, Pugh JA. Assessing the quality of a diagnostic test evaluation. *J Gen Intern Med* 1989;**4**:288–95.
22 Reid MC, Lachs MS, Feinstein AR. Use of methodological standards in diagnostic test research. *JAMA* 1995;**274**:645–51.
23 Devillé W, Yzermans N, Bouter LM, Bezemer PD, van der Windt. Heterogeneity in systematic reviews of diagnostic studies. *Proc 2nd symp systematic reviews: beyond the basics.* Oxford, 1999 [Abstract]. Available at http://www.ihs.ox.ac.uk/csm/talks.html#p21
24 Smith-Bindman R, Kerlikowske K, Feldstein VA, *et al.* Endovaginal ultrasound to exclude endometrial cancer and other endometrial abnormalities. *JAMA* 1998;**280**:1510–17.
25 Midgette AS, Stukel TA, Littenberg B. A meta-analytical method for summarizing diagnostic test performance: receiver-operating characteristic-curve point estimates. *Med Decis Making* 1993;**13**:253–7.
26 Shapiro DE. Issues in combining independent estimates of the sensitivity and specificity of a diagnostic test. *Acad Radiol* 1995;**2**:S37–S47.
27 Owens DK, Holodniy M, Garber AM, *et al.* Polymerase chain reaction for the diagnosis of HIV infection in adults. A meta-analysis with recommendations for clinical practice and study design. *Ann Intern Med* 1996;**124**:803–15.
28 Campbell MJ, Daly LE, Machin D. Special topics. In: Altman DG, Machin D, Bryant TN, Gardner MJ (eds). *Statistics with confidence*, 2nd edn. London: BMJ Books, 2000:153–67.
29 McCullagh P, Nelder JA. *Generalised linear models*, 2nd edn. London: Chapman and Hall, 1989.
30 Simel DL, Samsa GP, Matchar DB. Likelihood ratios with confidence: sample size estimation for diagnostic test studies. *J Clin Epidemiol* 1991;**44**:763–70.
31 Moses LE, Littenberg B, Shapiro D. Combining independent studies of a diagnostic test into a summary ROC curve: data-analytical approaches and some additional considerations. *Stat Med* 1993;**12**:1293–316.
32 Kardaun JWPF, Kardaun OJWF. Comparative diagnostic performance of three radio-

logical procedures for the detection of lumbar disk herniation. *Meth Info Med* 1990; **29**:12–22.

33 Littenberg B, Moses LE. Estimating diagnostic accuracy from multiple conflicting reports: a new meta-analytical method. *Med Decis Making* 1993;**13**:313–21.

34 Hanley JA, McNeil BJ. The meaning and use of the area under the receiver operating characteristic (ROC) curve. *Radiology* 1982;**143**:29–36.

35 Zhou XH. Empirical Bayes' combination of estimated areas under ROC curves using estimating equations. *Med Decis Making* 1996;**16**:24–8.

36 Tosteson ANA, Begg CB. A general regression methodology for ROC curve estimation. *Med Decis Making* 1988;**8**:204–15.

37 Hellmich M, Abrams KR, Sutton AJ. Bayesian approaches to meta-analysis of ROC curves. *Med Decis Making* 1999;**19**:252–64.

38 Deeks JJ. Using evaluations of diagnostic tests: understanding their limitations and making the most of available evidence. *Ann Oncol* 1999;**10**:761–8.

39 Guyatt GH, Tugwell PX, Feeny DH, Haynes RB, Drummond M. A framework for clinical evaluation of diagnostic technologies. *Can Med Assoc J* 1986;**134**:587–94.

Part IV: Statistical methods and computer software

15 Statistical methods for examining heterogeneity and combining results from several studies in meta-analysis

JONATHAN J DEEKS, DOUGLAS G ALTMAN,
MICHAEL J BRADBURN

Summary points

- Meta-analysis is a two-stage process involving the calculation of an appropriate summary statistic for each of a set of studies followed by the combination of these statistics into a weighted average.
- Methods are available for combining odds ratios, risk ratios and risk differences for binary data, and hazard ratios for time to event data.
- Continuous data can be combined either as differences in means, or as standardised differences in means when a mixture of measurement scales has been used.
- Fixed effect models average the summary statistics, weighting them according to a measure of the quantity of information they contain. Several methods are available (inverse variance, Mantel–Haenszel and Peto) which differ mainly in the computations used to calculate the individual study weights.
- Random effects models incorporate an estimate of between study variation (heterogeneity) into the calculation of the common effect. One simple method is readily available (DerSimonian and Laird); other methods require more complex statistical computations.
- Selection of a meta-analysis method for a particular analysis should reflect the data type, choice of summary statistic (considering the consistency of the effect and ease of interpretation of the statistic), observed heterogeneity, and the known limitations of the computational methods.

An important step in a systematic review is the thoughtful consideration of whether it is appropriate to combine all (or perhaps some) of the studies in a meta-analysis, to yield an overall statistic (together with its confidence interval) that summarises the effectiveness of the treatment (see Chapter 2). Statistical investigation of the degree of variation between individual study results, which is known as heterogeneity, can often contribute to making decisions regarding the "combinability" of results. In this chapter we consider the general principles of meta-analysis, and introduce the most commonly used methods for performing meta-analysis and examining heterogeneity. We shall focus on meta-analysis of randomised trials evaluating therapies, but much the same principles apply to other comparative studies, notably case-control and cohort studies.

Meta-analysis

General principles

Meta-analysis is a two-stage process. In the first stage a summary statistic is calculated for each study. For controlled trials, these values describe the treatment effect observed in each individual trial. The summary statistics are usually risk ratios, odds ratios or risk differences for event data, differences in means for continuous data, or hazard ratios for survival time data. In the second stage the overall treatment effect is calculated as a weighted average of these summary statistics. The weights are chosen to reflect the amount of information that each trial contains. In practice the weights are often the inverse of the variance (the square of the standard error) of the treatment effect, which relates closely to sample size. The precision (confidence interval) and statistical significance of the overall estimate are also calculated. It is also possible to weight additionally by study quality, although this is not generally recommended (see Chapter 5). All commonly used methods of meta-analysis follow these basic principles. There are, however, some other aspects that vary between alternative methods, as described below.

In a meta-analysis we do not combine the data from all of the trials as if they were from a single large trial. Such an approach is inappropriate for several reasons and can give misleading results, especially when the number of participants in each group is not balanced within trials.[1]

Assessing heterogeneity

An important component of a systematic review is the investigation of the consistency of the treatment effect across the primary studies. As the trials will not have been conducted according to a common protocol, there will usually be variations in patient groups, clinical settings, concomitant care and the methods of delivery of the intervention. Whilst some

286

divergence of trial results from the overall estimate is always expected purely by chance, the effectiveness of the treatment may also vary according to individual trial characteristics, which will increase the variability of results. The possibility of excess variability between the results of the different trials is examined by the test of homogeneity (occasionally described as a test for heterogeneity).

Consistency of trial results with a common effect despite variation in trial characteristics provides important and powerful corroboration of the generalisation of the treatment effect, so that a greater degree of certainty can be placed on its application to wider clinical practice.[7] However, the test of homogeneity has low power to detect excess variation, especially when there are not many studies, so the possibility of a type II (false negative) error must always be considered. By contrast, if the test of homogeneity is statistically significant, the between trial variability is more than expected by chance alone. In these situations it is still possible for a treatment to be shown to have a real, if not constant, benefit. In particular, the extra variation can be incorporated into the analysis using a random effects model (see below).

Where the heterogeneity is considerable, the reviewer ought to consider an investigation of reasons for the differences between trial results (see Chapters 8–11)[3] or not reporting a pooled estimate. Stratified meta-analysis (described below) and special statistical methods of meta-regression (see Chapters 9 and 11, and STATA command `metareg` in Chapter 18) can be used to test and examine potential associations between study factors and the estimated treatment effect.

Formulae for estimates of effect from individual studies

We assume here that the meta-analysis is being carried out on summary information obtained from published papers. The case of individual patient data (see Chapter 6) is considered briefly.

Individual study estimates of treatment effect: binary outcomes

For studies with a binary outcome the results can be presented in a 2×2 table (Table 15.1) giving the numbers of people who do or do not experience the event in each of the two groups (here called intervention and control).

Table 15.1 Summary information when outcome is binary.

Study i	Event	No event	Group size
Intervention	a_i	b_i	n_{1i}
Control	c_i	d_i	n_{2i}

287

For the ith study we denote the cell counts as in Table 15.1, with $N_i = n_{1i} + n_{2i}$. Zero cells cause problems with computation of the standard errors so 0.5 is usually added to each cell (a_i, b_i, c_i, d_i) for such studies.[4]

The treatment effect can be expressed as either a relative or absolute effect. Measures of relative effect (odds ratios and risk ratios) are usually combined on the log scale. Hence we give the standard error for the log ratio measure.

The *odds ratio*[5] for each study is given by

$$OR_i = \frac{a_i d_i}{b_i c_i},$$

the standard error of the log odds ratio being

$$SE[\ln(OR_i)] = \sqrt{\frac{1}{a_i} + \frac{1}{b_i} + \frac{1}{c_i} + \frac{1}{d_i}},$$

where ln denotes logarithms to base e (natural logarithms).

The *risk ratio*[5] for each study is given by

$$RR_i = \frac{a_i / n_{1i}}{c_i / n_{2i}},$$

the standard error of the log risk ratio being

$$SE[\ln(RR_i)] = \sqrt{\frac{1}{a_i} + \frac{1}{c_i} - \frac{1}{n_{1i}} - \frac{1}{n_{2i}}}.$$

The *risk difference*[6] for each study is given by

$$RD_i = \frac{a_i}{n_{1i}} - \frac{c_i}{n_{2i}},$$

with standard error

$$SE(RD_i) = \sqrt{\frac{a_i b_i}{n_{1i}^3} + \frac{c_i d_i}{n_{2i}^3}}.$$

For the *Peto odds ratio* method[7] (see below) the individual odds ratios are given by

$$OR_i = \exp\left(\frac{a_i - E[a_i]}{v_i}\right),$$

with standard error

$$SE[\ln(OR_i)] = \sqrt{1/v_i},$$

where $E[a_i] = n_{1i}(a_i + c_i)/N_i$ (the expected number of events in the intervention group under the null hypothesis of no treatment effect) and

$$v_i = \frac{n_{1i}n_{2i}(a_i + c_i)(b_i + d_i)}{N_i^2(N_i - 1)},$$

the hypergeometric variance of a_i.

Individual study estimates of treatment effect: continuous outcomes

If the outcome is a continuous measure, we require the number of participants, the mean response and its standard deviation, for intervention and control groups (Table 15.2).

Table 15.2 Summary information when outcome is continuous.

Study i	Mean response	Standard deviation	Group size
Intervention	m_{1i}	SD_{1i}	n_{1i}
Control	m_{2i}	SD_{2i}	n_{2i}

We let $N_i = n_{1i} + n_{2i}$ be the total number of participants in study i, and

$$s_i = \sqrt{\frac{(n_{1i} - 1)SD_{1i}^2 + (n_{2i} - 1)SD_{2i}^2}{N_i - 2}}$$

be the pooled standard deviation of the two groups.

There are two summary statistics used for meta-analysis of continuous data. The *difference in means* can be used when outcome measurements in all trials are made on the same scale. The meta-analysis computes a weighted average of these differences in means, but is confusingly termed the *weighted mean difference* (WMD) method.

289

The *standardised difference* is used when the trials all assess the same outcome, but measure it in a variety of ways (for example, all trials measure depression but they use different psychometric scales). In this circumstance it is necessary to standardise the results of the trials to a uniform scale before they can be combined. The *standardised mean difference* method expresses the size of the treatment effect in each trial (again in reality a difference in means and not a mean difference) relative to the variability observed in that trial. The method assumes that the differences in standard deviations between trials reflect differences in measurement scales and not real differences in variability between trial populations. This assumption may be problematic in some circumstances where pragmatic and explanatory trials (which may differ in the risk of poor outcomes) are combined in the same review. The overall treatment effect can also be difficult to interpret as it is reported in units of standard deviation rather than in units of any of the measurement scales used in the review.

For a particular study the *difference in means* (denoted MD)[8] is given by

$$MD_i = m_{1i} - m_{2i},$$

with standard error

$$\mathrm{SE}(MD_i) = \sqrt{\frac{\mathrm{SD}_{1i}^2}{n_{1i}} + \frac{\mathrm{SD}_{2i}^2}{n_{2i}}}.$$

There are three popular formulations of effect size used in the standardised mean difference method. These formulations differ with respect to the standard deviation used in calculations and whether or not a correction for *small sample bias* is included. In statistics small sample bias is defined as the difference between the expected value of an estimate given a small sample and the expected value if the sample is infinite. Simulations show that the standardised mean difference tends to be overestimated with finite samples but the bias is substantial only if total sample size is very small (less than 10).[9]

Cohen's *d* [10] is given by

$$d_i = \frac{m_{1i} - m_{2i}}{s_i},$$

with standard error

$$\mathrm{SE}(d_i) = \sqrt{\frac{N_i}{n_{1i} n_{2i}} + \frac{d_i^2}{2(N_i - 2)}}.$$

Hedges' adjusted g[10] is very similar to Cohen's d but includes an adjustment to correct for the small sample bias mentioned above. It is defined as

$$g_i = \frac{m_{1i} - m_{2i}}{s_i}\left(1 - \frac{3}{4N_i - 9}\right),$$

with standard error

$$SE(g_i) = \sqrt{\frac{N_i}{n_{1i}n_{2i}} + \frac{g_i^2}{2(N_i - 3.94)}}.$$

Finally, **Glass's Δ**[11] takes the standard deviation from the control group as the scaling factor, giving

$$\Delta_i = \frac{m_{1i} - m_{2i}}{SD_{2i}},$$

with standard error

$$SE(\Delta_i) = \sqrt{\frac{N_i}{n_{1i}n_{2i}} + \frac{\Delta_i^2}{2(n_{2i} - 1)}}.$$

This method is preferable when the intervention alters the observed variability as well as potentially changing the mean value.

Both the weighted mean difference and standardised mean difference methods assume that the outcome measurements within each trial have a Normal distribution. When these distributions are skewed or severely non-Normal, the results of these methods may be misleading.

Formulae for deriving a summary (pooled) estimate of the treatment effect by combining trial results (meta-analysis)

The methods of meta-analysis described below all combine the individual study summary statistics described above, denoted generically by θ_i, each given a weight w_i which is usually related to $SE(\theta_i)$. All the methods described are available in the Stata routines described in Chapter 18. The summation notation indicates summation of the i trials included in the analysis.

Fixed effect and random effects methods

In fixed effect meta-analysis it is assumed that the true effect of treatment is the same value in each study, or *fixed*, the differences between study results being due solely to the play of chance. The assumption of a fixed effect can be tested using a test of homogeneity (see below).

In a random effects meta-analysis the treatment effects for the individual studies are assumed to vary around some overall average treatment effect. Usually the effect sizes θ_i are assumed have a Normal distribution with mean θ and variance τ^2. In essence the test of homogeneity described below tests whether τ^2 is zero. The smaller the value of τ^2 the more similar are the fixed and random effects analyses.

Peto describes his method for obtaining a summary odds ratio as assumption free,[7] arguing that it does not assume that all the studies are estimating the same treatment effect, but it is generally considered to be most similar to a fixed effect method.

There is no consensus about whether to use fixed or random effects models.[12] All of the methods given below are fixed effect approaches except the DerSimonian and Laird method.

Inverse variance method

Inverse variance methods may be used to pool either binary or continuous data. In the general formula below, the effect size, denoted θ_i, could be the log odds ratio, log relative risk, risk difference, difference in means or standardised mean difference from the ith trial.

The effect sizes are combined to give a pooled estimate by calculating a *weighted average* of the treatment effects from the individual trials:

$$\theta_{\text{IV}} = \frac{\sum w_i \theta_i}{\sum w_i}.$$

The weights are the reciprocals of the squared standard errors:

$$w_i = \frac{1}{\text{SE}(\theta_i)^2}.$$

Thus larger studies, which have smaller standard errors, are given more weight than smaller studies, which have larger standard errors. This choice of weight minimises the variability of the pooled treatment effect θ_{IV}.

The standard error of θ_{IV} is given by

$$\text{SE}(\theta_{\text{IV}}) = \frac{1}{\sqrt{\sum w_i}}.$$

The heterogeneity statistic is given by

$$Q - \sum w_i (\theta_i - \theta_{IV})^2.$$

The strength of this approach is its wide applicability. It can be used to combine any estimates that have standard errors available. Thus it can be used for estimates from many types of study, including standardised mortality ratios, diagnostic test indices (Chapter 14), hazard ratios (Chapter 6), and estimates from cross-over trials and cluster-randomised trials. It is also possible to use this method when crude 2×2 tables cannot be obtained for each study, but treatment effects and confidence intervals are available (see Stata commands **meta** and **metan** in Chapter 18).

Mantel–Haenszel methods

When data are sparse, both in terms of event rates being low and trials being small, the estimates of the standard errors of the treatment effects that are used in the inverse variance methods may be poor. Mantel–Haenszel methods use an alternative weighting scheme, and have been shown to be more robust when data are sparse, and may therefore be preferable to the inverse variance method. In other situations they give similar estimates to the inverse variance method. They are available only for binary outcomes (see Stata command **metan** in Chapter 18).

For each study, the effect size from each trial θ_i is given weight w_i in the analysis. The overall estimate of the pooled effect, θ_{MH} is given by:

$$\theta_{MH} = \frac{\sum w_i \theta_i}{\sum w_i}.$$

Unlike with inverse variance methods, relative effect measures are combined in their natural scale, although their standard errors (and confidence intervals) are still computed on the log scale.

For combining *odds ratios*, each study's OR is given weight[13,11]

$$w_i = \frac{b_i c_i}{N_i},$$

and the logarithm of OR_{MH} has standard error given by[15]

$$SE[\ln(OR_{MH})] = \sqrt{\frac{1}{2} \left(\frac{E}{R^2} + \frac{F+G}{R \times S} + \frac{H}{S^2} \right)},$$

293

where

$$R = \sum \frac{a_i d_i}{N_i}; \quad S = \sum \frac{b_i c_i}{N_i};$$

$$E = \sum \frac{(a_i + d_i) a_i d_i}{N_i^2}; \quad F = \sum \frac{(a_i + d_i) b_i c_i}{N_i^2};$$

$$G = \sum \frac{(b_i + c_i) a_i d_i}{N_i^2}; \quad H = \sum \frac{(b_i + c_i) b_i c_i}{N_i^2}.$$

For combining *risk ratios*, each study's RR is given weight[16]

$$w_i = \frac{c_i n_{1i}}{N_i},$$

and the logarithm of RR_{MH} has standard error given by

$$\mathrm{SE}[\ln(RR_{\mathrm{MH}})] = \sqrt{\frac{P}{R \times S}},$$

where

$$P = \sum \frac{(n_{1i} n_{2i}(a_i + c_i) - a_i c_i N_i)}{N_i^2}; \quad R = \sum \frac{a_i n_{2i}}{N_i}; \quad S = \sum \frac{c_i n_{1i}}{N_i}.$$

For *risk differences*, each study's RD has the weight[16]

$$w_i = \frac{n_{1i} n_{2i}}{N_i},$$

and RD_{MH} has standard error given by

$$\mathrm{SE}(RD_{\mathrm{MH}}) = \sqrt{\mathcal{J} / K^2},$$

where

$$\mathcal{J} = \sum \left(\frac{a_i b_i n_{2i}^3 + c_i d_i n_{1i}^3}{n_{1i} n_{2i} N_i^2} \right); \quad K = \sum \left(\frac{n_{1i} n_{2i}}{N_i} \right).$$

294

However, the test of homogeneity is based upon the inverse variance weights and not the Mantel–Haenszel weights. The heterogeneity statistic is given by

$$Q = \sum w_i (\theta_i - \theta_{MH})^2$$

where θ is the log odds ratio, log relative risk or risk difference.

Peto's odds ratio method

An alternative to the Mantel–Haenszel method is a method due to Peto (sometimes attributed to Yusuf, or to Yusuf and Peto).[7] The overall odds ratio is given by

$$OR_{Peto} = \exp\left(\frac{\sum w_i \ln(OR_i)}{\sum w_i}\right),$$

where the odds ratio OR_i is calculated using the approximate Peto method described in the individual trial section, and the weight w_i is equal to the hypergeometric variance of the event count in the intervention group, v_i.

The logarithm of the odds ratio has standard error

$$SE[\ln(OR_{Peto})] = \frac{1}{\sqrt{\sum v_i}}.$$

The heterogeneity statistic is given by

$$Q = \sum v_i (\ln OR_i - \ln OR_{Peto})^2.$$

The approximation upon which Peto's method relies has shown to fail when treatment effects are very large, and when the sizes of the arms of the trials are seriously unbalanced.[17] Severe imbalance, with, for example, four or more times as many participants in one group than the other, would rarely occur in randomised trials. In other circumstances, including when event rates are very low, the method performs well.[18] Corrections for zero cell counts are not necessary for this method (see Stata command **metan** in Chapter 18).

Extending the Peto method for pooling time-to-event data

Pooling of time-to-event outcomes can be achieved either by computing hazard ratios for each trial and pooling them using the inverse variance method (as explained above), or by exploiting a link between the log rank test statistic and the Peto method, as follows.

For each trial, the calculation of a log rank statistic involves dividing the follow-up period into a series of discrete time intervals. For each interval the number of events observed in the treated group O_{ij}, the number of events that would be expected in the treatment group under the null hypothesis E_{ij} and its variance v_{ij} are calculated (for formulae, see for example Altman[19]). The expected count and its variance are computed taking into account the number still at risk of the event within each time period. The log-rank test for the ith trial is computed from $\sum O_{ij}$, $\sum E_{ij}$ and $\sum v_{ij}$ summed over all the time periods, j.

Following the same format as the Peto odds ratio method, an estimate of the hazard ratio in each trial is given by[19]

$$HR_i = \exp\left(\frac{\sum O_{ij} - \sum E_{ij}}{\sum v_{ij}}\right),$$

with standard error

$$\mathrm{SE}[\ln(HR_i)] = \sqrt{1/\sum v_{ij}}\,.$$

The overall hazard ratio is given by the weighted average of the log hazard ratios

$$HR_{\mathrm{Peto}} = \exp\left(\frac{\sum w_i \ln(HR_i)}{\sum w_i}\right),$$

where the weights w_i are equal to the variances computed from the trials, $\sum v_{ij}$.

The logarithm of the overall hazard ratio has standard error

$$\mathrm{SE}[\ln(HR_{\mathrm{Peto}})] = \frac{1}{\sqrt{\sum w_i}}.$$

Computation of the components of the log-rank statistic $\sum O_{ij}$, $\sum E_{ij}$ and $\sum v_{ij}$ is straightforward if individual patient data are available. Methods have been proposed for indirectly estimating the log hazard ratio and its variance from graphical and numerical summaries commonly published in reports of randomised controlled trials.[20]

296

DerSimonian and Laird random effects models

Under the random effects model, the assumption of a common treatment effect is relaxed, and the effect sizes θ_i are assumed have a Normal distribution with mean and variance τ^2. The usual DerSimonian and Laird[21] estimate of τ^2 is given by

$$\tau^2 = \frac{Q - (k - 1)}{\sum w_i - \left(\dfrac{\sum w_i^2}{\sum w_i} \right)},$$

where Q is the heterogeneity statistic, with τ^2 set to zero if $Q < k - 1$, and the w_i are calculated as in the inverse variance method. The estimate of the combined effect for the heterogeneity may be taken as the inverse variance estimate, although the Mantel–Haenszel estimate may be preferred. Again, for odds ratios and risk ratios, the effect size is taken as the natural logarithm of the OR and RR. Each study's effect size is given weight

$$w_i' = \frac{1}{SE(\theta_i)^2 + \tau^2}.$$

The pooled effect size is given by

$$\theta_{DL} = \frac{\sum w_i' \theta_i}{\sum w_i'},$$

with standard error

$$SE(\theta_{DL}) = \frac{1}{\sqrt{\sum w_i'}}.$$

Note that when $\tau^2 = 0$, i.e. where the heterogeneity statistic Q is as small as or smaller than its degrees of freedom $(k - 1)$, the weights reduce to those given by the inverse variance method.

If the estimate of τ^2 is greater than zero then the weights in random-effects models ($w_i' = 1/(SE(\theta_i)^2 + \tau^2)$) will be smaller and more similar to each other than the weights in fixed effect models ($w_i = 1/SE(\theta_i)^2$). This means than random-effects meta-analyses will be more conservative (the confidence intervals will be wider) than fixed effect analyses[22] since the variance of the pooled effect is the inverse of the sum of the weights. It also means that random effects models give relatively more weight to smaller studies than the fixed effect model. This may not always be desirable (see Chapter 11).

The DerSimonian and Laird method has the same wide applicability as the inverse variance method, and can be used to combine any type of estimates provided standard errors are available (see Stata commands `meta` and `metan` in Chapter 18).

Confidence interval for overall effect

The $100(1 - \alpha)\%$ confidence interval for the overall estimate θ is given by

$$\theta - \left(z_{1-\alpha/2} \times \text{SE}(\theta)\right) \text{ to } \theta + \left(z_{1-\alpha/2} \times \text{SE}(\theta)\right),$$

where θ is the log odds ratio, log relative risk, risk difference, mean difference or standardised mean difference, and z is the standard Normal deviate. For example, if $\alpha = 0.05$, then $z_{1-\alpha/2} = 1.96$ and the 95% confidence interval is given by

$$\theta - \left(1.96 \times \text{SE}(\theta)\right) \text{ to } \theta + \left(1.96 \times \text{SE}(\theta)\right).$$

Confidence intervals for log odds ratios and log risk ratios are exponentiated to provide confidence intervals for the pooled OR or RR.

Test statistic for overall effect

In all cases a test statistic for the overall difference between groups is derived as

$$z = \frac{\theta}{\text{SE}(\theta)}$$

(where the odds ratio or risk ratio is again considered on the log scale). Under the null hypothesis that there is no treatment effect, z will follow a standard Normal distribution.

For odds ratios an alternative test statistic is given by comparing the number of observed and expected events in the treatment group given no difference is present between the groups. This test is given by

$$\chi^2 = \frac{\sum (a_i - E[a_i])^2}{\sum v_i},$$

where $E[a_i]$ and v_i are as defined above. Under the null hypothesis of no treatment effect, this statistic follows a chi-squared distribution on one degree of freedom.

Test statistics of homogeneity

For a formal test of homogeneity, the statistic Q will follow a chi-squared distribution on $k - 1$ degrees of freedom under the null hypothesis that the true treatment effect is the same for all trials.

Breslow and Day proposed an alternative test of the homogeneity of odds ratios,[14] based upon a comparison of the observed number of events in the intervention groups of each trial (a_i), with those expected when the common treatment effect OR is applied (calculation of these expected values involves solving quadratic expressions). The test statistic is given by

$$Q_{BD} = \sum \left(\frac{a_i - E[a_i \mid OR]}{v_i} \right),$$

where each trial's variance v_i is computed using the fitted cell counts

$$v_i = \frac{1}{E[a_i \mid OR]} + \frac{1}{E[b_i \mid OR]} + \frac{1}{E[c_i \mid OR]} + \frac{1}{F[d_i \mid OR]}.$$

Under the null hypothesis of homogeneity Q_{BD} also has a chi-squared distribution on $k - 1$ degrees of freedom.

Use of stratified analyses for investigating sources of heterogeneity

In a stratified analysis the trials are grouped according to a particular feature or characteristic and a separate meta-analysis carried out of the trials within each subgroup. The overall summaries calculated within each subgroup can then be inspected for evidence of variation in the effect of the intervention, which would suggest that the stratifying characteristic is an important source of heterogeneity and may moderate treatment efficacy.

Stratified analysis can be used when the trials can be grouped into a small number of categories according to the study characteristic; meta-regression (see Chapter 9) can be used when the characteristic is a continuous measure.

An inference that the treatment effect differs between two or more subsets of the trials should be based on a formal test of statistical significance. There are three methods to assess statistical significance.

Consider first a stratified analysis with the trials grouped into k subgroups. By performing separate meta-analyses within each subgroup, we obtain for the kth subgroup:

θ_k, an estimate of the overall effect within each group,

$SE(\theta_k)$, the standard error of these estimates,

Q_k, the heterogeneity observed within each group.

If there are only 2 groups, the significance of the difference between the two groups can be examined by comparing the z statistic

$$z = \frac{\theta_1 - \theta_2}{\sqrt{[SE(\theta_1)]^2 + [SE(\theta_2)]^2}},$$

with critical values of the Normal distribution.

An alternative test, which can be used regardless of the number of subgroups, involves explicitly partitioning the overall heterogeneity into that which can be explained by differences between subgroups, and that which remains unexplained within the subgroups. If the heterogeneity of the overall unstratified analysis is Q_T, the heterogeneity explained by differences between subgroups, Q_B, is given by:

$$Q_B = Q_T - \sum_k Q_k,$$

which can be compared with critical values of the chi-squared distribution with $k-1$ degrees of freedom.

The problem can also be formulated as a meta-regression (see Chapter 9), using $k-1$ dummy variables to indicate membership of the k subgroups, in the standard manner used in multiple regression. The meta-regression will also produce estimates of the differences between a baseline reference subgroup and each of the other subgroups. If the categories are ordered, meta-regression should be used to perform a test for trend by denoting group membership by a single variable indicating the ranked order of each subgroup.

The interpretation of comparisons between subgroups should be undertaken cautiously, as significant differences can easily arise by chance (a type I error), or are explicable by other factors. Even when the studies in the meta-analysis are randomised controlled trials, the investigation of differences between subgroups is a non-randomised comparison, and is prone to all of the difficulties in inferring causality in observational studies (see Chapter 12). Where multiple possible sources of heterogeneity are investigated, the chance of one of them being found to be statistically significant increases, so the number of factors considered should be restricted. Pre-specification (in a protocol) of possible sources of heterogeneity increases the credibility of any statistically significant findings, as there is evidence that the findings are not data-derived. Examples of stratified meta-analyses are shown in the Case studies 1 and 3 below.

Often the stratifying factor is the type of intervention. For example, a systematic review may include placebo controlled trials of several drugs, all for the same condition. The meta-analysis will be stratified by drug, and will provide estimates of treatment effect for each drug. Here a test of differences between subgroups is effectively an indirect comparison of the effects of the drugs. Although such a test can provide indirect evidence of relative treatment effects, it is much less reliable than evidence from randomised controlled trials which compare the drugs directly (head-to-head comparisons). Similar situations also arise with non-pharmacological interventions. Such indirect comparisons are considered by Bucher et al.[23] and Song et al.[24]

Meta-analysis with individual patient data

The same basic approaches and meta-analysis methods are used for meta-analyses of individual patient data (IPD)[25] (see Chapter 6). However, there are two principal differences between IPD analyses and those based on published summary statistics. Firstly, the IPD meta-analyst calculates the summary tables or statistics for each study, and therefore can ensure all data are complete and up-to-date, and that the same method of analysis is used for all trials. Secondly, summary statistics can be calculated for specific groups of participants enabling full intention-to-treat (see below) and subgroup analyses to be produced. Additionally, it is worth noting that IPD meta-analyses often combine time-to-event data rather than binary or continuous outcomes, the meta-analyst calculating the required components of the log rank statistic in the same manner for each of the trials.

Additional analyses

Additional analyses undertaken after the main meta-analysis investigate *influence*, *robustness* and *bias*. Influence and robustness can be assessed in sensitivity analyses by repeating the meta-analysis on subsets of the original dataset (see Chapter 2 for an example). The influence of each study can be estimated by deleting each in turn from the analysis and noting the degree

301

to which the size and significance of the treatment effect changes (see Stata command `metainf` in Chapter 18). Other sensitivity analyses can assess robustness to uncertainties and assumptions by removing or adding sets of trials, or by changing the data for individual trials. Situations where these may be considered include when some of the trials are of poorer quality (Chapter 5), when it is unclear whether some trials meet the inclusion criteria, or when the results of trials in the published reports are ambiguous and assumptions are made when extracting data. Methods for investigating bias, including publication bias, are described in detail in Chapter 11 (see also Stata command `metabias` in Chapter 18).

Some practical issues

Although it is desirable to include trial results from intention to treat analyses, this is not always possible given the data provided in published reports. Reports commonly omit participants who do not comply, receive the wrong treatment, or who drop out of the study. All of these individuals can easily be included in intention to treat analyses if follow-up data are available, and it is most important that they are included if the reasons for exclusion relate to the treatment that they received (such as drop-outs due to side-effects and poor tolerability of treatment). Occasionally full details of the outcomes of those excluded during the trial may be mentioned in the text of the report, but in many situations assumptions must be made regarding their fate. By inventive use of sensitivity analysis (using *worst case*, *best case* and *most likely case* scenarios for every trial) it is possible to assess the influence of these excluded cases on the final results. The issue is more problematic for continuous outcomes, where there is a continuum of possible scenarios for every excluded participant.

Other problems can occur when trials have no events in one or both arms. In these situations inverse variance, Mantel–Haenszel and DerSimonian and Laird methods require the addition of a small quantity (usually 0.5) to the cell counts to avoid division by zero errors. (Many software implementations of these methods automatically add this correction to all cell counts regardless of whether it is strictly needed.) When both groups have event rates of zero (there being no events in either arm) odds ratios and relative risks are undefined, and such trials must be excluded from the analysis. The risk difference in such situations is zero, so the trials will still contribute to the analysis. However, both inverse variance and Mantel–Haenszel methods perform poorly when event rates are very low, underestimating both treatment effects and statistical significance.[18] Peto's odds ratio method gives more accurate estimates of the treatment effects and their confidence intervals providing the sample sizes of the arms in the trials are not severely unbalanced.

Other methods of meta-analysis

The meta-analytical methods described above are straightforward and easy to implement in most statistical software and spreadsheet packages. Other more complex methods exist, and are implemented in specialist statistical software packages, such as Stata (see Chapter 18), SAS, and StatXact (see Box 17.1 in Chapter 17). Maximum likelihood logistic regression can also be used to perform fixed effect meta-analysis, and will give similar answers to the Mantel–Haenszel and inverse variance methods provided sample sizes are large. Maximum likelihood (ML) and restricted maximum likelihood (REML) estimation techniques also enable better estimation of the between trial variance τ^2,[26] and can estimate additional parameters, such as the standard error of τ^2.[27] Bayesian methods (see Chapter 2) can incorporate prior information from other sources, such as is available from qualitative research,[28] whilst exact methods[29] use challenging permutation algorithms to compute treatment effects and P values.

Case study 1 : support from caregivers during childbirth

Descriptive studies of women's childbirth experiences have suggested that women appreciate advice and information from their caregivers, comfort measures and other forms of tangible assistance to cope with labour, and the continuous presence of a sympathetic person. A systematic review included studies that evaluated the effects of intrapartum support from caregivers on a variety of childbirth outcomes, medical as well as psychosocial.[31] One outcome included in the review was the use of epidural anaesthesia during delivery. Six trials reported this outcome, four from America and two from Europe. In four of the six trials husbands, partners or other family members were also usually present. The person providing the support intervention was variously described in the trials as a midwife, nurse, *monitrice* and a *doula*. The results of the six studies are given in Table 15.3.

Ten alternative methods have been described in this chapter which can be used to perform a meta-analysis of these data. The results are shown in Table 15.4.

Table 15.3 Rates of use of epidural anaesthesia in trials of caregiver support.

Trial	Caregiver present Epidurals / N	Standard Care Epidurals / N
Bréart 1992 (France)	55/133	62/131
Bréart 1992 (Belgium)	281/656	319/664
Gagnon 1997 (Canada)	139/209	142/204
Hodnett 1989 (Canada)	30/72	43/73
Kennell 1991 (USA)	24/212	55/200
Langer 1998 (Mexico)	205/361	303/363

Table 15.4 Results of meta-analyses of epidural rates from trials of caregiver support.

Method	Estimate of effect (95% CI)	Significance of effect	Test for heterogeneity
Odds ratio			
Peto	0·59 (0·51 to 0·69)	$z = 7·05$, P < 0·0001	$\chi_5^2 = 38·5$, P < 0·001
Mantel–Haenszel	0·59 (0·51 to 0·69)	$z = 6·98$, P < 0·0001	$\chi_5^2 = 38·9$, P < 0·001
Inverse variance	0·60 (0·52 to 0·70)	$z = 6·70$, P < 0·0001	$\chi_5^2 = 38·8$, P < 0·001
DerSimonian			
and Laird	0·54 (0·34 to 0·85)	$z = 2·64$, P = 0·008	
Risk ratio			
Mantel–Haenszel	0·79 (0·74 to 0·85)	$z = 6·95$, P < 0·0001	$\chi_5^2 = 29·8$, P < 0·001
Inverse variance	0·80 (0·75 to 0·85)	$z = 7·14$, P < 0·0001	$\chi_5^2 = 29·7$, P < 0·001
DerSimonian			
and Laird	0·77 (0·64 to 0·92)	$z = 2·93$, P = 0·003	
Risk difference			
Mantel–Haenszel	−0·117 (−0·149 to −0·085)	$z = 7·13$, P < 0·0001	$\chi_5^2 = 33·1$, P < 0·001
Inverse variance	−0·127 (−0·158 to −0·095)	$z = 7·86$, P < 0·0001	$\chi_5^2 = 32·7$, P < 0·001
DerSimonian			
and Laird	−0·124 (−0·211 to −0·038)	$z = 2·81$, P = 0·005	

There are some notable patterns in the results in Table 15.4. First, there is substantial agreement between Peto, Mantel–Haenszel and inverse variance methods for odds ratios and for risk ratios, indicating that in this instance, where trials are large and event rates reasonably high, the choice of the fixed effect weighting method makes little difference to the results. Secondly, there are substantial differences between treatment effects expressed as odds ratios and risk ratios. Considering the Mantel–Haenszel results, the reduction in the odds of having an epidural with additional caregiver support is 41% ($100 \times (1 - 0·59)$), whilst the relative risk reduction is 21% ($100 \times (1 - 0·79)$), only around half the size. Where events are common (around half the women in the standard care groups received epidurals) odds and risks are very different, and care must be taken to ensure that a reader of the review is not misled into believing that benefits of intervention are larger than is truly the case.[32]

The tests of homogeneity were also statistically significant for odds ratios, risk ratios and risk differences. As a result the confidence intervals for the DerSimonian and Laird random effects estimates are wider than those calculated from fixed effect models. The estimates of the benefit of treatment expressed as relative risks and odds ratios also increase as the random effects model attributes proportionally greater weight to the smallest trials, which in this example report larger relative benefits of treatment.

The report mentions that the benefit of the intervention may be expected to be greater when partners or other family members are absent at the birth, which could explain the significant heterogeneity. Stratifying the analysis into 'accompanied' and 'unaccompanied' trials (partners were absent in the Kennell and Langer trials) does explain a large proportion of the heterogeneity. The relative risk reduction in the four trials where partners were also present is 11% (95% CI: 3 to 18%; heterogeneity test $\chi_3^2 = 2 \cdot 92$, P = $0 \cdot 4$), whilst in the two trials where partners were absent it is 36% (95% CI: 29 to 43%; heterogeneity test $\chi_1^2 = 5 \cdot 39$, P = $0 \cdot 02$). The differences between the subgroups is highly statistically significant (heterogeneity explained by the subgroups $\chi_1^2 = 29 \cdot 8 - (2 \cdot 92 + 5 \cdot 39) = 21 \cdot 5$: P < $0 \cdot 0001$).

The conclusion of the analysis is that the presence of a caregiver is of benefit in reducing the use of epidural analgesia in all situations, but that the benefit seems much greater in situations were partners are usually absent.

Case study 2 : Assertive community treatment for severe mental disorders

Assertive community treatment (ACT) is a multidisciplinary team based approach to care for the severely mentally ill in the community. It is assertive in that it continues to offer services to uncooperative and reluctant people, and places emphasis on treatment compliance with the aim of improving mental state. A systematic review comparing ACT to standard care (which consists of outpatient appointments and assistance from community mental health teams) found three trials that assessed mental state at around 12 months.[33] The results are shown in Table 15.5.

Table 15.5 Trials comparing mental state at 12 months between ACT and standard care.

Trial	ACT		Standard care		Assessment scale
	N	Mean (SD)	N	Mean (SD)	
Audini (London)	30	41·4 (14·0)	28	42·3 (12·4)	Brief psychiatric rating scale
Morse (St Louis)	37	0·95 (0·76)	35	0·89 (0·65)	Brief symptom inventory
Lehman (Baltimore)	67	4·10 (0·83)	58	3·80 (0·87)	Colorado symptom index

All three trials have used different scoring systems so the trial results require standardisation to a common scale before they can be combined. In addition, high scores on the Colorado symptom index indicate good outcomes, whilst high scores on the other two scales are poor outcomes, so the direction of the results for Lehman must be reversed before the data can be combined (this is easily accomplished by multiplying the means by –1). Six alternative models for combining the data were described above, and their results are given in Table 15.6.

In this situation, the differences between the analyses are minimal.

305

Table 15.6 Results of meta-analyses of mental status from trials of ACT.

Method	Estimate of effect (95% CI)	Significance of effect	Test for heterogeneity
Fixed effect models			
Cohen's d	−0·16 (−0·41 to 0·08)	$z = 1·29$, P = 0·20	$\chi_2^2 = 2·34$, P = 0·31
Hedges' adjusted g	−0·16 (−0·41 to 0·08)	$z = 1·29$, P = 0·20	$\chi_2^2 = 2·31$, P = 0·32
Glass's Δ	−0·16 (−0·40 to 0·09)	$z = 1·24$, P = 0·21	$\chi_2^2 = 2·28$, P = 0·32
Random effects models			
Cohen's d	−0·15 (−0·42 to 0·12)	$z = 1·12$, P = 0·26	
Hedges' adjusted g	−0·15 (−0·42 to 0·11)	$z = 1·12$, P = 0·26	
Glass's Δ	−0·15 (−0·42 to 0·12)	$z = 1·10$, P = 0·27	

Cohen's d and Hedges' adjusted g will only differ in very small samples. Glass's Δ will differ when the standard deviations vary substantially between treatment and control groups, which was not the case here. Very little heterogeneity was observed, so random and fixed effects analyses are very similar. The analysis can conclude that although all trials favoured ACT no significant change in mental status at 12 months was found with ACT. Also benefits of ACT larger than 0·5 standard deviations or more can probably be excluded as they are outside the lower limit of the confidence interval. To express the findings in a more accessible way consider the standard deviations from each of the trials. A change of 0·5 standard deviations can be estimated to be 6–7 points on the brief psychiatric rating scale, 0·45–0·5 points on the brief symptom inventory and 0·4–0·45 points on the Colorado symptom index.

Case study 3 : effect of reduced dietary sodium on blood pressure

Restricting the intake of salt in diet has been proposed as a method of lowering blood pressure, both in hypertensives and people with normal blood pressure. A systematic review of randomised studies of dietary sodium restrictions compared to control included 56 trials comparing salt lowering diets with control diets.[34] Only trials which assessed salt reduction through measurement of sodium excretion were included. Twenty-eight of the studies recruited hypertensive participants, and 28 recruited normotensive participants; 41 studies used a cross-over design, whilst 15 used a parallel group design.

The focus of interest in these trials is the difference in mean blood pressure (both diastolic and systolic) between the salt reducing diet and the control diet. As all measurements are in the same units (mmHg) the difference in means can be used directly as a summary statistic in the meta-analysis. The trials estimated this difference in mean blood pressure in four different ways:

(i) in a parallel group trial, as the difference in mean final blood pressure between those receiving the salt lowering diet and the control diet

(ii) in a parallel group trial, as the difference in mean change in blood pressure whilst on the diets, between those on the salt lowering diet and those on the control diet

(iii) in a cross-over trial, as the mean within person difference between final blood pressure at the end of the salt lowering diet and at the end of the control diet

(iv) in a cross-over trial, as the mean within person difference in the change in blood pressure whilst on the salt lowering diet compared to the control diet.

Results from these four different designs all estimate the same summary measure. However, it is likely that trials that use within person changes are more efficient than those that use final values, and that those which use cross-over designs are more efficient than those recruiting parallel groups. These differences are encapsulated in the standard errors of the estimates in differences in mean blood pressure between the two diets, provided appropriate consideration is given to the within person pairing of the data for change scores and cross-over trials in the analysis of those trials. As the standard inverse variance approach to combining trials uses weights inversely proportional to the square of these standard errors, it copes naturally with data of these different formats, so that the trials are given appropriate weightings according to the relative efficiency of their designs.

The authors of the review reported that they had had to use a variety of techniques to estimate these standard errors, as they were not always available in the original reports. If necessary standard errors can be derived directly from standard deviations, confidence intervals, t values and exact P values. However, when paired data (both for change scores and cross-over trials) are used it is occasionally necessary to make an assumption about the within participant correlation between two time-points if the analysis presented mistakenly ignores the pairings. Similarly, when results are reported simply either as significant or non-significant, particular P values must be assumed from which the standard errors can be derived. Such problems are common in meta-analyses of continuous data due to the use of inappropriate analyses and the poor standard of presentation commonly encountered in published trial reports.

Meta-analyses were undertaken separately for the trials in normotensive and hypertensive groups, and for systolic and diastolic blood pressure. The results are given in the Table 15.7.

The analysis shows statistically significant reductions of around 5–6 mmHg in systolic blood pressure in hypertensive participants, with a

307

Table 15.7 Impact of salt lowering diets on systolic and diastolic blood pressure.

Method	Estimated difference in blood pressure reduction (95% CI) (diet–control) (mmHg)	Test of overall effect	Test for heterogeneity
Normotensive trials			
Systolic			
Inverse variance	−1·2 (−1·6 to −0·8)	$z = 6·4$, P < 0·001	$\chi^2_{27} = 75·1$, P < 0·001
DerSimonian and Laird	−1·7 (−2·4 to −0·9)	$z = 4·2$, P < 0·001	
Diastolic			
Inverse variance	−0·7 (−1·0 to −0·3)	$z = 3·4$, P = 0·001	$\chi^2_{27} = 56·1$, P = 0·001
DerSimonian and Laird	−0·5 (−1·2 to 0·1)	$z = 1·63$, P = 0·10	
Hypertensive trials			
Systolic			
Inverse variance	−5·4 (−6·3 to −4·5)	$z = 12·0$, P < 0·001	$\chi^2_{27} = 99·2$, P < 0·001
DerSimonian and Laird	−5·9 (−7·8 to −4·1)	$z = 6·4$, P < 0·001	
Diastolic			
Inverse variance	−3·5 (−4·0 to −2·9)	$z = 11·6$, P < 0·001	$\chi^2_{27} = 57·3$, P = 0·001
DerSimonian and Laird	−3·8 (−4·8 to −2·9)	$z = 8·0$, P < 0·001	

smaller reduction in diastolic blood pressure. The size of the reductions observed in normotensive participants was much smaller, the differences between the hypertensive and normotensive subgroups being statistically significant for both systolic ($z = 4·12$: P < 0·0001) and diastolic ($z = 5·61$: P < 0·0001) measurements. The confidence intervals for the DerSimonian and Laird random effects analyses for all reductions are much wider than those of the inverse variance fixed effect analyses, reflecting the significant heterogeneity detected in all analyses. The authors investigated this further using methods of meta-regression (see Chapters 9 and 11 and Stata command **metareg** in Chapter 18) and showed that the heterogeneity between trials could in part be explained by a relationship between the reduction in blood pressure and the reduction in salt intake achieved in each trial. This regression analysis, and the possible presence of bias, is discussed in Chapter 11.

On the basis of these analyses the authors concluded that salt-lowering diets may have some worthwhile impact on blood pressure for hypertensive people but not for normotensive people, contrary to current recommendations for universal dietary salt reduction.

Discussion

We have outlined a variety of methods for combining results from several studies in a systematic review. There are three aspects of choosing the right method for a particular meta-analysis: identifying the data type (binary, continuous, time to event), choosing an appropriate summary statistic, and selecting a weighting method for combining the studies, as summarised below and in Box 15.1.

What is clearly required from a summary statistic is that it is as stable as possible over the trials in the meta-analysis and subdivisions of the population to which the treatment will be applied. The more consistent it is, the greater is the justification for expressing the effect of treatment in a single summary number.[30] A second consideration is that the summary statistic should be easily understood and applied by those using the review. For binary data the choice is not straightforward, and no measure is best in all circumstances. These issues are considered in detail in Chapter 16.

Selection of summary statistics for continuous data is principally determined by whether trials all report the outcome using the same scale. If

Box 15.1 Considerations in choosing a method of meta-analysis

Choice of summary statistic depends upon:
(a) the type of data being analysed (binary, continuous, time-to-event)
(b) the consistency of estimates of the treatment effect across trials and subgroups
(c) the ease of interpretation of the summary statistic.

Choice of weighting method depends upon:
(a) the reliability of the method when sample sizes are small
(b) the reliability of the method if events are very rare
(c) the degree of imbalance in allocation ratios in the trials.

Consideration of heterogeneity can affect:
(a) whether a meta-analysis should be considered, depending on the similarity of trial characteristics
(b) whether an overall summary can have a sensible meaning, depending on the degree of disagreement observed between the trial results
(c) whether a random effects method is used to account for extra between-trial variation and to modify the significance and precision of the estimate of overall effect
(d) whether the impact of other factors on the treatment effect can be investigated using stratified analyses and methods of meta-regression.

this is not the case use of a weighted mean difference method would be erroneous. However, the standardised mean difference method can be used for either circumstance. Differences in results between these two methods can reflect differences in both the treatment effects calculated for each study, and the study weights. Interpretation of a weighted mean difference is easier than that of a standardised mean difference as it is expressed in natural units of measurement rather than standard deviations.

For all types of outcome, the choice of weighting scheme involves deciding between random and fixed effect models, and for fixed effect analyses of binary outcome measures, between inverse variance, Mantel–Haenszel and Peto methods. There is no consensus regarding the choice of fixed or random effects models, although they differ only in the presence of heterogeneity, when the random effects result will usually be more conservative. It is important to be aware of circumstances in which Mantel–Haenszel, inverse variance and Peto methods give erroneous results when deciding between them. Inverse variance methods are poor when trials are small and are rarely preferable to Mantel–Haenszel methods. Both Mantel–Haenszel and inverse variance methods are poor when event rates are very low, and Peto's method can be misleading when treatment effects are large, and when there are severely unequal numbers of participants in treatment and control groups in some or all of the trials.[17] Some of these points are illustrated in the case studies discussed above.

It is important to note that none of the analyses described can compensate for any publication bias (see Chapter 11), nor can they account for bias introduced through poor trial design and execution.

Acknowledgements

We are grateful to Julian Midgley for allowing us access to the data on which the third case study is based.

1 Deeks JJ. Systematic reviews of published evidence: miracles or minefields? *Ann Oncol* 1998;**9**:703–9.
2 Cook DJ, Guyatt GH, Laupacis A, Sackett DL. Rules of evidence and clinical recommendations on the use of antithrombotic agents. *Chest* 1992;**102**:305S–311S.
3 Thompson SG. Why sources of heterogeneity in meta-analysis should be investigated. *BMJ* 1994;**309**:1351–5.
4 Haldane JBS. The estimation and significance of the logarithm of a ratio of frequencies. *Ann Hum Genet* 1955;**20**:309–14.
5 Morris JA, Gardner MJ. Epidemiological studies. In: Altman DG, Machin D, Bryant TN, Gardner MJ, eds. *Statistics with confidence*, 2nd edn. London: BMJ Books, 2000:57–72.
6 Newcombe RG, Altman DG. Proportions and their differences. In: Altman DG, Machin D, Bryant TN, Gardner MJ, eds. *Statistics with confidence*, 2nd edn. London: BMJ Books, 2000:45–56.
7 Yusuf S, Peto R, Lewis J, Collins R, Sleight P. Beta blockade during and after myocardial infarction: an overview of the randomized trials. *Prog Cardiovasc Dis* 1985;**27**:335–71.

8 Sinclair JC, Bracken MB. *Effective care of the newborn infant.* Oxford: Oxford University Press, 1992: chapter 2.
9 Hedges LV, Olkin I. *Statistical methods for meta-analysis.* San Diego: Academic Press 1985: chapter 5.
10 Rosenthal R. Parametric measures of effect size. In: Cooper H, Hedges LV, eds. *The Handbook of research synthesis.* New York: Russell Sage Foundation, 1994.
11 Glass GV. Primary, secondary, and meta-analysis of research. *Educat Res* 1976;5:3–8.
12 Thompson SG, Pocock SJ. Can meta-analyses be trusted? *Lancet* 1991;338:1127–30.
13 Mantel N, Haenszel W. Statistical aspects of the analysis of data from retrospective studies of disease. *J Natl Cancer Inst* 1959;22:719–48.
14 Breslow NE, Day NE. Combination of results from a series of 2 × 2 tables; control of confounding. In: *Statistical methods in cancer research, Vol. 1: The analysis of case-control data.* IARC Scientific Publications No.32. Lyon: International Agency for Health Research on Cancer, 1980.
15 Robins J, Greenland S, Breslow NE. A general estimator for the variance of the Mantel-Haenszel odds ratio. *Am J Epidemiol* 1986;124:719–23.
16 Greenland S, Robins J. Estimation of a common effect parameter from sparse follow-up data. *Biometrics* 1985;41:55–68.
17 Greenland S, Salvan A. Bias in the one-step method for pooling study results. *Stat Med* 1990;9:247–52.
18 Deeks JJ, Bradburn MJ, Localio R, Berlin J. Much ado about nothing: meta-analysis for rare events [abstract]. *6th Cochrane Colloquium.* Baltimore, MD, 1998.
19 Altman DG. *Practical statistics for medical research.* London: Chapman and Hall, 1991: 379.
20 Parmar MKB, Torri V, Stewart L. Extracting summary statistics to perform meta-analyses of the published literature for survival endpoints. *Stat Med* 1998;17:2815–34.
21 DerSimonian R, Laird N. Meta-analysis in clinical trials. *Controlled Clin Trials* 1986;7:177–88.
22 Berlin JA, Laird NM, Sacks HS, Chalmers TC. A comparison of statistical methods for combining events rates from clinical trials. *Stat Med* 1989;8:141–51.
23 Bucher HC, Guyatt GH, Griffith LE, Walter SD. The results of direct and indirect treatment comparisons in meta-analyses of randomized controlled trials. *J Clin Epidemiol* 1997;50:683–91.
24 Song F, Glenny A-M, Altman DG. Indirect comparison in evaluating relative efficacy of antimicrobial prophylaxis in colorectal surgery. *Controlled Clin Trials* 2000;21:488–97.
25 Stewart LA, Clarke MJ. Practical methodology of meta-analyses (overviews) using updated individual patient data. *Stat Med* 1995;14:2057–79.
26 Normand ST. Meta-analysis: formulating, evaluating, combining and reporting. *Stat Med* 1999;18:321–60.
27 Hardy RJ, Thompson SG. A likelihood approach to meta-analysis with random effects. *Stat Med* 1996;15:619–29.
28 Louis TA, Zelterman D. Bayesian approaches to research synthesis. In: Cooper H, Hedges LV, eds. *The handbook of research synthesis.* New York: Russell Sage Foundation, 1994.
26 Normand ST. Meta-analysis: formulating, evaluating, combining and reporting. *Stat Med* 1999;18:321–60.
27 Hardy RJ, Thompson SG. A likelihood approach to meta-analysis with random effects. *Stat Med* 1996;15:619–29.
28 Louis TA, Zelterman D. Bayesian approaches to research synthesis. In: Cooper H, Hedges LV, eds. *The handbook of research synthesis.* New York: Russell Sage Foundation, 1994.
29 Gart J. Point and interval estimation of the common odds ratio in the combination of 2 × 2 tables with fixed marginals. *Biometrika* 1970;38:141–9.
30 Hodnett ED. Caregiver support for women during childbirth (Cochrane Review). In: *The Cochrane Library,* Issue 4. Oxford: Update Software, 1999.
31 Sackett DL, Deeks JJ, Altman DG. Down with odds ratios! *Evidence-Based Med* 1996;1:164–6.
32 Marshall M, Lockwood A. Assertive community treatment for people with severe mental disorders. (Cochrane Review) In: *The Cochrane Library,* Issue 4. Oxford: Update Software, 1999.

311

33 Midgley JP, Matthew AG, Greenwood CMT, Logan AG. Effect of reduced dietary sodium on blood pressure: a meta-analysis of randomized controlled trials. *JAMA* 1996;**275**:1590–7.
34 Breslow NE, Day NE. Fundamental measures of disease occurrence and association. In: *Statistical methods in cancer research, Vol. 1: The analysis of case-control data.* IARC Scientific Publications No.32. Lyon: International Agency for Health Research on Cancer, 1980.

16 Effect measures for meta-analysis of trials with binary outcomes

JONATHAN J DEEKS, DOUGLAS G ALTMAN

Summary points

- Major considerations when choosing a summary statistic are consistency of effect across studies, mathematical properties and ease of interpretation.
- Four statistics – the odds ratio, the risk difference and risk ratios of beneficial and harmful outcomes – can be used as summary statistics in meta-analyses of binary outcomes.
- Consistency of summary measures for a given meta-analysis can be examined in L'Abbé plots and by tests of homogeneity. Empirical investigations suggest that risk differences on average are the least likely to be consistent, risk ratios and odds ratios being on average equally consistent.
- Numbers needed to treat, relative risk reductions (%) and relative odds reductions (%) do not have the mathematical properties required for performing meta-analyses, but can be derived from the other four summary statistics estimated by meta-analysis and used in the presentation of overall results.
- Odds and odds ratios are not easily interpreted and are best converted to risks and risk ratios when considering their application to particular scenarios. The differences between odds ratios and risk ratios from the same meta-analyses can be large, and misinterpretation of odds ratios as risk ratios usually overestimates the benefits and harms of an intervention.
- When considering the clinical significance of a treatment effect it is important to be aware of the expected probability of the outcome with or without the intervention, regardless of the chosen summary statistic.
- When applying the results of a systematic review to a clinical scenario, the predicted benefits of interventions (expressed in terms of the number of people who will benefit) may vary according to the summary statistic used in the meta-analysis.

313

The starting point of all meta-analyses involves the selection of the summary statistic (effect measure) used to describe the observed treatment effect in each trial, from which the overall meta-analytical summary can be calculated (see Chapter 15). This chapter considers the choice of a summary statistic when the outcome of interest has a binary form (where the outcome for every participant is one of two possibilities, for example, dead and alive). The most commonly encountered effect measures used in clinical trials for binary data are:

- the risk difference (RD) (also called the absolute risk reduction, ARR);
- the risk ratio (RR) (also called the relative risk);
- the odds ratio (OR);
- the number needed to treat (NNT).

(As events may occasionally be desirable rather than undesirable, we would prefer a more neutral term than risk (such as probability), but for the sake of convention we use the terms risk ratio and risk difference throughout.)

Details of the calculations of these measures are given in Box 16.1. In this chapter we review the interpretation of these measures, consider their properties, present empirical evidence about their suitability for meta-analysis, and offer guidance on how to choose an appropriate measure for a particular meta-analysis.

Although we will focus on point estimates of treatment effect, all measures of effect should be accompanied by confidence intervals. These are easily obtained in all cases (Chapter 15). We also note that the relative measures (RR, OR) are sometimes expressed as the percentage reduction in risk or odds. For example, the relative risk reduction is defined as RRR = $100(1-RR)\%$. While this representation can help interpretation, it does not affect the choice between different measures: meta-analysis will always be undertaken of the original ratio measures. Summary risk ratios and odds ratios estimated from meta-analyses can be converted into relative risk and relative odds reductions in exactly the same way as for individual clinical trials.

Criteria for selection of a summary statistic

What are the desirable attributes of a summary statistic used in a meta-analysis?

Consistency

First, we would like the estimated statistic to be applicable across the situations where the trial results will be used. To have this property,

314

Box 16.1 Calculation of OR, RR, RD and NNT from a 2 × 2 table

The results of a clinical trial can be displayed as a 2 × 2 table:

	Event	No event	Total
Intervention	a	b	$n_1 = a+b$
Control	c	d	$n_2 = c+d$

where a, b, c and d are the numbers of participants with each outcome in each group. The following summary statistics can be calculated:

$$\text{odds ratio} = \frac{\text{odds of event in intervention group}}{\text{odds of event in control group}} = \frac{a/b}{c/d} = \frac{ad}{bc}$$

$$\text{relative risk} = \frac{\text{risk of event in intervention group}}{\text{risk of event in control group}} = \frac{a/(a + b)}{c/(c + d)}$$

risk difference = risk of event in intervention group − risk of event in control group

$$= \frac{a}{a + b} - \frac{c}{c + d}$$

$$\text{number needed to treat} * = \frac{1}{|\text{risk difference}|} = \frac{1}{|a/(a + b) - c/(c + d)|}$$

* The vertical bars in the denominator of the number needed to treat formula are directions to *take the absolute (positive) value*. Numbers needed to treat cannot be negative, but it is important to be aware of whether the NNT is a number needed to treat for one person to *benefit*, or a number needed to treat for one person to be *harmed*.

estimates of the treatment effect have to be as stable as possible over the various populations from which the trials have been drawn, and to which the intervention will be applied. The more nearly constant the statistic is, the greater the justification for expressing the effect of the intervention as a single summary number.[1] In practice we can usually only assess the stability of an overall treatment effect across the trials included in the meta-analysis, although some trial reports include investigation of variability of the treatment effect across patient subgroups.

A set of trials will often display greater heterogeneity than is expected by chance alone, indicating that a single summary statistic may be an inadequate summary of the treatment effect. We can investigate whether

315

certain study characteristics explain some of this variation either using meta-regression (see Chapters 8–11) or stratified meta-analysis (see Chapter 15). However, in any meta-analysis it is likely that there is variation in the underlying event rate observed in the control groups across the trials. When this is the case, the risk difference, risk ratio and odds ratio cannot all be equally consistent summaries of the trial results. Table 16.1 shows the results of four hypothetical trials, all of which have different control group event rates. Trials 2–4 have, respectively, the same odds ratio, the same relative risk and the same risk difference as trial 1. However, it is clear that when two trials have the same value for one of the measures, they will differ on the other two measures. The only situation where this relationship does not hold is when there is no treatment effect. The heterogeneity observed between the trials may thus in part be an artefact of a poor choice of summary statistic, and be reduced or even disappear when an alternative summary statistic is used.

Table 16.1 Results of four hypothetical trials with varying control group events

Trial	Relation to trial 1	Control	Treatment	OR	RR	RD
1	–	24/100	16/100	**0·60**	**0·67**	**0·08**
2	Same OR	32/100	22/100	**0·60**	0·69	0·10
3	Same RR	42/100	28/100	0·54	**0·67**	0·14
4	Same RD	42/100	34/100	0·71	0·81	**0·08**

Mathematical properties

Second, the summary statistic must have the mathematical properties required for performing a valid meta-analysis. The most important of these is the availability of a reliable variance estimate. The last measure shown in Box 16.1, the number needed to treat, does not have a variance estimator and is therefore not a valid statistic to use in meta-analysis. As discussed in depth in Chapter 20, in most situations the number needed to treat is best obtained by computing an overall risk ratio or odds ratio and applying this to a typical event rate without treatment. Our main focus here will be on the other three measures shown in Box 16.1.

Ease of interpretation

Lastly, a summary statistic should present a summary of the effect of the intervention in a way that helps readers to interpret and apply the results appropriately. "The essence of a good data analysis is the effective communication of clinically relevant findings",[2] so the ability of general readers of a review to understand and make logical decisions based on the reported summary statistic must not be overlooked.

Odds and risks

In general conversation the words "odds" and "risks" are used interchangeably (together with the words "chances", and "likelihood"), as if they describe the same quantity. In statistics, however, odds and risks have particular meanings, and are calculated in different ways (Box 16.1). When the difference between them is ignored the results of a systematic review may be misinterpreted.

Risk is the concept more familiar to patients and health professionals. Risk describes the probability with which a health outcome (usually an adverse event) will occur. In research risk is commonly expressed as a decimal number between 0 and 1, although these are occasionally converted into percentages. As "risk" is synonymous with "event rate" it is simple to grasp the relationship between a risk and the likely occurrence of events: in a sample of 100 people the number of events observed will be the risk multiplied by 100. For example, when the risk is 0·1, 10 people out of every 100 will develop the event, when the risk is 0·5, 50 people out of every 100 will develop the event.

Odds is a concept that is more familiar to gamblers than health professionals. The odds is the probability that a particular event will occur divided by the probability that it will not occur, and can be any number between 0 and infinity. In gambling, the odds describes the ratio of the size of the potential winnings to the gambling stake; in health care it is the ratio of the number of people with the event to the number without. It is commonly expressed as a ratio of two integers. For example, an odds of 0·01 is often written as 1:100, odds of 0·33 as 1:3, and odds of 3 as 3:1. Odds can be converted to risks, and risks to odds, using the formulae:

$$risk = \frac{odds}{1 + odds} ; \quad odds = \frac{risk}{1 - risk}.$$

The practical application of an odds is more complicated than for a risk. The best way to ensure that the interpretation is correct is to first convert the odds into a risk. For example, when the odds are 1 to 10, or 0·1, one person will have the event for every 10 who do not, and, using the above formula, the risk of the event is $0·1/(1 + 0·1) = 0·091$. In a sample of 100, about nine individuals will have the event and 91 will not. When the odds are equal to 1, one person will have the event for every one who does not, so in a sample of 100, $100 \times 1/(1 + 1) = 50$ will have the event and 50 will not.

The difference between odds and risk is small when the event rate is low, as shown in the above example. When events are common the differences between odds and risks are large. For example, a risk of 0·5 is equivalent to

317

an odds of 1; a risk of 0·9 is equivalent to odds of 9. Similarly, a ratio of risks (the risk ratio) is similar to a ratio of odds (the odds ratio) when events are rare, but not when events are common (unless the two risks are very similar) (see Box 2.2 in Chapter 2 and Case study 1 in Chapter 15).

Many epidemiological studies investigate rare events, and here it is common to see the phrases and calculations for risks and odds used interchangeably. However, in randomised controlled trials event rates are often in the range where risks and odds are very different, and, as discussed below, risk ratios and odds ratios should not be used interchangeably.

Measure of absolute effect – the risk difference

The estimated risk difference is the difference between the observed event rates (proportions of individuals with the outcome of interest) in the two groups. This effect measure is often the most natural statistic to use when considering clinical significance, and is often used when carrying out sample size calculations for randomised trials. The risk difference can be calculated for any trial, even when there are no events in either group. The risk difference is straightforward to interpret. It describes the actual difference in the event rate that was observed with treatment; for an individual it describes the estimated change in the probability of experiencing the event. However, the clinical importance of a risk difference may depend on the underlying event rate. For example, a risk difference of 2% may represent a small clinically insignificant change from a risk of 58 to 60% but a proportionally much larger and potentially important change from 1 to 3%. Although there are some grounds to claim that the risk difference provides more complete information than relative measures[3,4] it is still important to be aware of the underlying event rates and consequences of the events when interpreting a risk difference.

The risk difference is naturally constrained, which may create difficulties when applying results to other patient groups and settings. For example, if a trial or meta-analysis estimates a risk difference of −10%, then for a group with an initial risk of less than 10% the outcome will have an impossible negative probability. Similar scenarios occur at the other end of the scale with increases in risk. Such problems arise when the results are applied to patients with different expected event rates from those observed in the trial(s).

As noted earlier, the risk difference is sometimes called the absolute risk reduction. The adjective "absolute" is used here to distinguish this measure from measures of relative effect, but it should be recognised that this usage is different from the mathematical usage of "absolute" to mean the size of the effect regardless of the sign. Retaining the sign of the difference is of course vital as it distinguishes trials that are estimating a beneficial effect from those that are estimating a harmful effect.

Measures of relative effect – the risk ratio and odds ratio

Measures of relative effect express the outcome in one group relative to that in the other. The risk ratio (relative risk) is the ratio of two event rates whereas the odds ratio is the ratio of the odds of an event in the two groups (Box 16.1). Neither the risk ratio nor the odds ratio can be calculated for a trial if there are no events (or all participants experience events) in one of the groups. In this situation it is customary to add one half to each cell of the 2×2 table (Chapter 15). In the case where no events (or all events) are observed in both groups the trial provides no information about relative event rates and must be omitted from the meta-analysis.

Interpretation of risk ratios is not difficult as they describe the multiplication of the risk (or the event rate) that occurs with use of the intervention. For example, a risk ratio of 3 implies that the event rate with treatment is three times higher than the event rate without treatment (or alternatively that treatment increases the event rate by $100 \times (RR-1)\% = 200\%$. Similarly a risk ratio of 0·25 is interpreted as the event rate associated with treatment being one-quarter of that without treatment (or alternatively that treatment decreases event rates by $100 \times (1-RR)\% = 75\%$). Again, the interpretation of the clinical importance of a given risk ratio cannot be made without knowledge of the typical event rate without treatment: a risk ratio of 0·75 could correspond to a clinically important reduction in events from 80% to 60%, or a small, less clinically important reduction from 4% to 3%.

The value of the observed risk ratio is constrained to lie between 0 and $100/ p_c$, where p_c is the event rate in the control group. This means that for common events large values of risk ratio are impossible. For example, when the event rate in the control group is 66% then the observed risk ratio cannot exceed 1·5. This problem only applies for increases in event rates, and could be circumvented by considering all trials – whether treatment or prevention – as designed to reduce the risk of a bad outcome.[5] In other words, instead of considering the increase in success rate one could consider the decrease in failure rate.

Odds ratios, like odds, are somewhat more difficult to interpret.[6,7] Odds ratios describe the multiplication of the odds of the outcome that occur with use of the intervention. To understand what an odds ratio means in terms of changes in numbers of events it is best to first convert it into a risk ratio, and then interpret the risk ratio in the context of a typical event rate without treatment, as outlined above. Formulae for converting an odds ratio to a risk ratio, and *vice versa*, are:

319

$$RR = \frac{OR}{1 - p_c(1 - OR)} \; ; \quad OR = \frac{RR(1 - p_c)}{1 - p_c RR},$$

where p_c is the typical event rate without treatment (see Case study 1 for an example of the interpretation of an odds ratio).

The non-equivalence of the risk ratio and odds ratio does not indicate that either is wrong – both are entirely valid. Problems may arise, however, if the odds ratio is interpreted directly as a risk ratio.[8,9] For treatments that increase event rates, the odds ratio will be larger than the risk ratio, so the misinterpretation will tend to overestimate the treatment effect, especially when events are common (with, say, event rates more than 30%). For treatments that reduce event rates, the odds ratio will be smaller than the risk ratio, so that again it overestimates the effect of treatment. This error in interpretation is quite common in published reports of systematic reviews.

The odds ratio has several mathematical properties that may be advantageous for use as a summary statistic in a meta-analysis.[10] The behaviour of odds ratio methods does not rely on which of the two outcome states is coded as the event (in contrast to the risk ratio). The odds ratio also has the advantage over the risk ratio of being "unbounded" – this means that it can take values anywhere from 0 to infinity regardless of underlying event rates. On the logarithmic scale the odds ratio is unbounded in both directions which is one reason why regression models for binary outcomes usually use log odds ratios (logistic regression). The odds ratio is also the measure obtained from Peto's approach to the meta-analysis of randomised trials.

Meta-analyses of risk ratios and odds ratios differ in the weights that are given to individual trials. For meta-analyses of risk ratios the proportional weights given to trials of the same sample size estimating the same effect increase with increasing event rates (Chapter 15). The relationship becomes particularly strong when event rates are above 50%, and any trials with event rates higher than 95% totally dominate risk ratio meta-analyses unless they have particularly small sample sizes. This reflects the precision with which estimates of risk ratios are made across different event rates. For odds ratios the pattern is similar to that for risk ratios when event rates are less than 50%, with weights for trials of the same sample size and effect size increasing as event rates rise to 50%, but then decreasing in a symmetrical pattern as the rates rise towards 100%. These differences in trial weights are another reason why results from meta-analyses using risk ratios or odds ratios may differ. The contrast will be most marked in meta-analyses with very variable or very high event rates.

What is the event?

Most health care interventions are intended either to reduce the risk of occurrence of an adverse outcome or increase the chance of a good outcome. These may be seen broadly as prevention and treatment interventions respectively. All of the effect measures described above apply equally to both types of outcome.

In many situations it is natural to talk about one of the outcome states as being an *event*. For example, in treatment trials participants are generally ill at the start of the trial, and the event of interest is recovery or cure. In prevention trials participants are well at the beginning of the trial and the event is the onset of disease or perhaps even death. This distinction is oversimplistic, however, as trials do (and should) investigate both good and bad outcomes. For example, trials of therapy will look at both intended beneficial effects and unintended adverse effects. Because the focus is usually on the intervention group, a trial in which a treatment reduces the occurrence of an adverse outcome will have an odds ratio and risk ratio less than one, and a negative risk difference. A trial in which a treatment increases the occurrence of a good outcome will have an odds ratio and risk ratio greater than one, and a positive risk difference (see Box 16.1).

However, as already mentioned, it is also possible to switch events and non-events and consider instead the proportion of patients not recovering or not experiencing the event. For meta-analyses using risk differences or odds ratios the impact of this switch is of no great consequence: the switch simply changes the sign of a risk difference, whilst for odds ratios the new odds ratio is the reciprocal ($1/x$) of the original odds ratio. (Similar considerations apply when a trial compares two active treatments, and it is unclear which is being compared with which as neither is a "control" treatment.) By contrast, switching the outcome can make a substantial difference for risk ratios, affecting the effect size, its significance and observed heterogeneity.[11] In a meta-analysis the effect of this reversal cannot be predicted mathematically. An example of the impact the switch can make is given in Case study 1 below. The *a priori* identification of which risk ratio is more likely to be a consistent summary statistic is an area that requires further empirical investigation.

Lastly, a simple binary outcome may hide considerable variation in the time from the start of treatment to the event, and many treatments can only aim to delay rather than prevent an event. Such data are best analysed using methods for the analysis of time-to-event or survival data, the appropriate summary statistic being the "hazard ratio". Meta-analysis of such studies ideally needs individual patient data (see Chapter 6), although it may be possible to extract adequate summary information from some papers.[12] If variation in time to event is ignored, then variation in average length of follow-up may vary across trials and could be an important source of heterogeneity. Neither the risk ratio nor the odds ratio will be the same as the hazard ratio.

The L'Abbé plot

The most common graphical display associated with a meta-analysis is the forest plot (Chapter 2). This plot cannot help with the question of whether an effect measure is an appropriate summary. A more useful graph here is the L'Abbé plot, in which the event rates in each treatment group are plotted against each other.[13] Examples are shown in the case studies below.

The L'Abbé plot is a helpful adjunct to a "standard" meta-analysis. It has several useful features, including the explicit display of the range of variation in event rates in treatment and control groups.[14]

In the present context the particular value of the L'Abbé plot is that it is simple to superimpose contours of constant treatment effect according to each possible measure – risk difference, RR, or OR.[15,16] Such plots are shown in Figure 16.1. The L'Abbé plot for a given set of trials may thus shed light on whether a chosen effect measure is likely to be a good overall summary for a meta-analysis, as illustrated in the case studies below.

Empirical evidence of consistency

A L'Abbé plot is not the only way to assess the consistency of results with the overall summary statistic: it is routine in meta-analysis to evaluate the consistency of results with the summary estimate using tests of homogeneity (see Chapter 15). Rather than visually investigating the appropriateness of different summary statistics it is possible to undertake the meta-analysis using risk ratio, odds ratio and risk difference measures, and to choose the one which gives the lowest heterogeneity statistic. However, there are problems in this procedure as the decision is data-derived and usually based on very few data points (and thus vulnerable to the play of chance).

We have undertaken an empirical investigation to assess the consistency of estimates of odds ratio, risk ratio and risk difference across a large sample of meta-analyses.[16] The analysis considered all the meta-analyses of binary outcomes published on the Cochrane Library in the Spring issue of 1997.[17] In total, 1889 analyses were considered which combined data from more than one trial. Meta-analyses were performed using Mantel–Haenszel risk difference, risk ratio and odds ratio methods (described in Chapter 15) on each data set. The consistency of the results for each meta-analysis was measured using the standard heterogeneity statistic, computing a weighted sum of the squares of the differences between the trial estimates and the overall

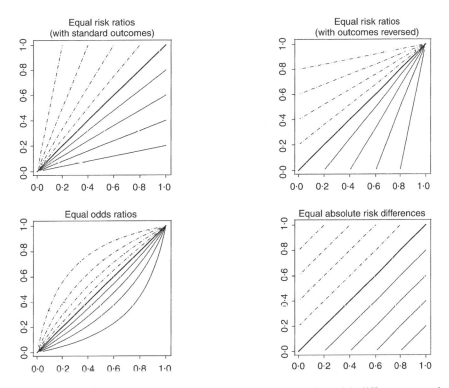

Figure 16.1 L'Abbé plots demonstrating constant odds ratios, risk differences, and risk ratios for standard and reversed outcomes. Lines are drawn for risk ratios and odds ratios of 0·2, 0·4, 0·6, 0·8, 1, 1·25, 1·67, 2·5 and 5, and for risk differences of −0·8 to +0·8 in steps of 0·2. The bold solid line marks the line of no treatment effect (RR = 1, OR = 1, RD = 0). The solid lines indicate treatments where the event rate is reduced (or the alternative outcome is increased). The dashed lines indicate interventions where the event rate is increased (or the alternative outcome is decreased). In each case, the further the lines are from the diagonal line of no effect, the stronger is the treatment effect.

estimate. The three summary statistics for each analysis were then compared.

Plots of the heterogeneity statistics for comparisons of risk difference with risk ratio, and of risk ratio with odds ratio are given in Figure 16.2. It is clear from the first plot that analyses of risk differences tend to have higher heterogeneity than risk ratios (more points are above the diagonal line than below it), whilst in the second plot there is little difference on average between heterogeneity for odds ratios and risk ratios. This is clear in the summary of median heterogeneity statistics for these analyses presented in Table 16.2.

It therefore appears that the risk difference is likely to be the poorest

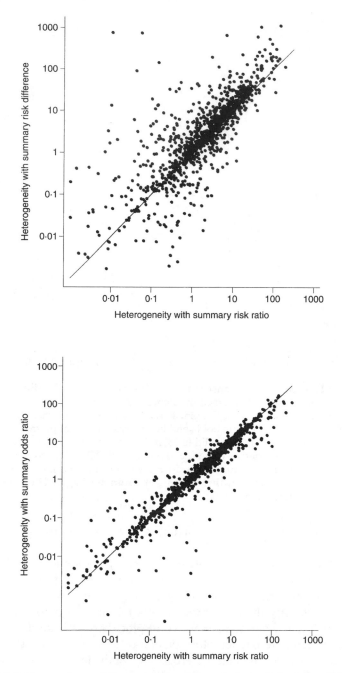

Figure 16.2 Comparison of heterogeneity (χ^2 statistics) of the same 1889 meta-analyses using RD, RR and OR summary statistics.

Table 16.2 Average heterogeneity statistics for different outcome measures.

	Median heterogeneity statistic	
	Analyses with average control group event rates <20% $N = 1179$	Analyses with average control group event rates ≥20% $N = 710$
Risk ratio	1·9	2·7
Odds ratio	1·9	2·7
Risk difference	2·4	3·6

summary in terms of consistency, whilst there is little difference between odds ratios and risk ratios. Even for meta-analyses with high event rates in the control group (275 had average event rates above 50%), there was little difference in median heterogeneity scores for the two measures of relative effect (median scores for odds ratio 3·3, for risk ratio 3·2). These findings do not mean that the risk difference should never be used. As Figure 16.2 shows, some meta-analyses demonstrate less heterogeneity with the risk difference than the risk ratio. An example of a situation where the risk difference is the most consistent summary statistic is given in Case study 2 below.

In these analyses we did not consider the impact of switching the selected event for the risk ratio analyses; we took the reviewers' original selections of the event for the computation of all risk ratios. It should also be noted that the heterogeneity statistics in the analyses are computed using the standard methods, which use different weights for risk ratio, odds ratio and risk difference analyses, although all are considered to approximate to a chi-squared distribution of k-1 degrees of freedom where k is the number of studies contributing to the meta-analysis.

Empirical evidence of ease of interpretation

Several studies have examined whether different ways of expressing numerical results of clinical trial results (such as choice of summary statistics) may influence perceptions about the worth of a treatment. McGettigan et al. undertook a systematic review of the published literature on the effects of information "framing" on the practices of physicians.[18] Among twelve randomised trials, most studies compared the effect of presenting results in terms of relative risk reduction, absolute risk reductions or the number needed to treat. Overall, the studies found that, in simple clinical scenarios, expressing treatment effects in terms of a risk ratio (or relative risk reduction) was more likely to elicit use of the intervention than expression of the same results in terms of risk differences or numbers needed to treat.

Several factors were found to reduce the impact of framing. These included the risk of causing harm, pre-existing prejudices about treatments, the type of decision, the therapeutic yield, clinical experience, and costs.

Importantly, no study had investigated the effect of framing on actual clinical practice. McGettigan *et al.* were critical of the methodology of many of the trials. It is noteworthy that none of these trials investigated the use of the odds ratio as a measure of treatment effect. However, based on the results for risk ratios, and noting the evidence that odds ratios are often misinterpreted as risk ratios and that they exaggerate treatment benefit, it seems reasonable to surmise that presentations of odds ratios is even more likely to elicit use of interventions than presentation of risk ratios.

Due to subjective components in clinical decisions these studies cannot assess whether switching summary statistics leads to clinical decisions being more or less rational, only that different decisions are made when the same findings are presented in different ways.

Case studies

Many of the issues mentioned in the preceding sections are illustrated by two case studies. Case study 1 shows results from a meta-analysis of eradication of *Helicobacter pylori* in non-ulcer dyspepsia. Case study 2 shows results from a meta-analysis of trials of vaccines to prevent influenza.

Case study 1: eradication of *H. pylori* in non-ulcer dyspepsia

H. pylori is a bacterium that inhabits the stomach and has been linked to the development of peptic ulcer; eradication of the bacterium with antibiotics is an effective cure for most ulcer disease. *H. pylori* is also considered to have a possible causal role in the development of non-ulcer dyspepsia. A meta-analysis of the five relevant trials reported a small reduction in dyspepsia rates 12 months after eradication, which was just statistically significant.[19] The effect measure used in the published analysis was the relative risk of remaining dyspeptic 12 months after eradication. This was chosen as it was thought to be the most clinically relevant outcome and had been pre-stated in the review protocol. No alternative effect measures were considered.

Eight alternative meta-analyses are presented in Table 16.3. Results are shown using fixed and random effects analyses for odds ratios, risk differences and the two risk ratios of dyspepsia recovery and remaining dyspeptic. (Estimates of the odds ratios and risk differences of remaining dyspeptic rather than of dyspepsia cure can be determined from the cure results by taking reciprocals and by multiplying by −1 respectively, as explained earlier in the chapter). In the following we consider the interpretation of these results, considering random effects analyses when the significance of the test of homogeneity is less than 0·1.

The tests of homogeneity clearly indicate that the authors' chosen effect measure, the risk ratio of remaining dyspeptic, is the most consistent

Table 16.3 Alternative analyses of eradication trials for non-ulcer dyspepsia.

Measure	Effect	95% CI	Test of homogeneity
Odds ratio of cure			
Fixed effect model	1·31	1·03 to 1·68	$Q = 10·8$, df = 4, P = 0·03
Random effects model	1·38	0·90 to 2·11	
Risk difference for cure			
Fixed effect model	0·05	0·01 to 0·09	$Q = 8·3$, df = 4, P = 0·08
Random effects model	0·06	−0·01 to 0·12	
Risk ratio for cure			
Fixed effect model	1·21	1·02 to 1·43	$Q = 12·7$, df = 4, P = 0·01
Random effects model	1·28	0·92 to 1·77	
Risk ratio for remaining dyspeptic			
Fixed effect model	0·93	0·88 to 0·99	$Q = 6·4$, df = 4, P = 0·18
Random effects model	0·92	0·85 to 0·99	

estimator across all the trials, with significant heterogeneity being detected for the three alternative summary statistics. In fact, the statistical significance of the overall estimates crucially depends on this choice of summary statistic: the random effects analyses for odds ratios, risk differences and the risk ratio for cure are all not statistically significant at the $P = 0·05$ level. Inspection of the L'Abbé plot in Figure 16.3 also suggests that the pattern of the trial estimates is consistent with the risk ratio for the reversed outcome of remaining dyspeptic, although this is somewhat hard to discern with so few data points. However, selection of the risk ratio of remaining dyspeptic on the basis of minimal heterogeneity and maximum statistical significance would be a data driven decision. Where the interpretation of the analysis so critically depends on the choice of effect measure it is essential for the effect measure to be pre-stated before the analysis (as was the case in this review), the selection being based on clinical and scientific argument.

It is also of interest to consider the consistency (or otherwise) of the estimates of treatment benefit across the different analyses. The choice of effect measure can lead to different predictions of benefit. The risk ratio for cure of 1·21 can be interpreted as the chances of recovery increasing by 21% (around one-fifth) with treatment, or that recovery is 1·2 times more likely with treatment. This effect may be important if symptomatic recovery commonly occurs without treatment, but not if it is rare. It is necessary to obtain an estimate of this typical recovery rate, p_c, to gauge the likely impact of the effect in terms of numbers of patients recovering. In the review there was considerable variation of baseline recovery rates between 10% and 50%, as shown in the L'Abbé plot in Figure 16.3. Consider a scenario where the spontaneous recovery rate is 10%: for every 100 people receiving eradication therapy, $100 \times (0·1 \times 1·21) = 12$ will not have dyspeptic symptoms later this year, 10 of whom would have recovered without treatment, and 2 due to treatment.

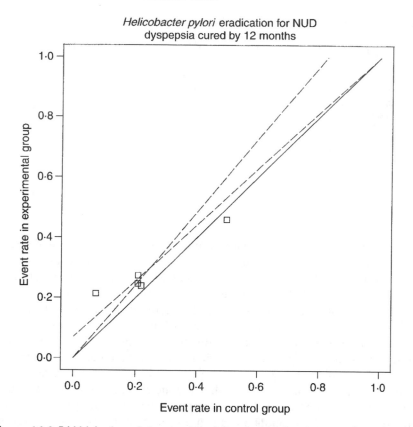

Figure 16.3 L'Abbé plot of the results of the five trials of *H. pylori* eradication therapy in the treatment of non-ulcer dyspepsia. The dashed line ascending from the point (0,0) corresponds to a risk ratio for dyspepsia cured at 12 months of 1·21 (Mantel–Haenszel fixed effect estimate; test for heterogeneity: $Q = 12·7$, df $= 4$, $P = 0·01$). The dashed line descending from the point (1,1) corresponds to a risk ratio for remaining dyspeptic at 12 months of 0·93 (Mantel–Haenszel fixed effect estimate; test for heterogeneity: $Q = 6·4$, df $= 4$, $P = 0·18$).

Alternatively the risk difference analysis estimated an absolute increase in recovery rates of 0·05, or 5%. This can be interpreted as showing that the chance of recovery increases by 5 percentage points, regardless of baseline recovery rates. Thus for every 100 people treated, 5 will recover as a result of treatment, regardless of how many recover anyway.

The estimate of the odds ratio of 1·38 is interpreted as showing that eradication treatment increases the odds of cure by 38%, or that the odds are about 1·4 times higher. To understand the effect that this odds ratio describes it is necessary first to convert it into a risk ratio. Taking the same

328

spontaneous recovery rate of 10%, the equivalent risk ratio is 1·33, which leads to an estimate of three additional people being cured for every 100 treated.

The fourth option differs, in that the event being described is *remaining dyspeptic*. The estimate suggests that the rate of dyspepsia with treatment will be 93% of the rate without treatment, or that the rate has decreased by 7%. In terms of numbers of people remaining dyspeptic, this should be considered in the context of the reversed event rate. We estimate the proportion remaining dyspeptic at 12 months to be 0·9, to fit in with the previous scenario. Using this value, for every 100 people receiving eradication therapy, $100 \times (0·9 \times 0·93) = 84$ will still be dyspeptic at the end of follow-up, 6 fewer than would be the case without treatment.

The choice of summary statistic therefore also makes a difference to the estimated benefit of treatment in a particular scenario, the number of people benefiting from treatment varying between 2 and 6 per 100 depending on the chosen summary statistic. These discrepancies are less for projections at typical event rates close to the mean of those observed in the trials. The pattern of predictions of absolute benefit according to placebo response rates for the four effect measures are shown in Figure 16.4.

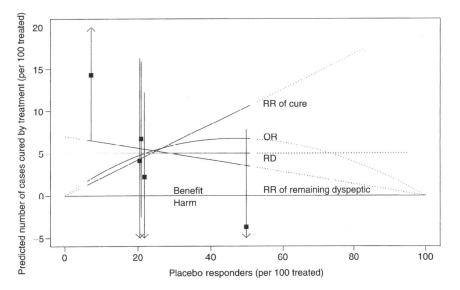

Figure 16.4 Predictions of treatment benefit at 6–12 months using *H. pylori* eradication therapy in non-ulcer dyspepsia. Solid lines indicate predictions within the range of the trial data, dotted lines indicate predictions beyond the observed range. The black boxes and vertical lines indicate the point estimates and confidence intervals of the five trials.

329

Case study 2 : prevention of influenza through vaccination

Only a small proportion of cases of clinical influenza are caused by the influenza A virus, the target of most vaccines which protect against influenza. This means that in clinical trials of influenza vaccines a large proportion of the cases of clinical influenza would not be prevented even by a totally efficacious vaccine. Also, the proportion of clinical influenza cases unrelated to influenza A fluctuates between trials according to seasonal and geographical variations in other viral infections which cause "flu like illnesses".

In a systematic review of the efficacy of influenza vaccines[20] it was argued that, in this situation, the risk difference is the most appropriate summary statistic if the proportion of participants acquiring influenza A cases is more stable than the proportion acquiring of non-other influenza like viruses across the trials. Inspection of a L'Abbé plot (Figure 16.5) and heterogeneity statistics (Table 16.4) indicate that this is the case. However, the statistical significance of the heterogeneity remains whichever summary statistic is used. This may in part be explained by the test of homogeneity being powerful enough to detect small variations in treatment effects in reviews with large samples (more than 30 000 participants were included in this review). However, it may also be explained through variation in the formulation of the vaccine used in the different trials, and to changes in circulating influenza A viral subtypes. For this situation it does not make clinical sense to reverse the outcome and consider the risk ratio for remaining free of clinical influenza. Such a model would predict the largest absolute benefit of vaccination in a population where rates of influenza like illnesses are very low, and no benefit in a population where rates are very high (see the patterns of risk ratios in Figure 16.4).

Table 16.4 Alternative analyses of influenza vaccination trials

Measure	Effect	95% CI	Test of homogeneity
Odds ratio for clinical illness			
Random effects model	0·66	0·53 to 0·81	$Q = 84·75$, df = 19, P < 0·001
Risk difference for clinical illness			
Random effects model	−0·051	−0·078 to −0·023	$Q = 57·86$, df = 19, P < 0·001
Risk ratio for clinical illness			
Random effects model	0·75	0·65 to 0·86	$Q = 86·98$, df = 19, P < 0·001

Discussion

All of the summary statistics considered in this chapter are equally valid measures of the treatment effect for a randomised controlled trial – the question we have considered here is their suitability for summarising a set

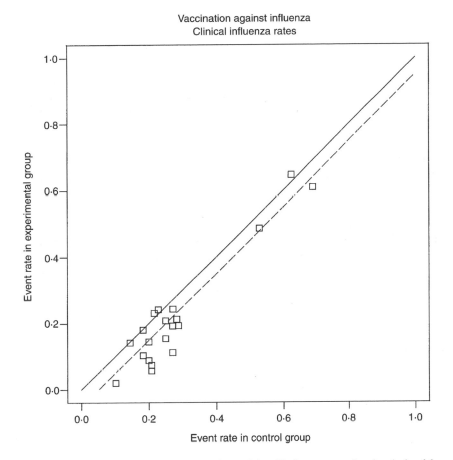

Figure 16.5 L'Abbé plot of the results of 20 trials of influenza vaccination in healthy adults. The dashed line indicates the summary risk difference of −5·1%.

of trials included in a formal meta-analysis within a systematic review. We have considered three criteria on which the selection of a measure should be based: consistency, mathematical behaviour, and ease of comprehension. No single measure is uniformly best, so that the choice inevitably involves a compromise.

The odds ratio has the strongest mathematical properties, but is the hardest to comprehend and to apply in practice. There are many published examples where odds ratios from meta-analyses have been misinterpreted by authors as if they were risk ratios.[8,9] Indeed, Schwartz et al. observed that "odds ratios are bound to be interpreted as risk ratios".[21] There must always be some concern that routine presentation of the results of systematic

331

reviews as odds ratios will lead to frequent overestimation of the benefits and harms of treatments when the results are applied in clinical practice.

The common use of the odds ratio as the summary measure for a systematic review may have arisen for reasons of history and convenience. The Mantel–Haenszel odds ratio method was published as a statistical method for the stratified analysis of case-control studies,[22] for which the odds ratio is the only valid summary measure of association. When meta-analyses of clinical trials were first undertaken in health care, the analogy between pooling trials and pooling strata was noted, and the method was reconceived as a meta-analytical method. The widespread use of the method was supported by the availability of software to undertake the calculation, and the simplification and extension of the method by Richard Peto for pooling data from survival analyses (see Chapter 15). Since then, meta-analytic methods have been developed for summarising risk ratios and risk differences.[23] While there are strong advocates of the odds ratio,[10] some statisticians and epidemiologists have argued that the odds ratio is often not the most suitable choice of summary statistic for summarising the results of randomised trials and systematic reviews.[7,24,25]

A presentation based on risks appears on the surface to be more likely to be correctly interpreted than one based on odds. The risk difference is the easiest measure to understand but is the measure least likely to be consistent across a set of trials. Its use is problematic when it is applied to real patients with widely ranging expected risks, as treatment benefit often relates to baseline risk. The risk ratio has some undesirable mathematical properties, but these apply only to those analyses where event rates are very high and risk ratios are much greater than unity. For other meta-analyses the risk ratio may be a wise choice as it is relatively easy to comprehend, and our empirical study shows that it as likely to be consistent across trials as an odds ratio. However, there are two "opposing" risk ratios which can be considered for any analysis, according to how we define outcome, and selecting the "wrong" one can dramatically alter the results of the systematic review, as shown in the Case study 1.

Another possible approach is to use one statistic to analyse the data and present the results using another. The choice of statistic for analysis might be based on considerations of mathematics and consistency, whilst an easily interpreted statistic could be used for presentation. This approach might, for example, indicate the use of the odds ratio for analysis with results converted to a risk ratio or a number needed to treat for presentation (see Box 16.2). A difficulty here is that conversions from odds ratios to other statistics are sensitive to the typical event rate without treatment (p_c), which will vary greatly according to the situation to which the results are applied. An average value for p_c is often estimated from the control groups of the clinical trials, but as trials are rarely designed to provide a valid

Box 16.2 The number needed to treat

The number needed to treat is considered at some length in Chapter 20. Here we show how to estimate the number needed to treat from estimates of risk difference, risk ratio or odds ratio as summaries of treatment effect from a meta-analysis (although their application to a clinical trial is identical).

The number needed to treat is estimated from a summary risk difference simply as $NNT = 1/RD$. This calculation gives a single number with no way of adapting it to reflect variations in underlying event rates. It is only sensible, therefore, when there is evidence that the risk difference is relatively constant across different studies and different event rates.

Numbers needed to treat can be computed directly from summary odds ratios (OR) or risk ratios (RR) according to the following formulae:

$$NNT = \frac{1}{p_c(1 - RR)} \; ; \quad NNT = \frac{1 - p_c(1 - OR)}{p_c\,(1 - p_c)(1 - OR)}$$

where p_c is the typical event rate without treatment for the scenario to which they will be applied.

As the typical event rate increases, the NNT based on a summary risk ratio will decrease. The NNT based on a summary odds ratio, however, will decrease as the event rate increases to 50%, and increases thereafter. This pattern for the odds ratio echoes the symmetry in the weights given to the trials in the meta-analysis (see main text).

estimate of this value this estimate may be inappropriate when applying the results of the review. A better approach might be to choose p_c based on clinical experience.

The impact of the choice of summary statistic can also be considered in sensitivity analyses, repeating the analysis for odds ratios, risk ratios and risk differences. Clearly we would hope that the interpretation of the results would be consistent irrespective of the summary statistic, indicating that the broad qualitative conclusions of the review do not depend on the use of a particular effect measure. However, we have seen that this will not always be the case (see Case study 1). In some situations changing the effect measure can have a large effect on the interpretation of the results, especially where the size as well as the direction of the effect is critical.

Although our investigations of heterogeneity statistics have been helpful in providing empirical evidence of the relative suitability of odds ratios, risk ratios and risk differences on average, their use in selecting a summary statistic for a particular analysis is limited. Selection of a summary measure on the basis of minimising heterogeneity is a somewhat data derived approach which can generate spurious (over-optimistic) findings. Also, in practice there are often too few trials for a L'Abbé plot or heterogeneity statistics to give clear guidance on which measure is most suitable.

A priori specification of the model on clinical or scientific grounds undoubtedly seems preferable to a *post hoc* selection based on comparisons of analyses. But how could such an *a priori* selection be determined? The choice of a summary statistic may best be viewed as a choice between different mathematical models of the relationship between control group event rates and event rates with treatment. The underlying patterns for these models are shown in the L'Abbé plots in Figure 16.1 (which show contours of constant effect for each measure) or more clearly in the plot of treatment benefit against control group event rates in Figure 16.4 (which shows predictions of actual benefit of treatment for the results of the first case study). Significant variation in control group event rates between trials must reflect variation in patient characteristics, control group interventions, outcome measures, study quality, or variation in length of follow-up (event rates usually increasing with time). If the causes of variation in control group event rates between the trials can be identified, and if the shape of the relationship between these event rates and treatment benefit can be hypothesised, it may be possible to choose the summary statistic which most closely fits the predicted patterns of these relationships. Clearly, the practical application of this approach to a particular meta-analysis is not straightforward, and there is a need for more research into these issues and the reliability of this approach.

Acknowledgements

We are grateful for the assistance of Gordon Dooley in undertaking the empirical investigation of Cochrane reviews, and thank Iain Chalmers, Dave Sackett and Chris Cates for commenting on a previous version of this chapter.

1 Breslow NE, Day NE. Combination of results from a series of 2 × 2 tables; control of confounding. In: *Statistical methods in cancer research*, volume 1: *The analysis of case-control data*. IARC Scientific Publications No. 32. Lyon: International Agency for Health Research on Cancer, 1980: 55.
2 Pocock SJ. *Clinical trials: a practical approach*. Chichester: Wiley, 1983: 210.
3 Sackett DL, Richardson WS, Rosenberg W, Haynes BR. *Evidence-based medicine: how to practice and teach EBM*. Edinburgh: Churchill Livingstone, 1997: 136.
4 Laupacis A, Sackett DL, Roberts RS. An assessment of clinically useful measures of the consequences of treatment. *N Engl J Med* 1988; **318**: 1728–33.
5 Altman DG, Deeks JJ, Sackett DL. Odds ratios revisited [author response]. *Evidence-Based Med* 1998;3:71–2.
6 Sackett DL, Deeks JJ, Altman DG. Down with odds ratios! *Evidence-Based Med* 1996;**1**: 164–6.

7 Sinclair JC, Bracken MB. Clinically useful measures of effect in binary analyses of randomized trials. *J Clin Epidemiol* 1994;47:81–90.

8 Deeks JJ. When can odds ratios mislead? *BMJ* 1998;317:1155–6.

9 Altman DG, Deeks JJ, Sackett DL. Odds ratios should be avoided when events are common. *BMJ* 1998;317:131.

10 Senn S, Walter S, Olkin I. Odds ratios revisited. *Evidence-Based Med* 1998;3:71.

11 Cates C. Calculation of numbers needed to treat from systematic reviews: point estimate and confidence intervals using six different methods [abstract]. *Proc 7th Cochrane Colloquium*, Rome, 1999.

12 Parmar MKB, Torri V, Stewart L. Extracting summary statistics to perform meta-analyses of the published literature for survival endpoints. *Stat Med* 1998; 17: 2815–34.

13 L'Abbé KA, Detsky AS, O'Rourke K. Meta-analysis in clinical research. *Ann Intern Med* 1987;107:224–33.

14 Song F. Exploring heterogeneity in meta-analysis: is the l'Abbé plot useful? *J Clin Epidemiol* 1999; 52: 725–30.

15 Jiménez FJ, Guallar E, Martin-Moreno JM. A graphical display useful for meta-analysis. *Eur J Public Health* 1997;7:101–5.

16 Deeks JJ, Altman DG, Dooley G, Sackett DL. Choosing an appropriate dichotomous effect measure for meta-analysis: empirical evidence of the appropriateness of the odds ratio and relative risk [abstract]. *Contr Clin Trials* 1997;18 (3S): 84S–85S.

17 *The Cochrane Library*, Issue 2, 1997. Oxford: Update Software.

18 McGettigan P, Sly K, O'Connell D, Hill S, Henry D. The effects of information framing on the practices of physicians. *J Gen Intern Med* 1999;14:633–42.

19 Moayyedi P, Soo S, Deeks J, *et al.* on behalf of the Dyspepsia Review Group. A systematic review and economic evaluation of H.pylori eradication therapy for non-ulcer dyspepsia. *BMJ* 2000 (forthcoming).

20 Demicheli V, Rivetti D, Deeks JJ, Jefferson TO. Vaccines for preventing influenza in healthy adults (Cochrane Review). In: *Cochrane Library*, Issue 1, 2000. Oxford: Update Software.

21 Schwartz LM, Woloshin S, Welch HG. Misunderstandings about the effects of race and sex on physicians' referrals for cardiac catheterization. *New Engl J Med* 1999;341:279–83.

22 Mantel N, Haenszel W. Statistical aspects of the analysis of data from retrospective studies of disease. *J Natl Cancer Inst* 1959; 22: 719–48.

23 Greenland S, Robins J. Estimation of a common effect parameter from sparse follow-up data. *Biometrics* 1985; 41: 55–68.

24 Fleiss JL. *Statistical methods for rates and proportions*. 2nd edn. New York: Wiley, 1981: 90–3.

25 Feinstein AR. Indexes of contrast and quantitative significance for comparisons of two groups. *Stat Med* 1999; 18: 2557–81.

17 Meta-analysis software

JONATHAN A C STERNE, MATTHIAS EGGER,
ALEXANDER J SUTTON

Summary points

- Both commercial and freely available meta-analytic software is available.
- Freely available software is generally DOS based and less user-friendly with more limited graphics.
- For commercial software, the main choice is between specialist meta-analysis software and general statistical packages with meta-analysis routines available.

A wide range of software to perform meta-analysis has become available in recent years. In addition to fairly expensive commercial software (which may be entirely devoted to meta-analysis or include meta-analytic procedures – sometimes using add-on macros) a number of meta-analysis packages are distributed free of charge. The purpose of this chapter is to provide a brief guide to free and commercial meta-analysis software. It updates a previous review published on the BMJ's web site.[1]

We started our search for meta-analysis software with packages listed in the previous review.[1] Authors and distributors of the packages were contacted to find out whether their software was still available and, if so, whether new facilities had been added. We then conducted internet searches using the phrase "meta-analysis software". Results of such searches produce very different results depending on the search engine and precise search specification. For example, using www.google.com in December 1999, searching for "meta-analysis software" (enclosed in quotation marks to limit the search to the exact phrase) gave 35 web pages but a search for meta-analysis software (without quotes) resulted in 3500 web pages. Using a number of different search engines we located some hundreds of possibly relevant web pages. These were checked further to see if they referred to relevant software, or to sites listing meta-analysis software.

Because the specification, price and availability of software changes rapidly (much more rapidly, we hope, than the lifetime of this book), we list web sites for the software packages and recommend that these be checked for up-to-date information. All versions of the software that we reviewed

336

were for Windows or MS DOS. We apologise for any omissions and would encourage authors of packages that we missed, or of packages released since writing this chapter, to contact us. A web page http://www.prw.le.ac.uk/epidemio/personal/ajs22/meta/ describing meta-analysis software is currently maintained by one of the authors and may be updated with new developments.

Although we do not formally rate the packages for quality, we describe the software that we considered particularly useful in more detail. We wish to emphasise that we have *not* thoroughly tested all the packages and cannot guarantee that their meta-analytic procedures work as claimed. Finally, little background information will be given on the meta-analytic procedures performed by the different software. Readers should consult Chapter 1 and Chapter 2 for the basic principles of meta-analysis, cumulative meta-analysis and forest plots, Chapter 11 for funnel plots and radial plots, Chapter 14 for meta-analysis of diagnostic studies and Chapter 15 for the statistical basis of meta-analysis.

We have categorised the software as follows: (i) commercial software exclusively for meta-analysis; (ii) freely available meta-analysis software; and (iii) general statistical software (commercial) which includes facilities for meta-analysis or for which meta-analysis routines have been written.

Commercial meta-analysis software

We found four commercial meta-analysis software packages, of which two were awaiting full release. The main advantage of these packages is that they are Windows-based (except for DSTAT), and thus allow easy transfer of data, results and graphics from and to other packages. The features of the commercial meta-analysis packages are described below and summarized in Table 17.1.

Metaxis version 1
(http://www.update-software.com/metaxis/metaxis-frame.html)

At the time of writing, this Windows-based program was awaiting full release. Metaxis is designed to perform all aspects of a systematic review, including meta-analysis. Management of the review is based on a set of tasks, from defining the review questions and study eligibility criteria to data extraction and analysis. Reference management is also available. Data can be imported directly from spreadsheets such as Excel. A full range of meta-analytic routines and graphics is available, including fixed effects and random effects models, forest plots and funnel plots. These routines are written in a scripting language which can be edited by users, who can thus change existing routines or write new ones. Once all tasks are completed, the program will produce a Word document for final editing into a manuscript for publication.

337

Table 17.1 Summary of features of commercial meta-analysis software packages.

	Comprehensive Meta-analysis	DSTAT	Metaxis	Meta-Win
Operating system	Windows	DOS	Windows	Windows
Distributor	Biostat	Lawrence Erlbaum Assoc.	Update Software Ltd	Sinauer and Associates Inc.
Data input	Spreadsheet format, or 2 × 2 tables	Within package (1 line per study)	Spreadsheet format	Spreadsheet format
Input format for binary outcomes	2 × 2 tables	2 × 2 tables	Either 2 × 2 tables or treatment effect and standard error	Either 2 × 2 tables or treatment effect and standard error
Input format for continuous outcomes	Mean, SD and sample size, or standardised mean difference and standard error, or t- or P value	Standardised mean differences may be entered directly, or derived from mean, SD and sample size	Mean, SD and sample size, or standardised mean difference and variance	Mean, SD and sample size, or standardised mean difference and variance
Statistical models	Fixed and random effects	Fixed effects only	Fixed and random effects	Fixed and random effects
Effect measures for binary outcomes	Odds ratio, relative risk, risk difference	Standardised difference	Odds ratio, relative risk, risk difference, sensitivity and specificity	Odds ratio, rate difference, relative risk
Effect measures for continuous outcomes	Standardised mean difference, correlation	Standardised mean difference	Mean difference, standardised mean difference	Hedges' d, log response ratio, correlation
Test for homogeneity	Yes	Yes	Yes	Yes
Manual	Yes (plus help system)	Yes	Yes (plus help system)	Yes (plus help system)
Funnel plots	Yes	No	Yes	Yes
Advanced techniques	No	No	Cumulative meta-analysis Meta-regression	Radial plots. Cumulative meta-analysis. Rank correlation test for publication bias Resampling methods Meta-regression (mixed models)

**Comprehensive Meta-Analysis version 0.0.72
(http://www.meta-analysis.com)**

This Windows-based program has recently been released. The user is able to create a database of studies, including abstracts and references. Data can be entered in a spreadsheet, or may be imported directly from Microsoft Excel. Different outcome measures, and groups of studies for analysis, may be specified. The program does fixed and random effects meta-analyses using a range of weighting schemes. Meta-analyses may be grouped according to covariates such as type of intervention or methodological quality of component studies. Forest plots and funnel plots can be displayed and exported to other Windows progams.

MetaWin version 2.0 (http://www.metawinsoft.com)

MetaWin is a Windows based package. Data is entered in a spreadsheet, and Excel files may be imported directly. For each study summary statistics are calculated from the numbers of patients with and without disease, or the mean and standard deviation of the response in each group. Fixed and random effects models are available to combine these summary statistics, and additionally nonparametric resampling tests and confidence intervals can be computed.[2] Cumulative meta-analysis and radial plots to assess heterogeneity and diagnose publication bias are available. Exploring heterogeneity by including study level covariates in a mixed model is also possible. At the time of writing, MetaWin was relatively inexpensive compared to Metaxis and Comprehensive Meta-Analysis.

DSTAT version 1.11 (http://www.erlbaum.com)

DSTAT was developed for meta-analysis in the psychological sciences. The data are entered as 2×2 tables (for binary outcomes), correlation coefficients, test statistics, P values or mixtures. These statistics are then converted into a standardised (scale-free) effect measure. Clinically more relevant quantities such as the difference in risk, the relative risk or the odds ratio cannot be calculated with DSTAT. Also, results cannot be graphically displayed. These drawbacks severely limit the usefulness of DSTAT for meta-analysis in medical research.

Freely available meta-analysis software

Other than RevMan (see below) all the freely available packages are DOS-based. This means that importing data from other packages such as Excel is more difficult than for the Windows-based commercial packages. While most standard meta-analytic procedures can be performed using these packages, graphics produced by the DOS-based packages are less flexible than those by the Windows packages because they must be edited within the package and are often difficult to import into word processing software. Features of the freely available meta-analysis packages are described below and summarized in Table 17.2.

The Cochrane Collaboration's Review Manager (RevMan version 4.03) (http://www.cochrane.org/cochrane/revman.htm)

RevMan is a Windows-based software package designed to enter review protocols or completed reviews in Cochrane format.[3] This includes a structured text of the review and tables of included as well as excluded studies. Technical support is available to members of registered Cochrane review groups.

RevMan includes an analysis module, MetaView. Dichotomous or continuous data can be entered and analysed using fixed and random models on the outcome scales: odds ratio, relative risk, risk difference, mean difference and standardised mean difference. Different comparisons and outcomes can be accommodated in the same data sheet. Forest plots may be displayed with or without raw data, weights and year of individual studies. Forest plots and data displays may be sorted by various study characteristics. Funnel plots are also available. Forest plots (but not funnel plots) can be exported as bitmap files.

A possible disadvantage of using RevMan for meta-analysis is that, because it is designed to contain an entire review for inclusion into the Cochrane Database of Systematic Reviews, the user must first enter a good deal of information, such as the full bibliographic details of the studies, before any meta-analytic procedures can be conducted.

Meta-Analyst

Meta-analyst was written by Dr Joseph Lau, New England Medical Center, Box 63, 750 Washington St, Boston, MA 02111, USA. The program is DOS-based; a Windows version is under development. Interested readers should contact the author (joseph.lau@es.nemc.org) to obtain a copy. The program was developed for standard and cumulative meta-analysis of clinical trials with dichotomous outcomes only. Only one outcome can be entered at a time. The programme offers the widely used fixed effects and random effects models for combining odds ratios, relative risks and risk differences. Other variables such as the year of publication or quality features of component studies may be included in the data table. Cumulative meta-analysis can be performed in ascending or descending order by covariates such as study quality or year of publication. There is an option to send graphical output to an encapsulated PostScript file.

Table 17.2 Summary of features of freely available meta-analysis software packages.

	RevMan	EasyMA	Meta-Analyst	Meta-Test	Meta
Operating system	Windows	DOS	DOS	DOS	DOS
Distributor	The Cochrane Collaboration	M Cucherat	J Lau	J Lau	R Schwarzer
Data input	Data is entered within a comprehensive review management system	Within package (one line per study)	Within package (one line per study)	Within package (one line per study)	Text files in column format
Input format for binary outcomes	Number of patients and number of events in each group	Number of patients and number of events in each group	Number of patients and number of events in each group	2 × 2 tables	NA
Input format for continuous outcomes	Mean, SD and sample size	NA	NA	NA	Standardised mean differences may be entered directly, or derived from mean, SD and sample size
Statistical models	Fixed and random effects	Fixed and random effects	Fixed and random effects	Fixed and random effects	Fixed and random effects
Effect measures for binary outcomes	Odds ratio, relative risk, risk difference	Odds ratio, relative risk, risk difference	Odds ratio, relative risk, risk difference	Sensitivity and specificity	No
Effect measures for continuous outcomes	Mean difference, standardised mean difference	No	No	No	Effect sizes, correlations
Test for homogeneity	Yes	Yes	Yes	No	Yes
Manual	Yes	Yes	No	No	Yes
Funnel plots	Yes	Yes	No	No	No
Advanced techniques	No	Rank test for publication bias. Cumulative meta-analysis. L'Abbé plot. Radial plots	Cumulative meta-analysis	ROC curve analysis	No

Meta-Test (http://hiru.mcmaster.ca/cochrane/cochrane/sadt.htm and http://som.flinders.edu.au/FUSA/Cochrane/COCHRANE/sadt.htm)

This DOS-based package, also written by Dr Joseph Lau (see email address above) is the only package specifically designed for the meta-analysis of diagnostic test data, and hence has features which are unique within this review. Data for each study (true +, false −, false +, true −) together with study-level covariates, are entered within the package. The package displays sensitivity and specificity, separately for each study and pooled under both fixed and random-effects models. Summary receiver operator curve (ROC) analyses are also displayed. Forest plots of sensitivity and specificity, and summary accuracy curves, are available. Graphics can be saved using the encapsulated PostScript format.

Easy MA version 99 (http://www.spc.univ-lyon1.fr/~mcu/easyma/)

EasyMA is a DOS-based package which was developed by Michel Cucherat from the University of Lyon. All menu headings are written in English but contextual help is available only in French, however a paper-based manual translated into English and a paper[4] describing the program are available. EasyMA was developed for meta-analysis of clinical trials with one or several dichotomous outcomes. It is menu driven and offers fixed effects (e.g. Mantel–Haenszel, Yusuf–Peto) and random effects models for calculation of combined odds ratios, relative risks and risk differences. In the latter case the number of patients needed to treat to prevent one event (NNT) is also given. Other useful features include a table ranking studies according to control group event rates, and weighted and unweighted regression analysis of control group against treatment group rates. EasyMA produces forest plots both for standard and cumulative meta-analysis as well as radial and funnel plots.

Meta (http://www.RalfSchwarzer.de)

Written by Ralf Schwarzer from Free University of Berlin, this program runs under DOS, and is designed for the meta-analysis of effect sizes (standardized mean differences). The program can be used to plot a stem-and-leaf display of correlation coefficients, but high quality graphics are not available.

General statistical software which includes facilities for meta-analysis, or for which meta-analysis routines have been written

For readers who are already familiar with and who have access to a commercial statistical software package, using its facilities for meta-analysis is likely to be the most convenient way to perform meta-analysis. Details of general packages are given in Box 17.1. The packages marked with an asterix do not provide ready-made meta-analysis routines but programs for meta-analysis have been written by users and made freely available. While the addresses of some useful websites are given in Box 17.1; to find further information, we recommend an internet search for "meta-analysis"

Box 17.1 General statistical software which includes facilities for meta-analysis, or for which meta-analysis routines are available

Stata* (http://www.stata.com)
Stata is a general purpose statistical package. A comprehensive range of meta-analytic procedures, which have been written by users and make available the vast majority of techniques and graphs possible in the commercial packages, can be downloaded from the internet. Meta-analysis in Stata is described in detail in Chapter 18.

SAS* (http://www.sas.com)
SAS is widely used for data management and statistical analysis. A whole book dedicated to the use of SAS for carrying out meta-analysis is available,[5] and the code routines described therein are available for downloading. Additionally, a further suite of SAS macros have been written and described[6] which carry out fixed and random effect analyses as well as several plots. These are available at:
http://www.prw.le.ac.uk/epidemio/personal/ajs22/meta/macros.sas.
References to SAS routines for more specialized methods can be found at:
http://www.prw.le.ac.uk/epidemio/personal/ajs22/meta/routines.html

Unfortunately, the relatively poor quality of the graphics produced by SAS (compared to other commercial packages listed here) seriously undermines its potential for meta-analysis, especially if high quality plots are desired for inclusion in a publication.

S-Plus* (http://www.mathsoft.com/splus) / R (http://cran.r-project.org)
S-Plus is a commercial statistical package based on the S programming language. Recently developed statistical methods are often made available as functions in S-Plus. Examples of routines for meta-analysis can be found at:
http://www.prw.le.ac.uk/epidemio/personal/ajs22/meta/routines.html, and
http://www.research.att.com/~dumouchel/bsoft.html

R is a freely distributed statistical package also based on the S programming language. It is often possible to run routines written for S-plus using R with little or no modification. Additionally, basic meta-analysis routines have been written specifically for R; available at:
http://cran.r-project.org

A particular strength of S-Plus/R is their graphical capabilities.

StatsDirect (http://www.camcode.com)
StatsDirect is a Windows-based general statistical package which includes facilities for meta-analysis. Data is contained in a spreadsheet-type editor and may be pasted from packages such as Excel. Meta-analysis is performed by clicking on menu options to specify columns corresponding to the total patients, and number of events, in each group. Output includes fixed and random effects models, forest plots and funnel plots.

BUGS and WinBUGS* (http://www.mrc-bsu.cam.ac.uk/bugs)
BUGS and WinBUGS (the Windows version of BUGS) are used for Bayesian analysis of complex statistical models. Bayesian methods are an alternative to the more common classical statistical methods (used exclusively in the other software described here, with the exception of a Bayesian routine written for S-Plus), however, they are often computationally demanding which made them impractical until recent advances in computer software and processing power. BUGS code for random effects meta-analysis is given by Smith et al.[7] The relative advantages and disadvantages of Bayesian models over classical methods are a matter of ongoing debate; see chapter 2 for a brief discussion of Bayesian meta-analysis and Smith et al.[7] and Sutton et al.[8] for more detailed descriptions.

BUGS software may be downloaded freely, but its use requires substantial expertise. BUGS provides a flexible platform to implement complex, non-standard, meta-analysis models: one useful extension is the ability to estimate associations between treatment effects and underlying risk (see chapter 10),[9] which is not possible using any of the other software reviewed. Additionally, Spiegelhalter et al.[10] have described how an alternative approach to meta-analysis, called the Confidence Profile Method[11] can be implemented using BUGS.

StatXact (http://www.cytel.com/products/statxact/statxact1.html)
StatXact is a specialist statistical package which provides exact nonparametric statistical inference on continuous or categorical data. It includes facilities for fixed-effects meta-analysis which provide exact and asymptotic tests of homogeneity of odds ratios, and exact and asymptotic tests and confidence intervals for the combined odds ratio, and may thus be of particular use in meta-analyses based on small numbers of events.

True Epistat (http://ic.net/~biomware/biohp2te.htm)
This is a comprehensive statistics package which includes meta-analysis. Studies using dichotomous outcomes or continuous outcomes can be analysed by inverse-variance-weighted fixed effects models or random effects models. Correlation coefficients can also be combined, and forest plots and funnel plots can be drawn. The latest version (5.3) is still DOS based but a Windows version is under development.

* No built-in meta-analysis routines available.

together with the name of the desired package. For example, to find information on meta-analysis routines using SAS, search on "meta-analysis SAS". For a detailed review of code routines available to do specialist meta-analysis procedures in several statistical packages including SAS, see Sutton et al.[12]

Conclusions

Software for meta-analysis has developed rapidly over the past five years, and it would appear that it will continue to do so. We consider no one software solution to be indisputably superior. The difficulty in choosing the best software is compounded by the fact that one of the commercial packages (Metaxis) is not fully released yet, and its full capabilities not finalised. However, it would appear that the specialist commercial packages Metaxis, Comprehensive Meta-Analysis and MetaWin will all provide a powerful and easy to use solution for most meta-analysts' needs. Metaxis, RevMan, and, to some extent, Comprehensive Meta-Analysis provide assistance in all aspects of a systematic review. It should also be noted that these packages are all under continued development and further facilities may be added in the future.

The freely available software is generally less polished and easy to use than the commercial packages. However most standard analyses and graphs can be obtained, although perhaps with more difficulty than for the commercial packages. The authors have also had problems getting these DOS programs to run under new operating systems such as Windows NT.

The most difficult choice is between buying commercial software specifically for meta-analysis, or choosing more general statistical software with meta-analysis facilities. The "learning curve" required to perform meta-analysis is likely to be steeper for general statistical software than for a specialist package. However the data manipulation and graphical facilities of the general packages may be of use to meta-analysts. Of the general software Stata has the most comprehensive, easy to use and well-documented meta-analysis macros; offering a range of options which compares favourably to the specifically designed commercial packages (see Chapter 18). While many different analyses and graphs are possible with other general packages, meta-analysis facilities are less comprehensive, and generally the user interfaces are less intuitive than the specifically designed menu driven Windows packages.

1 Egger M, Sterne JAC, Davey Smith G. Meta-analysis software. http://www.bmj.com/archive/7126/7126ed9.htm. (accessed 21.11.2000.)
2 Adams DC, Gurevitch J, Rosenberg MS. Resampling tests for meta-analysis of ecological data. *Ecology* 1997;**78**:1277–83.

3 *Cochrane Reviewer's Handbook* (updated July 1999). In: *The Cochrane Library* (database on disk and CDROM). *The Cochrane Collaboration*. Oxford: Update Software, 1999.

4 Cucherat M, Boissel JP, Leizorovicz A, Haugh MC. EasyMA: a program for the meta-analysis of clinical trials. *Comput Meth Programs Biomed* 1997;**53**:187–90.

5 Wang MC, Bushman BJ. *Integrating results through meta-analytic review using SAS(R) software*. Cary, NC: SAS Institute, 1999.

6 Kuss O, Koch A. Metaanalysis macros for SAS. *Computat Stat Data Anal* 1996;**22**:325–33.

7 Smith TC, Spiegelhalter DJ, Thomas A. Bayesian approaches to random-effects meta-analysis: a comparative study. *Stat Med* 1995;**14**:2685–99.

8 Sutton AJ, Abrams KR, Jones DR, *et al*. *Methods for meta-analysis in medical research*. London: Wiley, 2000.

9 Thompson SG, Smith TC, Sharp SJ. Investigating underlying risk as a source of heterogeneity in meta-analysis. *Stat Med* 1997;**16**:2741–58.

10 Spiegelhalter DJ, Miles JP, Jones DR, Abrams KR. Bayesian methods in health technology assessment. *Health Technol Assess* (in press).

11 Eddy DM, Hasselblad V, Shachter R. *Meta-analysis by the confidence profile method*. San Diego: Academic Press, 1992.

12 Sutton AJ, Lambert PC, Hellmich M, *et al*. Meta-analysis in practice: a critical review of available software. In: Berry DA, Stangl DK, eds. *Meta-analysis in medicine and health policy*. New York: Marcel Dekker, 2000.

18 Meta-analysis in Stata™

JONATHAN A C STERNE, MICHAEL J BRADBURN,
MATTHIAS EGGER

Summary points

- Stata™ is a general-purpose, command-line driven, programmable statistical package.
- A comprehensive set of user-written commands is freely available for meta-analysis.
- Meta-analysis of studies with binary (relative risk, odds ratio, risk difference) or continuous outcomes (difference in means, standardised difference in means) can be performed.
- All the commonly used fixed effect (inverse variance method, Mantel–Haenszel method and Peto's method) and random effect (DerSimonian and Laird) models are available.
- An influence analysis, in which the meta-analysis estimates are computed omitting one study at a time, can be performed.
- Forest plots, funnel plots and L'Abbé plots can be drawn and statistical tests for funnel plot asymmetry can be computed.
- Meta-regression models can be used to analyse associations between treatment effect and study characteristics.

We reviewed a number of computer software packages that may be used to perform a meta-analysis in Chapter 17. In this chapter we show in detail how to use the statistical package Stata both to perform a meta-analysis and to examine the data in more detail. This will include looking at the accumulation of evidence in cumulative meta-analysis, using graphical and statistical techniques to look for evidence of bias, and using meta-regression to investigate possible sources of heterogeneity.

Getting started

Stata is a general-purpose, command-line driven, programmable statistical package in which commands to perform several meta-analytic methods

All data sets described in this Chapter are available from the book's website: <www.systematicreviews.com>.

Box 18.1 Downloading and installing user-written meta-analysis commands

As a first step we recommend that you make sure that your installation is up-to-date by typing **update all** in the command window. Stata will automatically connect to www.stata.com and update the core package. It will also download brief descriptions of all user-written commands published in the Stata Technical Bulletin. Those relating to meta-analysis can be displayed by typing **search meta**. The most convenient way to install user-written commands is from within Stata. Go into the "Help" menu and click on the "STB and User-Written Programs" option. Now click on http://www.stata.com and then on stb (for Stata Technical Bulletins). The meta-analysis routines described in this chapter can then be downloaded as follows:

Click on...	... then click on	to install commands
stb45	sbe24.1	**metan, funnel, labbe**
stb43	sbe16.2	**meta**
stb42	sbe22	**metacum**
stb56	sbe26.1	**metainf**
stb58	sbe19.3	**metabias**
stb42	sbe23	**metareg**

Note that these are the latest versions as of December 2000 and you should check whether updated versions or new commands have become available (**update all, search meta**).

are available. Throughout this chapter, Stata commands appear in **bold font,** and are followed by the Stata output that they produce. Users should note that the commands documented here do not form part of the "core" Stata package, but are all user-written "add-ons" which are freely available on the internet. In order to perform meta-analyses in Stata, these routines need to be installed on your computer by downloading the relevant files from the Stata web site (www.stata.com). See Box 18.1 for detailed instructions on how to do this.

We do not attempt to provide a full description of the commands: interested readers are referred to help files for the commands, and to the relevant articles in the *Stata Technical Bulletin* (STB, see reference list). To display the help file, type **help** followed by the command (for example **help metan**) or go into the "Help" menu and click on the "Stata command..." option. Bound books containing reprints of a year's Stata

Technical Bulletin articles are also available and are free to university libraries. The articles referred to in this chapter are available in STB reprints volumes 7: (STB 38 to STB 42) and 8 (STB 43 to 48). The Stata website gives details of how to obtain these. All the output shown in this chapter was obtained using Stata version 6. Finally, we assume that the data have already been entered into Stata.

Commands to perform a standard meta-analysis

Example 1: intravenous streptokinase in myocardial infarction

The following table gives data from 22 randomised controlled trials of streptokinase in the prevention of death following myocardial infarction.[1-3]

Table 18.1

Trial number	Trial name	Publication year	Intervention group		Control group	
			Deaths	Total	Deaths	Total
1	Fletcher	1959	1	12	4	11
2	Dewar	1963	4	21	7	21
3	1st European	1969	20	83	15	84
4	Heikinheimo	1971	22	219	17	207
5	Italian	1971	19	164	18	157
6	2nd European	1971	69	373	94	357
7	2nd Frankfurt	1973	13	102	29	104
8	1st Australian	1973	26	264	32	253
9	NHLBI SMIT	1974	7	53	3	54
10	Valere	1975	11	49	9	42
11	Frank	1975	6	55	6	53
12	UK Collaborative	1976	48	302	52	293
13	Klein	1976	4	14	1	9
14	Austrian	1977	37	352	65	376
15	Lasierra	1977	1	13	3	11
16	N German	1977	63	249	51	234
17	Witchitz	1977	5	32	5	26
18	2nd Australian	1977	25	112	31	118
19	3rd European	1977	25	156	50	159
20	ISAM	1986	54	859	63	882
21	GISSI-1	1986	628	5860	758	5852
22	ISIS-2	1988	791	8592	1029	8595

These data were saved in Stata dataset **strepto.dta** which is available from the book's website (http://www.systematicreviews.com). We can list the variables contained in the dataset, with their descriptions (variable labels) by using the **describe** command:

describe

```
Contains data from strepto.dta
 obs:   22                        Streptokinase after MI
 vars:   7
 size: 638 (99.7% of memory free)
```

```
  1. trial      byte    %8.0g     Trial number
  2. trialnam   str14   %14s      Trial name
  3. year       int     %8.0g     Year of publication
  4. pop1       int     %12.0g    Treated population
  5. deaths1    int     %12.0g    Treated deaths
  6. pop0       int     %12.0g    Control population
  7. deaths0    int     %12.0g    Control deaths
```

```
Sorted by: trial
```

The metan command

The **metan** command[4] provides methods for the meta-analysis of studies with two groups. With binary data the effect measure can be the difference between proportions (sometimes called the risk difference or absolute risk reduction), the ratio of two proportions (risk ratio or relative risk), or the odds ratio. With continuous data both observed differences in means or standardised differences in means can be used. For both binary and continuous data either fixed effects or random effects models can be fitted.

For analysis of trials with binary outcomes, the command requires variables containing the number of individuals who did and did not experience disease events, in intervention and control groups. Using the streptokinase data, the variables required can be created as follows:

generate alive1=pop1-deaths1
generate alive0=pop0-deaths0

In the following, we use the **metan** command to perform a meta-analysis on relative risks, derive the summary estimate using Mantel–Haenszel methods, and produce a forest plot. The options (following the comma) that we use are:

rr	perform calculations using relative risks
xlab(.1,1,10)	label the *x*-axis
label(namevar=trialnam)	label the output and vertical axis of the graph with the trial name. The trial year may also be added by specifying **yearvar=year**.

Display the help file for a complete list of options. The command and output in our analysis are as follows (note that all commands are typed on one line although they may be printed on two):

```
metan deaths1 alive1 deaths0 alive0, rr xlab(.1,1,10)
label(namevar=trialnam)
```

Study	RR	[95% Conf Interval]		% Weight
Fletcher	.229167	.030012	1.74987	.177945
Dewar	.571429	.196152	1.66468	.298428
1st European	1.3494	.742948	2.45088	.63566
Heikinheimo	1.22321	.668816	2.23714	.74517
Italian	1.0105	.551044	1.85305	.784121
2nd European	.702555	.533782	.924693	4.0953
2nd Frankfurt	.457066	.252241	.828213	1.22434
1st Australian	.778646	.478015	1.26835	1.39327
NHLBI SMIT	2.37736	.648992	8.70863	.126702
Valere	1.04762	.480916	2.28212	.413208
Frank	.963636	.33158	2.80052	.260532
UK Collab	.895568	.626146	1.28092	2.25043
Klein	2.57143	.339414	19.4813	.051901
Austrian	.608042	.417252	.886071	2.67976
Lasierra	.282051	.033993	2.3403	.138556
N German	1.16088	.840283	1.60379	2.24179
Witchitz	.8125	.26341	2.5062	.235214
2nd Australian	.849654	.536885	1.34463	1.28713
3rd European	.509615	.33275	.78049	2.11133
ISAM	.880093	.619496	1.25031	2.65037
GISSI-1	.827365	.749108	.913797	32.3376
ISIS-2	.768976	.704392	.839481	43.8613
M-H pooled RR	.79876	.754618	.845484	

```
Heterogeneity chi-squared = 30.41 (d.f. = 21) p = 0.084
Test of RR=1 : z= 7.75 p = 0.000
```

The output shows, for each study, the treatment effect (here, the relative risk) together with the corresponding 95% confidence interval and the percentage weight contributed to the overall meta-analysis. The summary (pooled) treatment effect (with 95% CI and P value) and the heterogeneity test are also shown. By default, new variables containing the treatment effect size, its standard error, the 95% CI and study weights and sample sizes are added to the dataset.

The **metan** command also automatically produces a forest plot (see Chapter 2). In a forest plot the contribution of each study to the meta-analysis (its weight) is represented by the area of a box whose centre represents the size of the treatment effect estimated from that study (point estimate). The confidence interval for the treatment effect from each study is also shown. The summary treatment effect is shown by the middle of a diamond whose left and right extremes represent the corresponding confidence interval.

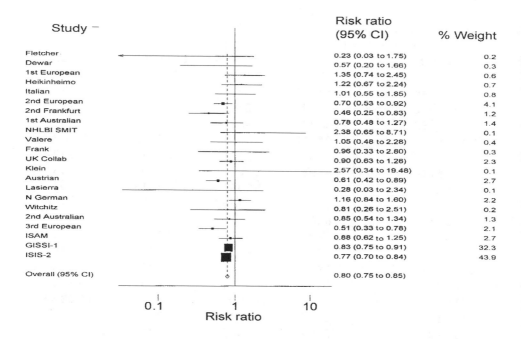

Study		Risk ratio (95% CI)	% Weight
Fletcher		0.23 (0.03 to 1.75)	0.2
Dewar		0.57 (0.20 to 1.66)	0.3
1st European		1.35 (0.74 to 2.45)	0.6
Heikinheimo		1.22 (0.67 to 2.24)	0.7
Italian		1.01 (0.55 to 1.85)	0.8
2nd European		0.70 (0.53 to 0.92)	4.1
2nd Frankfurt		0.46 (0.25 to 0.83)	1.2
1st Australian		0.78 (0.48 to 1.27)	1.4
NHLBI SMIT		2.38 (0.65 to 8.71)	0.1
Valere		1.05 (0.48 to 2.28)	0.4
Frank		0.96 (0.33 to 2.80)	0.3
UK Collab		0.90 (0.63 to 1.28)	2.3
Klein		2.57 (0.34 to 19.48)	0.1
Austrian		0.61 (0.42 to 0.89)	2.7
Lasierra		0.28 (0.03 to 2.34)	0.1
N German		1.16 (0.84 to 1.60)	2.2
Witchitz		0.81 (0.26 to 2.51)	0.2
2nd Australian		0.85 (0.54 to 1.34)	1.3
3rd European		0.51 (0.33 to 0.78)	2.1
ISAM		0.88 (0.62 to 1.25)	2.7
GISSI-1		0.83 (0.75 to 0.91)	32.3
ISIS-2		0.77 (0.70 to 0.84)	43.9
Overall (95% CI)		0.80 (0.75 to 0.85)	

Both the output and the graph show that there is a clear effect of streptokinase in protecting against death following myocardial infarction. The meta-analysis is dominated by the large GISSI-1[2] and ISIS-2[3] trials which contribute 76·2% of the weight in this analysis. If required, the text showing the weights or treatment effects may be omitted from the graph (options **nowt** and **nostats**, respectively). The **metan** command will perform all the commonly used fixed effects (inverse variance method, Mantel–Haenszel method and Peto's method) and random effects (DerSimonian and Laird) analyses. These methods are described in Chapter 15. Commands **labbe** to draw L'Abbé plots (see Chapters 8 and 10) and **funnel** to draw funnel plots (see Chapter 11) are also included.

The meta command

The **meta** command[5-7] uses inverse-variance weighting to calculate fixed and random effects summary estimates, and, optionally, to produce a forest plot. The main difference in using the **meta** command (compared to the **metan** command) is that we require variables containing the effect estimate and its corresponding standard error for each study. Commands **metacum, metainf, metabias** and **metareg** (described later in this chapter) also require these input variables. Here we re-analyse the streptokinase data to demonstrate **meta**, this time considering the outcome on the odds ratio scale. For odds ratios or risk ratios, the **meta** command works on the log scale. So, to produce a summary odds ratio we need to calculate the log of the ratio and its corresponding standard error for each study. This is straightforward for the odds ratio. The log odds ratio is calculated as

```
generate logor=log((deaths1/alive1)/(deaths0/alive0))
```

and its standard error, using Woolf's method, as

```
generate selogor=sqrt((1/deaths1)+(1/alive1)+
(1/deaths0)+(1/alive0))
```

Chapter 15 gives this formula, together with the standard errors of the risk ratio and other commonly used treatment effect estimates. The output can be converted back to the odds ratio scale using the **eform** option to exponentiate the odds ratios and their confidence intervals. Other options used in our analysis are:

graph(f)	display a forest plot using a fixed-effects summary estimate. Specifying **graph(r)** changes this to a random-effects estimate
cline	draw a broken vertical line at the combined estimate
xlab(.1,1,10)	label the x-axis at odds ratios $0\cdot1$, 1 and 10
xline(1)	draw a vertical line at 1
id(trialnam)	label the vertical axis with the trial name contained in variable **trialnam**
b2title(Odds ratio)	label the x-axis with the text "Odds ratio".
print	output the effect estimates, 95% CI and weights for each study

The command and output are as follows:

```
meta logor selogor, eform graph(f) cline xline(1)
xlab(.1,1,10) id(trialnam) b2title(Odds ratio) print
```

Meta-analysis (exponential form)

Method	Pooled Est	95% CI Lower	Upper	Asymptotic z_value	p_value	No. of studies
Fixed	0.774	0.725	0.826	-7.711	0.000	22
Random	0.782	0.693	0.884	-3.942	0.000	

Test for heterogeneity: Q= 31.498 on 21 degrees of freedom (p= 0.066)
Moment-based estimate of between studies variance = 0.017

Study	Weights Fixed	Random	Study Est	95% CI Lower	Upper
Fletcher	0.67	0.67	0.16	0.01	1.73
Dewar	1.91	1.85	0.47	0.11	1.94
1st European	6.80	6.10	1.46	0.69	3.10
Heikinheimo	8.72	7.61	1.25	0.64	2.42
Italian	8.18	7.19	1.01	0.51	2.01
2nd European	31.03	20.39	0.64	0.45	0.90
2nd Frankfurt	7.35	6.54	0.38	0.18	0.78
1st Australian	12.75	10.50	0.75	0.44	1.31
NHLBI SMIT	1.93	1.87	2.59	0.63	10.60
Valere	3.87	3.63	1.06	0.39	2.88
Frank	2.67	2.55	0.96	0.29	3.19
UK Collab	20.77	15.39	0.88	0.57	1.35
Klein	0.68	0.67	3.20	0.30	34.59
Austrian	20.49	15.24	0.56	0.36	0.87
Lasierra	0.65	0.64	0.22	0.02	2.53
N German	21.59	15.84	1.22	0.80	1.85
Witchitz	2.06	1.99	0.78	0.20	3.04
2nd Australian	10.50	8.92	0.81	0.44	1.48
3rd European	13.02	10.68	0.42	0.24	0.72
ISAM	27.13	18.63	0.87	0.60	1.27
GISSI-1	303.12	49.69	0.81	0.72	0.90
ISIS-2	400.58	51.76	0.75	0.68	0.82

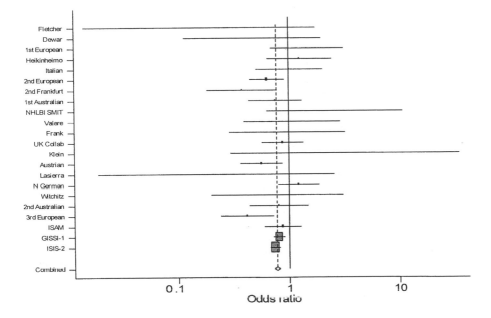

Note that **meta** performs both fixed and random effects analyses by default and the tabular output includes the weights from both analyses. It is clear that the smaller studies are given relatively more weight in the random effects analysis than with the fixed effect model. Because the **meta** command requires only the estimated treatment effect and its standard error, it will be particularly useful in meta-analyses of studies in which the treatment effect is not derived from the standard 2 × 2 table. Examples might include crossover trials, or survival trials, when the treatment effect might be measured by the hazard ratio derived from Cox regression.

Example 2: intravenous magnesium in acute myocardial infarction

The following table gives data from 16 randomised controlled trials of intravenous magnesium in the prevention of death following myocardial infarction. These trials are a well-known example where the results of a meta-analysis[8] were contradicted by a single large trial (ISIS-4)[9-11] (see also Chapters 3 and 11).

Table 18.2

Trial number	Trial name	Publication year	Intervention group		Control group	
			Deaths	Total	Deaths	Total
1	Morton	1984	1	40	2	36
2	Rasmussen	1986	9	135	23	135
3	Smith	1986	2	200	7	200
4	Abraham	1987	1	48	1	46
5	Feldstedt	1988	10	150	8	148
6	Schechter	1989	1	59	9	56
7	Ceremuzynski	1989	1	25	3	23
8	Bertschat	1989	0	22	1	21
9	Singh	1990	6	76	11	75
10	Pereira	1990	1	27	7	27
11	Schechter 1	1991	2	89	12	80
12	Golf	1991	5	23	13	33
13	Thogersen	1991	4	130	8	122
14	LIMIT-2	1992	90	1159	118	1157
15	Schechter 2	1995	4	107	17	108
16	ISIS-4	1995	2216	29 011	2103	29 039

These data were saved in Stata dataset **magnes.dta**.

describe

```
Contains data from magnes.dta
   obs:          16                Magnesium and CHD
  vars:           7
-----------------------------------------------------------------------
  1. trial    int      %8.0g    Trial number
  2. trialnam str12    %12s     Trial name
  3. year     int      %8.0g    Year of publication
  4. tot1     long     %12.0g   Total in magnesium group
  5. dead1    double   %12.0g   Deaths in magnesium group
  6. tot0     long     %12.0g   Total in control group
  7. dead0    long     %12.0g   Deaths in control group
-----------------------------------------------------------------------
Sorted by: trial
```


The discrepancy between the results of the ISIS-4 trial and the earlier trials can be seen clearly in the graph produced by the **metan** command. Note that because the ISIS-4 trial provides 89·7% of the total weight in the meta-analysis, the overall (summary) estimate using fixed-effects analysis is very similar to the estimate from the ISIS-4 trial alone.

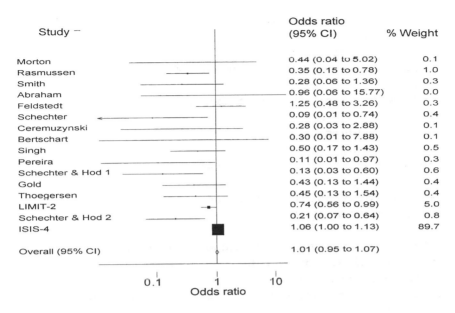

Study

	Odds ratio (95% CI)	% Weight
Morton	0.44 (0.04 to 5.02)	0.1
Rasmussen	0.35 (0.15 to 0.78)	1.0
Smith	0.28 (0.06 to 1.36)	0.3
Abraham	0.96 (0.06 to 15.77)	0.0
Feldstedt	1.25 (0.48 to 3.26)	0.3
Schechter	0.09 (0.01 to 0.74)	0.4
Ceremuzynski	0.28 (0.03 to 2.88)	0.1
Bertschart	0.30 (0.01 to 7.88)	0.1
Singh	0.50 (0.17 to 1.43)	0.5
Pereira	0.11 (0.01 to 0.97)	0.3
Schechter & Hod 1	0.13 (0.03 to 0.60)	0.6
Gold	0.43 (0.13 to 1.44)	0.4
Thoegersen	0.45 (0.13 to 1.54)	0.4
LIMIT-2	0.74 (0.56 to 0.99)	5.0
Schechter & Hod 2	0.21 (0.07 to 0.64)	0.8
ISIS-4	1.06 (1.00 to 1.13)	89.7
Overall (95% CI)	1.01 (0.95 to 1.07)	

Odds ratio

Dealing with zero cells

When one arm of a study contains no events – or, equally, all events – we have what is termed a "zero cell" in the 2×2 table. Zero cells create problems in the computation of ratio measures of treatment effect, and the standard error of either difference or ratio measures. For trial number 8 (Bertschart), there were no deaths in the intervention group, so that the estimated odds ratio is zero and the standard error cannot be estimated. A common way to deal with this problem is to add 0·5 to each cell of the 2×2 table for the trial. If there are no events in either the intervention or control arms of the trial, however, then any measure of effect summarised as a ratio is undefined, and unless the absolute (risk difference) scale is used instead, the trial has to be discarded from the meta-analysis.

The **metan** command deals with the problem automatically, by adding 0·5 to all cells of the 2×2 table before analysis. For the commands which require summary statistics to be calculated (**meta, metacum, metainf, metabias** and **metareg**) it is necessary to do this, and to drop trials with no events or in which all subjects experienced events, before calculating the treatment effect and standard error.

To drop trials with no events or all events:
```
drop if dead1==0&dead0==0
drop if dead1==tot1&dead0==tot0
```

357

To add 0·5 to the 2 × 2 table where necessary:

```
gen trzero=0
replace trzero=1 if
dead1==0|dead0==0|dead1==tot1|dead0==tot0
(1 real change made)
replace dead1=dead1+0·5 if trzero==1
(1 real change made)
replace dead0=dead0+0·5 if trzero==1
(1 real change made)
replace tot1=tot1+1 if trzero==1
(1 real change made)
replace tot0=tot0+1 if trzero==1
(1 real change made)
```

To derive summary statistics needed for meta-analysis:

```
generate alive0=tot0-dead0
generate alive1=tot1-dead1
generate logor=log((dead1/alive1)/(dead0/alive0))
generate
selogor=sqrt((1/dead1)+(1/alive1)+(1/dead0)+(1/alive0))
```

To use the **meta** command to perform a meta-analysis:

```
meta logor selogor, eform id(trialnam) print
```

```
Meta-analysis (exponential form)
```

Method	Pooled Est	95% CI Lower	Upper	Asymptotic z_value	p_value	No. of studies
Fixed	1.015	0.956	1.077	0.484	0.629	16
Random	0.483	0.329	0.710	-3.706	0.000	

Test for heterogeneity: Q= 47.059 on 15 degrees of freedom (p= 0.000)
Moment-based estimate of between studies variance = 0.224

Study	Weights Fixed	Random	Study Est	95% CI Lower	Upper
Morto	0.64	0.56	0.44	0.04	5.02
Rasmussen	5.83	2.53	0.35	0.15	0.78
Smith	1.53	1.14	0.28	0.06	1.36
Abraham	0.49	0.44	0.96	0.06	15.77
Feldstedt	4.18	2.16	1.25	0.48	3.26
Schechter	0.87	0.73	0.09	0.01	0.74
Ceremuzynski	0.70	0.61	0.28	0.03	2.88
Bertschart	0.36	0.34	0.30	0.01	7.88
Singh	3.48	1.96	0.50	0.17	1.43
Pereira	0.81	0.69	0.11	0.01	0.97
Schechter & Hod 1	1.64	1.20	0.13	0.03	0.60
Gold	2.61	1.65	0.43	0.13	1.44
Thoegersen	2.55	1.62	0.45	0.13	1.54
LIMIT-2	46.55	4.08	0.74	0.56	0.99
Schechter & Hod 2	3.03	1.81	0.21	0.07	0.64
ISIS-4	998.78	4.45	1.06	1.00	1.13

Note the dramatic difference between the fixed and random effects summary estimates, which arises because the studies are weighted much more equally in the random effects analysis. Also, the test of heterogeneity is highly significant. We will return to this example later.

Cumulative meta-analysis

The **metacum** command[12] performs and graphs cumulative meta-analyses,[13,14] in which the cumulative evidence at the time each study was published is calculated. This command also requires variables containing the effect estimate and its corresponding standard error for each study (see above). To perform a cumulative meta-analysis of the streptokinase trials, we first create a character variable of length 20 containing both trial name and year, and then sort by year:

```
gen str21 trnamyr=trialnam+" ("+string(year)+")"
```

```
sort year
```

The options for the **metacum** command are similar to those for the **meta** command, except:

359

effect(f)	perform all calculations using fixed-effects meta-analysis. Specifying **effect(r)** changes this to a random-effects estimate
graph	produce a cumulative meta-analysis graph

The command and output are as follows:

metacum logor selogor, effect(f) eform graph cline xline(1) xlab(.1,1,10) id(trnamyr) b2title(Odds ratio)

Cumulative fixed-effects meta-analysis of 22 studies
(exponential form)

Trial	Cumulative estimate	95% CI Lower	Upper	z	P value
Fletcher (1959)	0.159	0.015	1.732	-1.509	0.131
Dewar (1963)	0.355	0.105	1.200	-1.667	0.096
1st European (1969)	0.989	0.522	1.875	-0.034	0.973
Heikinheimo (1971)	1.106	0.698	1.753	0.430	0.667
Italian (1971)	1.076	0.734	1.577	0.376	0.707
2nd European (1971)	0.809	0.624	1.048	-1.607	0.108
2nd Frankfurt (1973)	0.742	0.581	0.946	-2.403	0.016
1st Australian (1973)	0.744	0.595	0.929	-2.604	0.009
NHLBI SMIT (1974)	0.767	0.615	0.955	-2.366	0.018
Valere (1975)	0.778	0.628	0.965	-2.285	0.022
Frank (1975)	0.783	0.634	0.968	-2.262	0.024
UK Collab (1976)	0.801	0.662	0.968	-2.296	0.022
Klein (1976)	0.808	0.668	0.976	-2.213	0.027
Austrian (1977)	0.762	0.641	0.906	-3.072	0.002
Lasierra (1977)	0.757	0.637	0.900	-3.150	0.002
N German (1977)	0.811	0.691	0.951	-2.571	0.010
Witchitz (1977)	0.810	0.691	0.950	-2.596	0.009
2nd Australian (1977)	0.810	0.695	0.945	-2.688	0.007
3rd European (1977)	0.771	0.665	0.894	-3.448	0.001
ISAM (1986)	0.784	0.683	0.899	-3.470	0.001
GISSI-1 (1986)	0.797	0.731	0.870	-5.092	0.000
ISIS-2 (1988)	0.774	0.725	0.826	-7.711	0.000

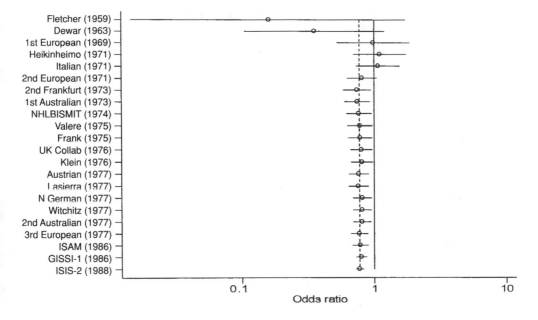

By the late 1970s, there was clear evidence that streptokinase prevented death following myocardial infarction. However it was not used routinely until the late 1980s, when the results of the large GISSI-1 and ISIS-2 trials became known (see Chapter 1). The cumulative meta-analysis plot makes it clear that although these trials reduced the confidence interval for the summary estimate, they did not change the estimated degree of protection.

Examining the influence of individual studies

The influence of individual studies on the summary effect estimate may be displayed using the **metainf** command.[15] This command performs an influence analysis, in which the meta-analysis estimates are computed omitting one study at a time. The syntax for **metainf** is the same as that for the **meta** command. By default, fixed-effects analyses are displayed. Let's perform this analysis for the magnesium data:

```
metainf logor selogor, eform id (trialnam)
```

361

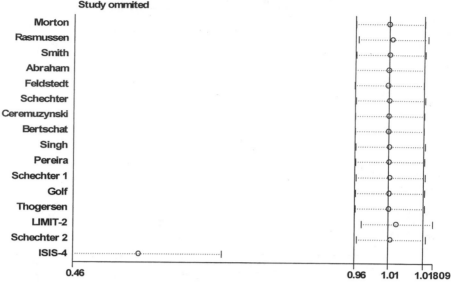

The label above the vertical axis indicates that the treatment effect estimate (here, log odds ratio) has been exponentiated. The meta-analysis is dominated by the ISIS-4 study, so omission of other studies makes little or no difference. If ISIS-4 is omitted then there appears to be a clear effect of magnesium in preventing death after myocardial infarction.

Funnel plots and tests for funnel plot asymmetry

The **metabias** command[16,17] performs the tests for funnel-plot asymmetry proposed by Begg and Mazumdar[18] and by Egger *et al.*[11] (see Chapter 11). If the **graph** option is specified the command will produce either a plot of standardized effect against precision[11] (**graph(egger)**) or a funnel plot (**graph(begg)**). For the magnesium data there is clear evidence of funnel plot asymmetry if the ISIS-4 trial is included. It is of more interest to know if there was evidence of bias *before* the results of the ISIS-4 trial were known. Therefore in the following analysis we omit the ISIS-4 trial:

```
metabias logor selogor if trial<16, graph(begg)
```

Note: default data input format (theta, se_theta) assumed.

```
  if trialno < 16
```

Tests for Publication Bias

Degg's Test

```
adj. Kendall's Score (P-Q) =       -3
        Std. Dev. of Score =    20.21
        Number of Studies =       15
                        z  =    -0.15
                Pr > |z|  =    0.882
                        z  =     0.10  (continuity corrected)
                Pr > |z|  =    0.921  (continuity corrected)
```

Egger's test

Std_Eff	Coef.	Std. Err.	t	P>|t|	[95% Conf. Interval]
slope	-.1512257	.1674604	-0.903	0.383	-.5130019 .2105505
bias	-1.192429	.3751749	-3.178	0.007	-2.002945 -.3819131

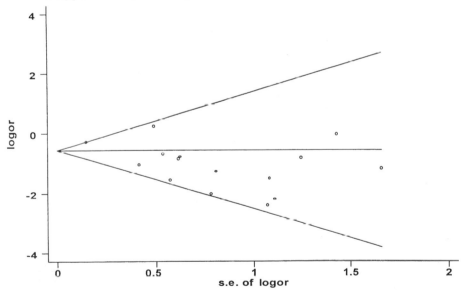

Begg's funnel plot with pseudo 95% confidence limits

The funnel plot appears asymmetric, and there is evidence of bias using the Egger (weighted regression) method (P for bias 0·007) but not using the Begg (rank correlation method). This is compatible with a greater statistical power of the regression test, as discussed in Chapter 11. The horizontal line in the funnel plot indicates the fixed-effects summary estimate (using

The funnel plot appears asymmetric, and there is evidence of bias using the Egger (weighted regression) method (P for bias 0·007) but not using the Begg (rank correlation method). This is compatible with a greater statistical power of the regression test, as discussed in Chapter 11. The horizontal line in the funnel plot indicates the fixed-effects summary estimate (using inverse-variance weighting), while the sloping lines indicate the expected 95% confidence intervals for a given standard error, assuming no heterogeneity between studies.

Meta-regression

If evidence is found of heterogeneity in the effect of treatment between studies, then meta-regression can be used to analyse associations between treatment effect and study characteristics. Meta-regression can be done in Stata by using the **metareg** command.[19]

Example 3: trials of BCG vaccine against tuberculosis

The following table is based on a meta-analysis by Colditz et al.[20] which examined the efficacy of BCG vaccine against tuberculosis.

Table 18.3

Trial	Trial name	Authors	Start year	Latitude*	Intervention group		Control group	
					TB cases	Total	TB cases	Total
1	Canada	Ferguson & Simes	1933	55	6	306	29	303
2	Northern USA	Aronson	1935	52	4	123	11	139
3	Northern USA	Stein & Aronson	1935	52	180	1541	372	1451
4	Chicago	Rosenthal et al.	1937	42	17	1716	65	1665
5	Chicago	Rosenthal et al.	1941	42	3	231	11	220
6	Georgia (School)	Comstock & Webster	1947	33	5	2498	3	2341
7	Puerto Rico	Comstock et al.	1949	18	186	50634	141	27338
8	UK	Hart & Sutherland	1950	53	62	13598	248	12867
9	Madanapalle	Frimont-Moller et al.	1950	13	33	5069	47	5808
10	Georgia (Community)	Comstock et al.	1950	33	27	16913	29	17854
11	Haiti	Vandeviere et al.	1965	18	8	2545	10	629
12	South Africa	Coetzee & Berjak	1965	27	29	7499	45	7277
13	Madras	TB prevention trial	1968	13	505	88391	499	88391

* Expressed in degrees from equator.

The data were saved in Stata dataset **bcgtrial.dta**.

describe

```
Contains data from bcgtrial.dta
  obs:          13
  vars:          9
  size:        754 (99.9% of memory free)
-------------------------------------------------------------------------
  1. trial       byte     %8.0g
  2. trialnam    str19    %19s
  3. authors     str19    %19s
  4. startyr     int      %8.0g
  5. latitude    byte     %8.0g
  6. cases1       int      %8.0g
  7. tot1        long     %12.0g
  8. cases0       int      %8.0g
  9. tot0        long     %12.0g
-------------------------------------------------------------------------

Sorted by: trial
```

Scientists had been aware of discordance between the results of these trials since the 1950s. The clear heterogeneity in the protective effect of BCG between trials can be seen in the forest plot (we analyse this study using risk ratios):

gen h1=tot1-cases1
gen h0=tot0-cases0

metan cases1 h1 cases0 h0, xlab(.1,1,10)
label(namevar=trialnam)

365

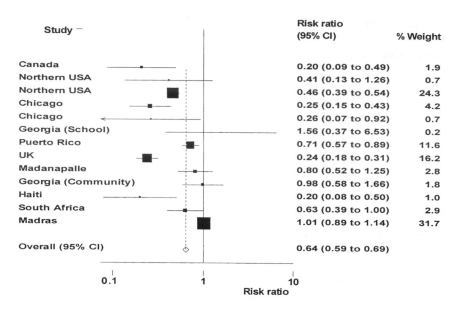

To use the **metareg** command, we need to derive the treatment effect estimate (in this case log risk ratio) and its standard error, for each study.

```
generate logrr=log((cases1/tot1)/(cases0/tot0))
generate  selogrr=sqrt((1/cases1)-(1/tot1)+(1/cases0)-
(1/tot0))
```

In their meta-analysis, Colditz *et al.* noted the strong evidence for heterogeneity between studies, and concluded that a random-effects meta-analysis was appropriate:

```
meta logrr selogrr, eform
```
Meta-analysis (exponential form)

Method	Pooled Est	95% CI Lower	Upper	Asymptotic z_value	p_value	No. of studies
Fixed	0.650	0.601	0.704	-10.625	0.000	13
Random	0.490	0.345	0.695	-3.995	0.000	

Test for heterogeneity: Q= 152.233 on 12 degrees of freedom (p= 0.000)
Moment-based estimate of between studies variance = 0.309

(The different weight of studies under the fixed and random effects assumption is discussed in Chapter 2).

The authors then examined possible explanations for the clear differences in the effect of BCG between studies. The earlier studies may have produced different results than later ones. The latitude at which the studies were conducted may also be associated with the effect of BCG. As discussed by Fine,[21] the possibility that BCG might provide greater protection at higher latitudes was first recognised by Palmer and Long,[22] who suggested that this trend might result from exposure to certain environmental mycobacteria, more common in warmer regions, which impart protection against tuberculosis.

To use **metareg**, we provide a list of variables, the first of which is the treatment effect (here, the log risk ratio) and the rest of which are (one or more) study characteristics (covariates) hypothesized to be associated with the treatment effect. In addition, the standard error or variance of the treatment effect must be provided, using the **wsse** (within-study standard error) or **wsvar** (within-study variance) option. It is also possible to specify the method for estimating the between-study variance: here we use the default; restricted maximum-likelihood (reml). To look for an association with start year and latitude:

metareg logrr startyr latitude, wsse(selogrr)

```
Iteration 1: tau^2 = 0
Iteration 2: tau^2 = .02189942
:
:
Iteration 9: tau^2 = .1361904
Iteration 10: tau^2 = .13635174


Meta-analysis regression          No of studies =  13
                                  tau^2 method    reml
                                  tau^2 estimate = .1364

Successive values of tau^2 differ by less than 10^-4 :con-
vergence achieved
```

	Coef.	Std. Err.	z	P>|z|	[95% Conf.Interval]	
startyr	-.004966	.0162811	-0.305	0.760	-.0368763	.0269444
latitude	-.0270477	.0118195	-2.288	0.022	-.0502135	-.0038819
_cons	9.890987	32.02516	0.309	0.757	-52.87717	72.65914

The regression coefficients are the estimated increase in the log risk ratio per unit increase in the covariate. So in the example the log risk ratio is estimated to decrease by 0·027 per unit increase in the latitude at which the study is conducted. The estimated between-study variance has been reduced from 0·31 (see output from the **meta** command) to 0·14. While there is strong evidence for an association between latitude and the effect of BCG, there is no evidence for an association with the year the study started. The estimated treatment effect given particular values of the covariates may be derived from the regression equation. For example, for a trial beginning in 1950, at latitude 50°, the estimated log risk ratio is given by:

Log risk ratio = $9·891 - 0·00497 \times 1950 - 0·0270 \times 50 = -1·1505$

which corresponds to a risk ratio of $\exp(-1·1505) = 0·316$

The use of meta-regression in explaining heterogeneity and identifying sources of bias in meta-analysis is discussed further in Chapters 8–11.

1 Yusuf S, Collins R, Peto R, *et al.* Intravenous and intracoronary fibrinolytic therapy in acute myocardial infarction: overview of results on mortality, reinfarction and side-effects from 33 randomized controlled trials. *Eur Heart J* 1985;**6**:556–85.
2 Gruppo Italiano per lo Studio della Streptochinasi nell'Infarto Miocardico (GISSI). Effectiveness of intravenous thrombolytic treatment in acute myocardial infarction. *Lancet* 1986;**1**:397–402.
3 ISIS-2 (Second International Study of Infarct Survival) Collaborative Group. Randomised trial of intravenous streptokinase, oral aspirin, both, or neither among 17,187 cases of suspected acute myocardial infarction: ISIS-2. *Lancet* 1988;**2**:349–60.
4 Bradburn MJ, Deeks JJ, Altman DG. sbe24: metan – an alternative meta-analysis command. *Stata Tech Bull* 1998;**44**:15.
5 Sharp S, Sterne J. sbe16: Meta-analysis. *Stata Tech Bull* 1997;**38**:9–14.
6 Sharp S, Sterne J. sbe16.1: New syntax and output for the meta-analysis command. *Stata Tech Bull* 1998;**42**:6–8.
7 Sharp S, Sterne J. sbe16.2: Corrections to the meta-analysis command. *Stata Tech Bull* 1998;**43**:15.
8 Teo KK, Yusuf S, Collins R, Held PH, Peto R. Effects of intravenous magnesium in suspected acute myocardial infarction: overview of randomised trials. *BMJ* 1991;**303**:1499–503.
9 ISIS-4 (Fourth International Study of Infarct Survival) Collaborative Group. ISIS-4: a randomised factorial trial assessing early oral captopril, oral mononitrate, and intravenous magnesium sulphate in 58,050 patients with suspected acute myocardial infarction. *Lancet* 1995;**345**:669–85.
10 Egger M, Smith GD. Misleading meta-analysis. Lessons from an "effective, safe, simple" intervention that wasn't. *BMJ* 1995;**310**:752–4.
11 Egger M, Smith GD, Schneider M, Minder C. Bias in meta-analysis detected by a simple, graphical test. *BMJ* 1997;**315**:629–34.
12 Sterne J. sbe22: Cumulative meta analysis. *Stata Tech Bull* 1998;**42**:13–16.
13 Lau J, Antman EM, Jimenez-Silva J, Kupelnick B, Mosteller F, Chalmers TC. Cumulative meta-analysis of therapeutic trials for myocardial infarction. *N Engl J Med* 1992;**327**:248–54.
14 Antman EM, Lau J, Kupelnick B, Mosteller F, Chalmers TC. A comparison of results of meta-analyses of randomized control trials and recommendations of clinical experts' Treatments for myocardial infarction. *JAMA* 1992;**268**:240–8.
15 Tobias A. sbe26: Assessing the influence of a single study in meta-analysis. *Stata Tech Bull* 1999;**47**:15–17.

16 Steichen T. sbe19: Tests for publication bias in meta-analysis. *Stata Tech Bull* 1998;**41**:9–15.
17 Steichen T, Egger M, Sterne J. sbe19.1: Tests for publication bias in meta-analysis. *Stata Tech Bull* 1998;**44**:3–4.
18 Begg CB, Mazumdar M. Operating characteristics of a rank correlation test for publication bias. *Biometrics* 1994;**50**:1088–101.
19 Sharp S. sbe23: Meta-analysis regression. *Stata Tech Bull* 1998;**42**:16–24.
20 Colditz GA, Brewer TF, Berkey CS, *et al.* Efficacy of BCG vaccine in the prevention of tuberculosis. Meta-analysis of the published literature. *JAMA* 1994;**271**:698–702.
21 Fine PEM. Variation in protection by BCG: implications of and for heterologous immunity. *Lancet* 1995;**346**:1339–45.
22 Palmer CE, Long MW. Effects of infection with atypical mycobacteria on BCG vaccination and tuberculosis. *Am Rev Respir Dis* 1966;**94**:553–68.

Part V: Using systematic reviews in practice

19 Applying the results of systematic reviews at the bedside

FINLAY A McALISTER

Summary points

Applying results from systematic reviews to an individual patient involves consideration of:

- *The applicability of the evidence to an individual patient*
  While some variation in treatment response between a patient and the patients in a systematic review is to be expected, the differences tend to be quantitative rather than qualitative.

  Outcomes research generally confirms that therapies found to be beneficial in a narrow range of patients have broader application in actual practice.

- *The feasibility of the intervention in a particular setting*
  Involves consideration of whether the intervention is available and affordable in that setting and whether the necessary expertise and resources are locally available.

- *The benefit: risk ratio in an individual patient*
  As a first step, the overall results must be summarised. In order to facilitate their extrapolation to a specific patient, formats which incorporate baseline risk and therapeutic effects (such as number needed to treat or number needed to harm) are preferable.

  Secondly, the results can be extrapolated to a specific patient by either considering results in the most relevant subgroup, or by multivariate risk prediction equations, or by using clinical judgement to determine a specific patient's risk status.

- *The incorporation of patient values and preferences*
  This is an evolving field and current techniques include patient decision support technology or the expression of likelihood to help or harm.

373

Systematic reviews provide the best estimates of the true effects (both beneficial and adverse) of medical interventions, and other chapters in this book have outlined criteria for their performance and critical appraisal. However, these effect estimates are derived by collating data from a diverse range of patients. In this chapter, we build upon previous work[1-4] and describe a framework for the clinician faced with deciding whether and how the results of a systematic review are applicable to a particular patient (see Summary points).

Determining the applicability of the evidence to an individual patient

Rather than pouring over the inclusion and exclusion criteria of the included studies to determine whether a particular patient would have been eligible, this question is better approached by asking "is the underlying pathobiology in my patient so different that the study cannot give any guidance?".[3,4] This involves consideration of the pathogenesis of the disease process as well as patient-specific biology and environmental exposures. While the potential challenges to the applicability of a systematic review described below may seem daunting, it is helpful to keep in mind that "differences between our patients and those we read about in trials tend to be quantitative (e.g. matters of degree in risk and responsiveness) rather than qualitative (no response or adverse response)".[4] For example, although randomised clinical trials had clearly established that beta-blockers were beneficial in reducing mortality risk in acute myocardial infarction (MI),[5] these drugs have been systematically under-used in MI patients as clinicians have tended to restrict their use to "ideal patients" who would have fulfilled trial entry criteria.[6] However, observational studies in the real-world setting have suggested that beta-blockers are just as beneficial in patients who would have been excluded from the original trials because of perceived contra-indications (such as peripheral vascular disease, diabetes mellitus, congestive heart failure, or chronic obstructive airways disease).[7] Moreover, such outcomes research has confirmed that the relative survival benefits are in the order of 30–40% in all major patient subgroups, including those traditionally under-represented in trials (such as women, blacks, or the elderly).[7]

However, there are some exceptions to this general rule. First, while disease pathophysiology is usually similar in two or more patients with the same diagnosis, this may not always be the case. To the extent that differences exist, a systematic review's applicability may be limited. For example, although the vast majority of the patients enrolled in the trials of angiotensin-converting enzyme (ACE) inhibitors in heart failure had systolic dysfunction, population-based cohort studies[8,9] suggest that

374

30–40% of all patients with heart failure have diastolic dysfunction. Thus, while a systematic review of these trials[10] demonstrated a marked survival benefit from ACE inhibitor therapy, it is uncertain whether the benefits extend to heart failure patients with diastolic dysfunction (indeed outcomes research[11] has failed to find any mortality advantage with ACE inhibitors in diastolic dysfunction). While the resolution of this clinical dilemma awaits further research, this example serves to highlight the necessity for a sound understanding of disease pathophysiology in order to properly interpret research evidence. Second, several patient-related factors can also impact upon the applicability of research results. For example, differences in drug metabolism (such as acetylation rates) or immune responsiveness among patients, arising from genetic polymorphism, may modulate the effects of interventions.[12,13] Third, environmental factors may influence treatment effects (for instance, the frequency of thyroid dysfunction with amiodarone varies with environmental iodine intake).[14] Finally, the balance between benefit and harm from an intervention may differ if an individual patient is less (or more) compliant than those in the studies: for example, non-compliant patients are at higher risk of bleeding with chronic warfarin therapy than their compliant peers (relative risk 2·3, $P = 0·003$).[15]

Given these myriad influences on the applicability of research evidence, one should expect some variation in treatment response between patients in one's practice and those described in systematic reviews. However, these variations are not always important (for example, the management of cataracts is generally similar despite the varied pathogenesis) or non-remediable (the dose of a drug can be adjusted based on individual patient responsiveness).[3] To return to the example of bleeding with chronic warfarin therapy, cohort studies have shown that the complication rates seen in randomised trials can be achieved with compliant patients and clinicians in actual practice.[16–18] Thus, the assumption that study results are applicable to a broader range of patients than enrolled in the trials generally holds true and outcomes research in the cardiovascular field consistently demonstrates that less harm results from this assumption than from withholding efficacious therapies from subgroups of patients not investigated in randomised trials.[19]

Determining the feasibility of the intervention in a particular setting

In deciding whether the results of a systematic review can be extrapolated to an individual patient, the realities of local circumstance must also be considered. For example, is the intervention available and affordable in that setting? Thus, while there is little doubt that thrombolytic therapy confers significant benefits in patients with acute myocardial infarction,[20] the cost makes provision of this therapy prohibitive in many developing countries.[3] Secondly, one must consider whether the necessary monitoring facilities are available if the intervention is offered. For example, if there is no facility for monitoring prothrombin times, it would be unwise to prescribe warfarin for a patient with atrial fibrillation, despite the trial evidence[21] proving substantial efficacy. Finally, one must consider whether local expertise is sufficient to warrant provision of the intervention. For example, although a recent systematic review of carotid endarterectomy in patients with asymptomatic carotid stenosis concluded that surgery "unequivocally reduces the incidence of ipsilateral stroke",[22] the rate of perioperative complications in the trials was much lower than seen in audits of non-trial surgeons. As a result, carotid endarterectomy in centres with higher surgical complication rates will confer more harm than benefit.[23] Thus, the clinician may decide to refer eligible patients to a centre with lower perioperative morbidity rates.

Determining the benefit : risk ratio in an individual patient

If the results of a systematic review are judged applicable and feasible, the clinician must then evaluate the likely benefits and harms from the intervention. This involves two steps: deriving clinically useful estimates of the overall results and extrapolating from the overall results to derive estimates for the individual patient. To illustrate this process, an example is outlined in Box 19.1 (adapted from Glasziou et al.[4]) and will be referred to below.

Deriving clinically useful estimates from the overall results

Although the results of randomised clinical trials and systematic reviews with binary outcomes can be expressed in a number of ways, expressing the effects of treatment in terms of the number of patients one would need to treat to prevent one clinical event (NNT)[24] is gaining widespread acceptance as the most relevant format for extrapolating to patients, can be directly applied to patients who are at the average risk in the included trials, and quickly adjusted at the bedside for patients who are not.[25,26] The advantage to front line clinicians of the NNT over the more traditional reporting formats (such as relative risk reduction (RRR) or odds ratio (OR), which do not reflect baseline risk) is illustrated by considering the benefits of antihypertensive therapy for patients with varying degrees of blood pressure elevation (Table 19.1). As can be seen, the OR (and RRR) in all three blood pressure strata are approximately 40%, but the amount of effort required by clinicians and patients to prevent one stroke varies according to the baseline risk.[27]

While NNTs are easily calculated when relative and absolute risks are reported (the NNT is the inverse of the difference in absolute event rates

Box 19.1 Determining the benefit:risk ratio in an individual patient – the example of warfarin therapy

Hypothetical patient
A 76-year-old female with hypertension and asymptomatic nonvalvular atrial fibrillation for at least three months. Transthoracic echocardiogram showed an enlarged left atrium, suggesting that attempts at cardioversion would be unlikely to be successful.

Deriving clinically useful estimates of the overall results
Benefit (defined as prevention of embolic stroke)

• control event rate (CER)	4·5% per year
• experimental event rate (EER)	1·4% per year
• absolute risk reduction (ARR)	3·1% per year
• NNT to prevent one embolic stroke	33 per year

Harm (defined as major bleeding)

• control event rate (CER)	1·0% per year
• experimental event rate (EER)	1·4% per year
• absolute risk increase (ARI)	0·4% per year
• NNH (i.e. to cause one major bleed)	250 per year

Extrapolating to the individual patient
1 Subgroup analysis:
Benefit

• CER in relevant subgroup	8·1% per year
• EER in relevant subgroup	1·2% per year
• ARR in relevant subgroup	6·9% per year
• NNT in relevant subgroup	15 per year

Harm
• Event rates not reported in patient-specific subgroups.

2 Use of the *f* factor
Benefit
• patient estimated to be at twice the risk of embolic stroke of the average patient in the trials; thus, *f* factor = 2
• average NNT/*f* factor = patient-specific NNT; thus, patient-specific NNT = 33/2 = 17

Harm
• patient estimated to be at twice the risk of bleeding as the average patient in the trials; thus, *f* factor = 2
• average NNH/*f* factor = patient-specific NNH; thus, patient-specific NNH = 250/2 = 125

NNT= number needed to treat; NNH= number needed to harm.

Table 19.1 Methods of reporting the results of systematic reviews.

Patient strata (by diastolic blood pressure [DBP])	Stroke rates		Odds ratio	Relative risk reduction [RRR = $(P_c - P_A)/P_c$]	Absolute risk reduction [ARR = $P_c - P_A$]	Number needed to treat for five years to prevent one stroke (1/ARR)
	Control [P_c]	Treatment [P_A]				
DBP < 110 mm Hg	0·0148	0·0087	0·41	0·41	0·006	164
DBP ≤ 115 mm Hg	0·0201	0·0122	0·42	0·39	0·008	125
DBP > 115 mm Hg	0·0263	0·0156	0·41	0·41	0·011	91

Data from Collins et al.[27]

between the control and experimental arms, see Chapter 20), they cannot be easily calculated from ORs. Since the value of the OR does not always reflect the RR (particularly when disease incidence is above 10%, see also Chapter 2),[28] the clinician must employ a formula[26] or consult Table 19.2 to derive the overall NNT from systematic reviews which report only the OR. The NNT for the prevention of one embolic stroke with warfarin therapy in the average patient with non-valvular atrial fibrillation (as determined in a systematic review of the atrial fibrillation trials) is approximately 33 (Box 19.1).[21]

Analogous to the NNT, the number needed to harm (NNH) is an expression of the number of patients who would need to receive an intervention to cause one additional adverse event. The NNH is the inverse of the difference in absolute adverse event rates between the control and experimental arms. For example, the NNH (harm defined as a major bleed) for warfarin therapy was 250 in the systematic review of the atrial fibrillation trials (Box 19.1).[21]

Extrapolating to the individual patient

While the NNT and NNH are clinically useful estimates of the average treatment effects in patients at the average risk in the included trials, they may not be directly relevant to an individual patient; thus, the clinician must extrapolate in one of three ways.

First, if the systematic review presents estimates of treatment effects in various subgroups, the clinician can extrapolate using the NNT and/or NNH from the subgroup most relevant to their patient. For example, a systematic review of antiplatelet agents[29] for the prevention of non-fatal myocardial infarction revealed similar proportional treatment effects in trials of primary and secondary prevention (OR 29% and 35% respectively). However, the NNT varied markedly such that 200 patients without symptomatic cardiovascular disease would need treatment for five years to prevent one myocardial infarction while only 71 "high risk" patients (those with prior myocardial infarction, stroke, or other cardiovascular event) would require treatment for three years to have the same clinical impact. Returning to our running example, the systematic review of atrial fibrillation trials[21] provided estimates of risk and treatment effects in various subgroups defined by baseline clinical features; the patient with non-valvular atrial fibrillation outlined in Box 19.1 has a baseline risk of embolic stroke of approximately 8% per annum without treatment, and warfarin therapy is associated with an 85% relative risk reduction. Thus, the NNT for this patient would be approximately 15 (Box 19.1). Unfortunately, the infrequent nature of adverse events precluded the investigators from determining the NNH in patient-specific subgroups. In this situation, one

Table 19.2 Deriving the NNT from the odds ratio.

Control event rate	Preventive intervention									Treatment								
	0·5	0·55	0·6	0·65	0·7	0·75	0·8	0·85	0·9	1·5	2	2·5	3	3·5	4	4·5	5	10
0·05	41	46	52	59	69	83	104	139	209	43	22	15	12	9	8	7	6	3
0·1	21	24	27	31	36	43	54	73	110	23	12	9	7	6	5	4	4	2
0·2	11	13	14	17	20	24	30	40	61	14	8	5	4	4	3	3	3	2
0·3	8	9	10	12	14	18	22	30	46	11	6	5	4	3	3	3	3	2
0·4	7	8	9	10	12	15	19	26	40	10	6	4	4	3	3	3	3	2
0·5	6	7	8	9	11	14	18	25	38	10	6	5	4	4	3	3	3	2
0·7	6	7	9	10	13	16	20	28	44	13	8	7	6	5	5	5	5	4
0·9	12	15	18	22	27	34	46	64	101	32	21	17	16	14	14	13	13	11

Reproduced from McQuay and Moore,[26] with permission. The formula for determining the NNT for preventive interventions is $\{1-[\text{CER} \times (1-\text{OR})]\} / [(1 - \text{CER}) \times \text{CER} \times (1-\text{OR})]$. For treatment, the formula is $[\text{CER} (\text{OR}-1) + 1] / [\text{CER} (\text{OR}-1) \times (1-\text{CER})]$.
CER = control event rate, OR = odds ratio.

is left with using the overall results or using one of the other methods of extrapolation outlined below.

While the use of subgroup analyses seems intuitively appealing, we must sound a note of caution at this point. A full discussion of the limitations of subgroup analysis is beyond the scope of this chapter, but has been covered in full elsewhere.[30] In particular, one should be wary of systematic reviews which stratify patients by risk (as determined by *post-hoc* analysis of event rates in the control groups of the included trials) as these analyses may produce biased and inaccurate estimates of the relative treatment effects (see also Chapters 8 and 10).[31,32] Instead, subgroups should be based on measurable patient characteristics at baseline (for example, gender, age, or primary versus secondary prevention). Since the derivation of such subgroups is often not possible using published trial results, this is a key advantage of individual patient data meta-analyses (see also Chapter 6).[33]

Secondly, as an extension of the subgroup approach, one can use multivariate risk prediction equations to quantitate an individual patient's potential for benefit (and harm) from therapy.[34,35] For example, returning to the systematic review of endarterectomy for asymptomatic carotid stenosis referred to earlier,[22] investigators are working on a prognostic model to identify patients who are most likely to benefit from operative intervention. This model incorporates the risk of stroke without surgery (and thus the potential benefit from surgery) with the risk of stroke or other adverse outcome from surgery.[36] Application of this model to patients with symptomatic carotid stenosis enables clinicians to identify high-risk patients who benefit considerably from surgery (OR 0.12, 95% CI 0.05 to 0.29) from other patients with the same degree of stenosis but little to gain from surgery (OR 1.00, 95% CI 0.65 to 1.54).[36] While these multivariate risk prediction models can be derived from the clinical trial data included in the systematic review, it is preferable if they come from other datasets such as population-based cohort studies.[37] No multivariate risk prediction models have yet been published for chronic warfarin therapy in non-valvular atrial fibrillation.

Finally, in the absence of subgroup data or prognostic models, the clinician can employ clinical judgement by dividing the average NNT (or NNH) by a factor (f) which relates the risk of the individual patient to that of the average patient in the published reports.[38] This factor is expressed as a decimal such that patients judged to be at less baseline risk than those in the trials will be assigned an $f < 1$ and those at greater risk will be assigned an $f > 1$. For example, if we did not have the subgroup-specific data for atrial fibrillation discussed above, we may have estimated that, since they are older than the average patient in the atrial fibrillation trials and have hypertension (while less than half of the randomised trial patients did), the patient outlined in Box 19.1 is at twice the risk of embolic stroke than the average randomised trial patient. Thus, the patient-specific NNT would be about 17. By the same token, we may have estimated they were at twice the risk of major bleeding (because of their age). Thus, the patient-specific NNH would be 125.

While this method may appear overly subjective, recent empirical evidence suggests that clinicians are accurate in estimating relative differences in baseline risk (i.e. f) between patients (far exceeding our abilities to judge absolute baseline risks).[39] However, it should be recognised that this method implicitly assumes that the proportional treatment effects (RR or OR) from an intervention are constant across different baseline risks, an assumption that may not hold for all therapies.[31,32,34] Moreover, further research is needed into the basis for, and determinants of, clinical judgement.

Incorporating patient values and preferences

After deriving patient-centered estimates for the potential benefit and harm from an intervention, the clinician must integrate this with their patient's values and preferences about therapy. Indeed, active patient involvement in medical decision making improves their quality of life[40,41] and outcomes from treatment;[41-44] moreover, there is preliminary evidence that it may also reduce health care expenditures.[45,46] However, the optimal means of involving patients in treatment decisions has not yet been found and patient decision support technology is a rich vein for current research. Decision support technology is distinct from general patient education in its focus on the benefits and risks of alternatives (with explicit discussion of the probabilities and consequences of clinically important outcomes), the tailoring of the information to the particular patient's risk profile, the emphasis on choice and shared decision making, and explicit elicitation of patient values.[47]

Until the techniques of formal decision analysis have evolved to the stage that they are feasible to use at the bedside, interim techniques such as decision aids[47] or the expression of likelihood to help or harm (a formula weighting the ratio of NNT:NNH by patient values)[48] will serve this need.

Conclusion

While systematic reviews provide the best estimates of the true effects of an intervention, their application at the bedside is a "difficult, time-consuming, and incompletely studied skill".[49] In this chapter, we have outlined a framework for approaching this task and anticipate that ongoing research will greatly expand our understanding and performance of these steps.

Acknowledgements

FAM is supported by the Medical Research Council of Canada and the Alberta Heritage Foundation for Medical Research.

1 Sackett DL, Richardson WS, Rosenberg W, Haynes RB. *Evidence-based medicine. How to practice and teach EBM*. London: Churchill Livingstone, 1997.
2 Sackett DL. Applying overviews and meta-analyses at the bedside. *J Clin Epidemiol* 1995;**48**:61–6.
3 Dans AL, Dans LF, Guyatt GH, Richardson, S. Users' guides to the medical literature. XIV. How to decide on the applicability of clinical trial results to your patient. *JAMA* 1998;**279**:545–9.
4 Glasziou P, Guyatt GH, Dans AL, Dans LF, Straus S, Sackett DL. Applying the results of trials and systematic reviews to individual patients [EBM Note]. *Evidence-Based Med* 1998;**3**:165–6.
5 Yusuf S, Sleight P, Held P, McMahon S. Routine medical management of acute myocardial infarction. Lessons from overviews of recent randomized controlled trials. *Circulation* 1990;**82**(suppl II):II-117–34.
6 Rogers WJ, Bowlby LJ, Chandra NC, *et al*. Treatment of myocardial infarction in the United States (1990–1993). Observations from the National Registry of Myocardial Infarction. *Circulation* 1994;**90**:2103–14.
7 Gottlieb SS, McCarter RJ, Vogel RA. Effect of beta-blockade on mortality among high-risk and low-risk patients after myocardial infarction. *N Engl J Med* 1998;**339**:489–97.
8 Vasan RS, Benjamin EJ, Levy D. Prevalence, clinical features, and prognosis of diastolic heart failure: an epidemiologic perspective. *J Am Coll Cardiol* 1995;**26**:1565–74.
9 Senni M, Tribouilloy CM, Rodeheffer RJ, *et al*. Congestive heart failure in the community. A study of all incident cases in Olmsted County, Minnesota, in 1991. *Circulation* 1998;**98**:2282–9.
10 Garg R, Yusuf S, for the Collaborative Group on ACE Inhibitor Trials. Overview of randomized trials of angiotensin-converting enzyme inhibitors on mortality and morbidity in patients with heart failure. *JAMA* 1995;**273**:1450–6.
11 McAlister FA, Teo KK, Taher M, *et al*. Insights into the contemporary epidemiology and outpatient management of congestive heart failure. *Am Heart J* 1999;**138**:87–94.
12 Schaefer O. Adverse reactions to drugs and metabolic problems perceived in Northern Canadian Indians and Eskimos. *Progr Clin Biol Res* 1986;**214**:77–83.
13 Ward J, Brenneman G, Letson GW, Heyward WL. Limited efficacy of a *Haemophilus* type B conjugate vaccine in Alaska Native infants: the Alaska *H. influenzae* Vaccine Study Group. *N Engl J Med* 1990;**323**:1415–6.
14 Martino E, Safran M, Aghini-Lombardi F, *et al*. Environmental iodine intake and thyroid dysfunction during chronic amiodarone therapy. *Ann Intern Med* 1984;**101**:28–34.
15 Fihn SD, McDonell M, Martin D, *et al*. Risk factors for complications of chronic anticoagulation. A multicenter study. *Ann Intern Med* 1993;**118**:511–20.
16 Levine MN, Raskob G, Landefeld S, Kearon C. Hemorrhagic complications of anticoagulant treatment. *Chest* 1998;**114**(suppl):511S–523S.
17 McKenna CJ, Galvin J, McCann HA, Sugrue DD. Risks of long-term oral anticoagulation in a non-trial medical environment. *Irish Med J* 1996;**89**:144–5.
18 Palareti G, Leali N, Coccheri S, *et al*. Bleeding complications of oral anticoagulant treatment: an inception cohort, prospective collaborative study (ISCOAT). *Lancet* 1996;**348**:423–8.
19 McAlister FA, Taylor L, Teo KK, *et al*. The treatment and prevention of coronary heart disease in Canada: do older patients receive efficacious therapies? *J Am Geriatr Soc* 1999;**47**:811–18.
20 Fibrinolytic Therapy Trialists Collaborative Group. Indications for fibrinolytic therapy in suspected acute myocardial infarction: collaborative overview of early mortality and major morbidity results from all randomised trials of more than 1000 patients. *Lancet* 1994;**343**:311–22.

21 Risk factors for stroke and efficacy of antithrombotic therapy in atrial fibrillation. Analysis of pooled data from five randomized controlled trials. *Arch Intern Med* 1994;**154**:1449–57.
22 Benavente O, Moher D, Pham B. Carotid endarterectomy for asymptomatic carotid stenosis: a meta-analysis. *BMJ* 1998;**317**:1477–80.
23 Barnett HJ, Eliasziw M, Meldrum HE, Taylor DW. Do the facts and figures warrant a 10-fold increase in the performance of carotid endarterectomy on asymptomatic patients? *Neurology* 1996;**46**:603–8.
24 Laupacis A, Sackett DL, Roberts RS. An assessment of clinically useful measures of the consequences of treatment. *N Engl J Med* 1988;**318**:1728–33.
25 Sackett DL, Haynes RB. Summarising the effects of therapy: a new table and some more terms [EBM Note]. *Evidence-Based Med* 1997;**2**:103–4.
26 McQuay HJ, Moore RA. Using numerical results from systematic reviews in clinical practice. *Ann Intern Med* 1997;**126**:712–20.
27 Collins R, Peto R, MacMahon S, *et al*. Blood pressure, stroke, and coronary heart disease. Part 2, short-term reductions in blood pressure: overview of randomised drug trials in their epidemiological context. *Lancet* 1990;**335**:827–38.
28 Sackett DL, Deeks JJ, Altman DG. Down with odds ratios![EBM Note]. *Evidence-Based Med* 1996;**1**:164–6.
29 Antiplatelet Trialists' Collaboration. Collaborative overview of randomised trials of antiplatelet therapy – I: Prevention of death, myocardial infarction, and stroke by prolonged antiplatelet therapy in various categories of patients. *BMJ* 1994;**308**:81–106.
30 Yusuf S, Wittes J, Probstfield J, Tyroler HA. Analysis and interpretation of treatment effects in subgroups of patients in randomized clinical trials. *JAMA* 1991;**266**:93–8.
31 Davey Smith G, Egger M. Who benefits from medical interventions? Treating low risk patients can be a high risk strategy. *BMJ* 1994;**308**:72–4.
32 Sharp SJ, Thompson SG, Altman DG. The relation between treatment benefit and underlying risk in meta-analysis. *BMJ* 1996;**313**:735–8.
33 Stewart LA, Clarke MJ. Practical methodology of meta-analyses (overviews) using updated individual patient data. *Stat Med* 1995;**14**:2057–79.
34 Rothwell PM. Can overall results of clinical trials be applied to all patients? *Lancet* 1995;**345**:1616–19.
35 Glasziou PP, Irwig LM. An evidence based approach to individualising treatment. *BMJ* 1995;**311**:1356–9.
36 Rothwell PM, Warlow CP on behalf of the European Carotid Surgery Trialists' Collaborative Group. Prediction of benefit from carotid endarterectomy in individual patients: a risk-modelling study. *Lancet* 1999;**353**:2105–10.
37 Laupacis A, Wells G, Richardson WS, Tugwell P, for the Evidence-Based Medicine Working Group. User's guides to the medical literature. V. How to use an article about prognosis. *JAMA* 1994;**272**:234–7.
38 Cook RJ, Sackett DL. The number needed to treat: a clinically useful measure of treatment effect. *BMJ* 1995;**310**:452–4.
39 Grover SA, Lowensteyn I, Esrey KL, Steinert Y, Joseph L, Abrahamowicz M. Do doctors accurately assess coronary risk in their patients? Preliminary results of the coronary health assessment study. *BMJ* 1995;**310**:975–8.
40 Szabo E, Moody H, Hamilton T, Ang C, Kovithavongs C, Kjellstrand C. Choice of treatment improves quality of life: a study of patients undergoing dialysis. *Arch Intern Med* 1997;**157**:1352–6.
41 Greenfield S, Kaplan SH, Ware JE Jr, Yano EM, Frank HJL. Patients' participation in medical care: effects on blood sugar control and quality of life in diabetes. *J Gen Intern Med* 1988;**3**:448–57.
42 Kaplan SH, Greenfield S, Ware JE Jr. Assessing the effects of physician-patient interactions on the outcomes of chronic disease. *Med Care* 1989;**27**(suppl 3):S110–127.
43 Schulman BA. Active patient orientation and outcomes in hypertension treatment. Application of a socio-organizational perspective. *Med Care* 1979;**17**:267–80.
44 Stewart MA. Effective physician-patient communication and health outcomes: a review. *Can Med Assoc J* 1995;**152**:1423–33.
45 Vickery DM, Golaszewski TJ, Wright EC, Kalmer H. The effect of self-care inter-

ventions on the use of medical service within a Medicare population. *Med Care* 1988;**26**:580–8.

46 Gage BF, Cardinalli AB, Owens DK. Cost-effectiveness of preference-based antithrombotic therapy for patients with nonvalvular atrial fibrillation. *Stroke* 1998;**29**:1083–91.

47 O'Connor AM. Consumer/patient decision support in the new millenium: where should our research take us? *Can J Nurs Res* 1997;**29**:7–12.

48 Straus SE, Sackett DL. The likelihood of being helped versus harmed – a new method of presenting information to patients about the risks and benefits of therapy. *3rd Cochrane Colloquium*, Amsterdam, October 1997.

49 Ross JM. Commentary on applying the results of trials and systematic reviews to individual patients [EBM Note]. *Evidence-Based Med* 1998;**3**:167.

20 Numbers needed to treat derived from meta-analyses: pitfalls and cautions

SHAH EBRAHIM

Summary points

- Numbers needed to treat are commonly used to summarise the beneficial effects of treatment in a clinically relevant way, taking into account both baseline risk without treatment and the risk reduction achieved with treatment.
- Numbers needed to treat are sensitive to factors that change baseline risk: the outcome considered; characteristics of patients included in trials; secular trends in incidence and case-fatality; and the clinical setting.
- Pooled numbers needed to treat derived from meta-analyses of absolute risk differences are commonly presented and easily calculated but may be seriously misleading because baseline risk often varies markedly between trials included in meta-analyses.
- Meaningful numbers needed to treat are obtained by applying the pooled relative risk reductions calculated from meta-analyses or individual trials to the baseline risk relevant to specific patient groups.

Eight hundred and thirty-three. This is the number of mildly hypertensive people who must be treated with antihypertensives for a year to avoid one stroke.[1] The number needed to treat (NNT) is now widely used to describe treatment effects.[2] NNTs are increasingly being calculated by pooling absolute risk differences of trials included in meta-analyses.[3,4] Indeed, the option of pooling absolute risk differences is readily available in statistical software (see Chapter 17), and *The Cochrane Database of Systematic Reviews*.[5]

Are NNTs a good thing? Proponents of their use suggest that they aid translation of trial effects to clinical practice in terms that clinicians understand (see Chapter 19). High risk patients stand to gain more from treatment and this is reflected in a small NNT, whereas low risk patients will have a large NNT. As the absolute levels of risk are taken into account, the clinician can better weigh up the size of benefit with possible harms of treatment.[1] NNTs can, therefore, help in setting priorities. Moreover, the NNT gives some idea of the clinical workload required to achieve health benefits and is consequently valued by public health medicine as investment often seems disproportionate to the benefits obtained. NNTs are also thought to be more intuitive and easier for clinicians to understand than relative measures of treatment effects.

In this chapter NNTs derived from trials and meta-analyses of interventions for the prevention of cardiovascular disease are used to illustrate problems in use of NNTs, and in particular, those derived from meta-analyses of pooled absolute risk differences – pooled NNTs. A pooled NNT may be misleading because of variation in event rates in trials, differences in the outcomes considered, effects of geographic and secular trends on disease risk, and the clinical setting. It is assumed throughout that relative measures of treatment effects – the odds ratio or relative risk – are the most appropriate measure in meta-analyses of trials (see Chapter 16 for a discussion of summary statistics). NNTs should be derived by applying relative risk reductions on treatment estimated by trials or meta-analysis to populations of specified absolute high, medium and low risk to illustrate a range of possible NNTs.

Describing the effects of treatment

The effects of treatment are conventionally expressed in relative terms – the ratio of the event rate in the treatment group divided by the event rate in the control group – often called the relative risk or more accurately, the rate ratio. Ratios greater than one imply that treatment is harmful, less than one, that treatment is beneficial. This hides the fact that a small relative benefit for patients at very high risk will generate more lives saved (and non-fatal events avoided) than the same relative benefit applied to much lower risk patients. However, the relative treatment effect may be dependent on the baseline level of risk, which is estimated by the risk in the control group. For example, surgery for carotid endarterectomy is effective for high risk tight stenosis but not for low risk, smaller degrees of stenosis.[6] It cannot be assumed that treatment effects are constant across a wide range of baseline levels of risk.

The absolute effects of treatment are simply the difference between intervention and control group rates. From a clinical and public health standpoint it is useful to have some idea of the amount of effort – both in terms of time and money – required to avoid one adverse event. This is given by

Box 20.1 Calculation of number needed to treat

The number needed to treat (NNT) is the number of patients who must be treated over a defined period of time to prevent a specified bad outcome or to cause an unwanted side effect (number needed to harm, NNH). The NNT is the reciprocal of the absolute risk difference for an adverse outcome between those treated and the control or placebo group:

NNT = 1 / (risk of bad outcome in placebo group – risk of bad outcome in treated group)

The NNT can be calculated by applying the relative risk reduction obtained from a meta-analysis or a trial to a baseline risk without treatment that reflects the risk of the type of patients to be treated.

Treatment with statins is associated with a relative risk of 0·69 for all cardiovascular disease (CVD) events (see Table 20.1). The likely risk of CVD in a high risk group of patients might be as high as 5% per year. This can be estimated from studies of prognosis in relevant patient groups:

- baseline risk of CVD outcome without treatment = 5% = 0·05 per year
- risk of CVD outcome with treatment = 0·05 × 0·69 = 0·0345 per year
- risk difference = 0·05 – 0·0345 = 0·0155
- NNT = 1/ risk difference = 1/ 0·0155 = 64 people treated for one year to avoid one CVD outcome

Among a low risk group of patients, for example, in primary care, the risk of CVD without treatment might be as low as 0·5% per year. In this case:

- baseline risk of CVD outcome without treatment = 0·5% = 0·005
- risk of CVD outcome with treatment = 0·005 × 0·69 = 0·0035
- risk difference = 0·005 – 0·0035 = 0·0016
- NNT = 1/ 0·0016 = 645 people treated for one year to avoid one CVD outcome

the reciprocal of the absolute risk difference – the number needed to treat (see Box 20.1).[2] The absolute effect and the NNT will vary – often greatly – according to the baseline level of risk and this means that a single measure of effect applicable to different age groups, for example, cannot be derived.

The effect of choice of outcome

The effects of treatment with statins derived from the five major trials[7–11] are shown in Table 20.1. NNTs vary greatly depending on the outcome chosen. In communicating a "positive message", it is tempting to choose

Table 20.1 Major statin trials. Rate ratios and numbers needed to treat.

Trial	Number of participants	Control group CHD mortality risk/100 person years	Rate ratios			NNT (5 years)		
			Total mortality	CHD mortality	All CVD events	Total mortality	CHD mortality	All CVD events
Primary prevention								
AF/TexCAPS[7]	6605	0·1	1·04	1·36	0·69	—*	—*	28
WOSCOPS[8]	6595	0·4	0·78	0·67	0·70	118	182	28
Secondary prevention								
4S[9]	4444	1·6	0·71	0·59	0·64	33	31	8
CARE trial[10]	4159	1·2	0·92	0·81	0·75	133	95	11
LIPID[11]	9014	1·4	0·78	0·77	NA	41	64	NA
Pooled effects (95% CI)			0·80 (0·74 to 0·87)	0·73 (0·66 to 0·81)	0·69 (0·66 to 0·73)	113 (77 to 285)	500 (222 to –)†	20 (17 to 25)

NNT = number needed to treat to prevent one adverse event; AF/TexCAPS = Air Force/Texas Coronary Atherosclerosis Prevention Study; WOSCOPS = West of Scotland Coronary Prevention Study; 4S = Scandinavian Simvastatin Survival Study; CARE = cholesterol and recurrent events; LIPID = long-term intervention with Pravastatin in ischemic heart disease; 95% CI = 95% confidence interval; NA = data not available.
* AF/TexCAPS reported a non-significant increased total and CHD mortality in the intervention group, with confidence intervals of risk ratio including the possibility of harm as well as benefit.
† Upper confidence limit of NNT not calculated as confidence interval of pooled absolute risk difference included possibility of harm.

389

the smallest NNT, for example when the outcome chosen is "all bad things that can happen".[12] The combined "all vascular events" endpoint was made up of different proportions of event in the different trials. In the WOSCOP and AFCAP/TexCAP studies, coronary heart disease deaths made up 16% and 3% of the combined endpoint, respectively.

Ineffective treatments and adverse effects

A mathematical quirk of the NNT is that if the treatment appears to have no effect, that is the event rates are identical in both the treatment and control groups, then the absolute risk difference is zero, and 1/zero, the NNT, is infinity.[13] Furthermore, a treatment producing an adverse effect gives a number needed to harm (NNH), which is the number of people who need to receive treatment to harm one additional patient, rather than benefit one patient. If confidence intervals of absolute risk differences include zero, then the confidence intervals of the number of patients who need to be treated will set out from a negative value indicating benefit (NNT), include infinity, and stretch to a positive value indicating harm (NNH) at the upper border. It is rather confusing to have a measure of effect with confidence intervals that may include benefit, harm and infinity! What this means is that no matter how many patients are treated (even up to an infinite number), the trial result is consistent with no effect, benefit and harm.

This is illustrated by the AF/TexCAP trial[7] of lovastatin, the absolute coronary heart disease mortality rate difference was very close to zero, with 95% confidence intervals which included the possibility of benefit and also of harm. Figure 20.1 shows hypothetically how the NNT (vertical axis) might vary with different values of absolute risk difference (horizontal axis) found in different trials. The larger the absolute difference, the smaller the NNT if treatment is better than control and similarly, the smaller the NNH, if control is better than treatment.

The effect of variation in baseline risk

Interventions for secondary prevention following myocardial infarction[14-16] are shown in Table 20.2. While they all have very similar relative risk reductions, their NNTs are much more variable and have wide confidence intervals. For most interventions, the control group mortality rates (which estimate the baseline mortality rates) in the individual trials varied by at least an order of magnitude. These very large differences in absolute levels of risk in the individual trials reflect the participants selected for inclusion. In the trials of multiple risk factor interventions, applying the same relative risk reduction to the trials with the highest and lowest

390

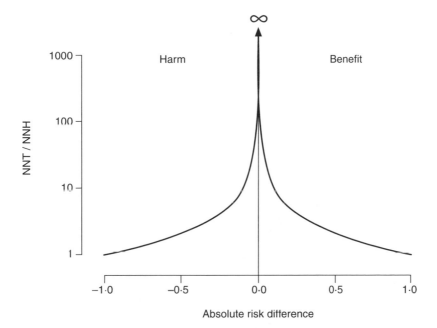

Figure 20.1 Relationship between absolute risk difference and number needed to treat to prevent an adverse event (NNT) or to cause an adverse event (number needed to harm, NNH). Adapted from Ebrahim and Davey Smith.[17]

coronary heart disease control group mortality rate resulted in five-year NNTs to benefit of 2 and 317 respectively.

The effects of geographical and secular trends

Geographic and secular trends in the baseline risk of cardiovascular diseases can be marked. For example, ischaemic heart disease and stroke mortality rates are about twice as high in the north as in the south of the Britain.[18] Consequently, the relevant cardiovascular disease baseline risk for a Scottish general practitioner will be twice that of an Oxford practitioner, resulting in an NNT for antihypertensive treatment that is twice as great in the south of England as in Scotland. Similarly, variation in cardiovascular disease between countries results in NNTs that differ in direct proportion to the underlying event rates.

Secular trends in stroke produce the same sort of effect. Stroke mortality rates are falling dramatically in most western countries[19] and with this fall, NNTs for antihypertensive treatment will rise over time. Table 20.3 shows the effects that may be expected on NNTs, assuming baseline event rates in

Table 20.2 Secondary prevention following myocardial infarction: effects on coronary heart disease mortality of different interventions.

Intervention	Pooled relative risk reduction (95% CI)	Range of mortality* in control groups (per 100 person-years)	Pooled absolute risk difference† per 100 person-years (95% CI)	Pooled NNT for 5 years derived from pooled absolute risk differences (95% CI)
Antiplatelet drugs[14]	0·15 (0·09 to 0·21)	2·8–13·9	0·4 (0·04 to 0·8)	50 (25 to 500)
Beta-blockers[15]	0·22 (0·13 to 0·29)	2·6–23·2	1·0 (0·6 to 1·5)	20 (13 to 33)
Statins, secondary prevention[9–11]	0·26 (0·17 to 0·34)	0·5–2·6	0·2 (0·1 to 0·3)	100 (67 to 200)
Multiple risk factor intervention[16]	0·19 (0·00 to 0·38)	0·3–10·0	0·3 (−0·1 to 0·7)	67 (29 to −)‡

NNT = number needed to treat to prevent one death.
* From cardiovascular disease or coronary heart disease.
† Risk difference is control group rate minus intervention group rate, hence positive differences indicate that intervention is better than control.
‡ Upper confidence limit of NNT to prevent one event not calculated as pooled absolute risk difference includes possibility of harm.

Table 20.3 Secular trends in stroke mortality and the effect on numbers needed to treat to avoid a stroke death (NNT) from 1971 to 1991.

Time period	Stroke mortality rate (ages 65–74) per 100 000		NNT for 5 years with antihypertensives to avoid one stroke death	
	Men	Women	Men	Women
1971	423	297	70	99
1981	300	213	98	138
1991	213	153	139	193

Calculations assume that stroke mortality rates in hypertensive people are twice those in the general population and that the relative risk reduction for stroke mortality on antihypertensive treatment is 33%.

hypertensives are twice those in the general population and that the relative risk reduction for stroke mortality on antihypertensive treatment is 33%. It is clear that NNTs vary widely over time, are higher in women than men – reflecting women's lower baseline risk – and are considerably lower than NNTs derived from participants in randomised controlled trials. Randomised controlled trial participants are selected and tend to be at lower than the typical general population risk of adverse outcomes. This point is discussed in more detail below.

If there are secular trends in case-fatality, perhaps due to changes in disease severity, such cautions in the uncritical use of NNTs may also apply to treatments used in secondary prevention.

The effect of clinical setting

Examining the effects of antihypertensive drug trials for elderly people[20] by clinical setting shows that the pooled relative risks for cardiovascular disease events are very similar for primary care and secondary care trials (Table 20.4). By contrast, the NNTs vary by two-fold depending on the setting. The total mortality relative risk reductions are 9% and 14% for primary and secondary care respectively and are more variable than for cardiovascular events. The greater relative risk reduction in secondary care probably reflects the higher event rates. Applying the NNTs derived from trials undertaken in one setting to patient care in another setting may be misleading. However the relative estimates of efficacy varied less across the different settings and could be generalised with more confidence.

Trial participants and patients in routine clinical practice

Randomised controlled trials aim to achieve internal validity through careful inclusion criteria of participants, random allocation to intervention

Table 20.4 Drug treatment of hypertension in the elderly. Rate ratios and numbers needed to treat (NNT) to prevent one event by setting of trial for different outcomes.

Setting	Total mortality			Cardiovascular morbidity and mortality		
	Number of participants	Rate ratio (95% CI)	NNT (95% CI)	Number of participants	Rate ratio (95% CI)	NNT (95% CI)
Primary care	6907	0·91 (0·80 to 1·03)	86 (35 to –)*	6907	0·75 (0·67 to 0·84)	23 (16 to 38)
Secondary care	4113	0·86 (0·79 to 0·94)	42 (27 to 109)	8738	0·71 (0·66 to 0·78)	13 (11 to 18)
All trials	21 020	0·88 (0·82 to 0·94)	51 (34 to 118)	15 645	0·73 (0·68 to 0·78)	17 (14 to 21)

Number of participants differ because specific outcome data not available for all trials.
* Upper confidence limit of NNT to prevent one event not calculated as rate ratio includes possibility of harm.

and blind ascertainment of end-points. In most randomised controlled trials, participants are at lower risk than might be expected because with given eligibility criteria healthier people are more likely to end up enrolled in trials. Thus trial event rates may not apply to clinical practice and NNTs will tend to be inflated. In the Medical Research Council (MRC) mild hypertension trial[21] event rates were much lower than in epidemiological studies and for fatal events were closer to those expected for normotensive men rather than hypertensive men. These differences reflect the selection bias mentioned above, and raise serious questions about the value of trial-derived NNTs (see Table 20.5). Selection bias may work in the opposite direction occasionally. In the Hypertension Detection and Follow Up Program – a comparison of careful stepped care versus usual care – the trial mortality rates were very high because the participants were predominately poor, and many were black.[22]

Pooling the trial event rates from several trials or calculating a pooled NNT does not help. Clinicians who want to use NNTs have to make a judgment about which baseline risk applies to their patients and without local epidemiological data this is difficult.

Pooling assumptions and NNTs

There are two main categories of statistical model for meta-analysis, fixed and random effect models. The fixed-effect models assume that all the studies are estimating the same "true" effect, and that the variation in effects seen between different trials is due only to the play of chance. The random-effects model assumes that the treatment effects from individual

Table 20.5 Variation in risk of events among men aged 35–64 in MRC mild hypertension trial and men aged 45–59 in British Regional Heart Study (BRHS).

Outcome	MRC placebo group	BRHS hypertensive	BRHS normotensive	NNT for 5 years derived from:	
				MRC trial	BRHS cohort
Stroke death	0·6	1·1	0·4	667	364
Coronary death	3·9	6·5	3·2	2608*	1200*
Fatal and non-fatal events	11·9	16·2	4·4	105	77

* Figures represent numbers needed to harm (NNH) as event rates were higher in treated group than placebo group for coronary deaths.
NNT = number needed to treat to prevent one event.
Rates per 1000 person-years are shown. Hypertension defined as diastolic blood pressure of 90–109 mmHg in MRC trial and systolic/diastolic of 160+ and/or 90+ in BRHS.

395

studies are a random sample from a "population" of different effect sizes that follows a normal distribution (see also Chapters 2 and 15).[23,24] There will almost always be differences in baseline risk of patients in trials carried out in different populations and at different times. Consequently, there is unlikely to be a single "true" absolute risk difference, as assumed in the fixed-effects models. Neither is the variation in risk difference between trials likely to represent a random sample from a symmetric distribution of effects. Decisions affecting the baseline risk of patients in a trial, such as inclusion and exclusion criteria or geographical setting, are not made in a random way.

Duration of treatment effect

Trials have different lengths of follow-up, but in order to produce, for example, a five-year NNT, all the absolute risk differences need to be standardised for five years if pooling of risk differences is undertaken. This standardisation requires an assumption of constancy of effect over time. This assumption may not be reasonable. For example in the Scandinavian Simvastatin Survival Study (4S), there was no effect on total mortality until one year of treatment, after which the absolute risk reduction gradually increased with duration of follow up.[9]

Care must be taken in calculating absolute risk differences in meta-analysis programmes. For example, most programs require the number of participants in each arm of a trial to be input as denominators. Since trials tend to have differing lengths of follow up, pooled absolute differences calculated using participants, rather than person-years as denominators, will assume equal length of follow up across trials, and result in false estimates of absolute risk differences. Duration of follow up is often not well reported and this may make it impossible to adjust for length of follow up in systematic reviews.[25]

Interpretation of NNTs

Calculating an overall NNT from a meta-analysis of pooled absolute risk differences achieves the feat of taking all the data from the trials, putting it together, and producing a less useful result than that provided by the individual trials. In the economic field, an incremental cost effectiveness analysis of an intervention at different levels of baseline risk will almost always be more informative than a summary of cost effectiveness based on a pooled NNT (see also Chapter 23).[26] The pooled NNT may also result in erroneous decisions about who should receive treatment if the concept of a threshold NNT, separating those who are likely to benefit from those who are not, is applied.

Deriving NNTs

It is preferable to derive NNTs by applying the relative risk reductions from trials or meta-analyses to estimates of prognosis from cohort studies (representative of the groups for whom treatment decisions are to be made), rather than from the trials and meta-analyses themselves.[24,27] If the relative risk reduction varies across different baseline risks, prognostic variables and regression techniques can be used to produce an estimate of treatment benefit to patients at different baseline risks.[28] This technique can be used for both individual trials[29] and for meta-analyses (see also Chapters 8 and 10).[30,31]

Alternative approaches have been used to derive absolute risk differences directly from the trials included in the meta-analyses[31,32] but these methods do not overcome the major differences between trial event rates – for example, a 10-fold difference between event rates in trials of beta-blockers after myocardial infarction.[32] Such trial derived NNTs cannot readily be applied to patients or policy decisions as the risk of trial participants is determined by design features of the trials, and is not representative of typical patients or populations.

Understanding of NNTs

The increasing use of NNTs is welcome in some respects for the reasons indicated at the outset, but caution is required. NNTs are no better understood than other measures.[33] The method of presenting results of studies influences health care decisions. Patients,[34] purchasers,[35] general practitioners,[36,37] and doctors in teaching hospitals[38] are all more likely to believe an intervention is desirable when effectiveness data is presented as a relative risk reduction than when data from the same studies is presented as an NNT. More effective methods of teaching about treatment effects are needed.

Conclusion

In spite of the reservations outlined in this chapter, NNTs have a place (see also Chapter 19). In the drug treatment of hypertension NNTs have been appropriately used to demonstrate the greater effectiveness in preventing cardiovascular events achieved when treating older rather than younger patients,[20] and treating moderate rather than mild hypertension.[1] When NNTs are presented, the intervention including the setting in which it occurred, the time period, the outcome and the baseline risk of the patients for whom the NNT is thought to be applicable, should be described.

Acknowledgements

I thank Professor Andy Haines, Dr Liam Smeeth and Professor George Davey Smith who contributed to earlier versions of this work.[39,17]

1 Cook RJ, Sackett DL. The number needed to treat: a clinically useful measure of treatment effect. *BMJ* 1995;**310**:452–4.
2 Laupacis A, Sackett DL, Roberts RS. An assessment of clinically useful measures of the consequences of treatment. *N Engl J Med* 1988;**318**:1728–33.
3 Rembold CM. Number-needed-to-treat analysis of the prevention of myocardial infarction and death by antidyslipidemic therapy. *J Fam Practice* 1996;**42**:577–86.
4 Review: statins prevent stroke, especially in patients with coronary heart disease. *Evidence-Based Med* 1998;**3**:10. Abstract of: Crouse JR III, Byington RP, Hoen HM, *et al.* Reductase inhibitor monotherapy and stroke prevention. *Arch Intern Med* 1997;**157**:1305–10.
5 *The Cochrane Database of Systematic Reviews.* Available in *The Cochrane Library* (database on disk and CDROM). *The Cochrane Collaboration* Issue 2. Oxford: Update Software, 1999.
6 Barnett HJ, Taylor DW, Eliasziw M, *et al.* for the North American Symptomatic Carotid Endarterectomy Trial Collaborators. Benefit of carotid endarterectomy in symptomatic patients with moderate or severe carotid stenosis. *N Engl J Med* 1998;**339**:1415–25.
7 Downs JR, Clearfield M, Weis S, *et al.* Primary prevention of acute coronary events with lovastatin in men and women with average cholesterol levels. Results of AFCAPS/TexCAPS. *JAMA* 1998;**279**:1615–22.
8 Shepherd J, Cobbe S, Ford E, *et al.* Prevention of coronary heart disease with pravastatin in men with hypercholesterolaemia. *N Engl J Med* 1995;**333**:1301–7.
9 4S Scandinavian Simvastatin Survival Group. Randomised trial of cholesterol lowering in 4444 patients with coronary heart disease: the Scandinavian Simvastatin Survival Study (4S). *Lancet* 1994;**344**:1383–9.
10 Sacks FM, Pfeffer MA, Moye LA, *et al.* The effect of pravastatin on coronary events after myocardial infarction in patients with average cholesterol levels. *N Engl J Med* 1996;**14**:1001–9.
11 The Long-Term Intervention with Pravastatin in Ischemic Heart Disease (LIPID) Study Group. Prevention of cardiovascular events and death with pravastatin in patients with coronary heart disease and a broad range of initial cholesterol levels. *N Engl J Med* 1998;**339**:1349–57.
12 Anonymous. Statins. *Bandolier* 1998;**47**:2–4.
13 Altman DG. Confidence intervals for the number needed to treat. *BMJ* 1998;**317**:1309–12.
14 Antiplatelet Trialists' Collaboration. Collaborative overview of randomized trials of antiplatelet therapy – I. Prevention of death, myocardial infarction, and stroke by prolonged antiplatelet therapy in various categories of patients. *BMJ* 1994;**308**:81–106.
15 Yusuf S, Peto R, Lewis J, Collins R, Sleight P. Beta blockade during and after myocardial infarction: an overview of the randomized trials. *Prog Cardiovasc Dis* 1985;**27**:335–71.
16 Ebrahim S, Davey Smith G. *Health promotion in older people for the prevention of coronary heart disease and stroke*. London: Health Education Authority, 1996.
17 Ebrahim S, Davey Smith G. The number needed to treat: does it help clinical decision making? *J Human Hypertens* 1999;**13**:721–4.
18 Shaper AG, Pocock SJ, Walker M, Cohen NM, Wale CJ, Thomson AG. British Regional Heart Study: cardiovascular risk factors in middle-aged men in 24 towns. *BMJ* 1981;**283**:179–86.
19 Charlton J, Murphy M, Khaw K-T, Ebrahim S, Davey Smith G. Cardiovascular diseases. In: Murphy M, Charlton J, eds. *Health of adult Britain 1841–1994*, vol 2. London: HMSO, 1997:60–81.
20 Mulrow C, Lau J, Cornell J, Brand B. Antihypertensive drug therapy in the elderly. *The Cochrane Library* Issue 2. Oxford: Update Software, 1998.

21 Medical Research Council Working Group. MRC Trial of mild hypertension: principal findings. *BMJ* 1985;**291**:97–104.
22 Hypertension Detection and Follow-up Program Cooperative Group. Five-year findings of the Hypertension Detection and Follow-up Program. II. Mortality by race-sex and age. *JAMA* 1979;**242**:2572–7.
23 Fleiss JL. The statistical basis of meta-analysis. *Stat Meth Med Res* 1993;**2**:121–45.
24 Egger M, Davey Smith G, Phillips AN. Meta-analysis: principles and procedures. *BMJ* 1997;**315**:1533–7.
25 D'Amico R, Deeks JJ, Altman DG. Poor reporting of length of follow up in clinical trials and systematic reviews. eBMJ 25 June 1999 http://www.bmj.com/cgi/eletters/318/7197/1548.
26 Morris S, McGuire A, Caro J, Pettitt D. Strategies for the management of hypercholesterolaemia: a systematic review of the cost-effectiveness literature. *J Health Serv Res Policy* 1997;**2**:231–50.
27 Jackson RT, Sackett DL. Guidelines for managing raised blood pressure. *BMJ* 1996;**313**:64–5.
28 Davey Smith G, Egger M, Phillips AN. Meta-analysis: beyond the grand mean? *BMJ* 1997;**315**:1610–14.
29 Rothwell PM. Can overall results of clinical trials be applied to all patients? *Lancet* 1995;**345**:1616–19.
30 Sharp SJ, Thompson SG, Altman DG. The relation between treatment benefit and underlying risk in meta-analysis. *BMJ* 1996;**313**:735–8.
31 Ioannidis JP, Cappelleri JC, Lau J, *et al*. Early or deferred zidovudine therapy in HIV-infected patients without AIDS defining illness. *Ann Intern Med* 1995;**122**:856–66.
32 Freemantle N, Cleland J, Young P, Mason J, Harrison J. Beta-blockade after myocardial infarction: systematic review and meta regression analysis. *BMJ* 1999;**318**:1730–7.
33 McColl A, Smith H, White P, Field J. General practitioners' perceptions of the route to evidence based medicine: a questionnaire survey. *BMJ* 1998;**316**:361–5.
34 Hux JE, Naylor CD. Communicating the benefits of chronic preventative therapy: does the format of efficacy data determine patients' acceptance of treatment? *Med Decis Making* 1995;**15**:152–7.
35 Fahey T, Griffiths S, Peters TJ. Evidence based purchasing: understanding results of clinical trials and systematic reviews. *BMJ* 1995;**311**:1056–60.
36 Bucher HC, Weinbacher M, Gyr K. Influence of method of reporting study results on decision of physicians to prescribe drugs to lower cholesterol concentration. *BMJ* 1994;**309**:761–4.
37 Cranney M, Walley T. Same information, different decisions: the influence of evidence on the management of hypertension in the elderly. *Br J Gen Pract* 1996;**46**:661–3.
38 Naylor CD, Chen E, Strauss B. Measured enthusiasm: does the method of reporting trial results alter perceptions of therapeutic effectiveness? *Ann Intern Med* 1992;**117**:916–21.
39 Smeeth L, Haines A, Ebrahim S. Numbers needed to treat derived from meta-analyses – sometimes informative, usually misleading. *BMJ* 1999;**318**:1548–51.

21 Using systematic reviews in clinical guideline development

MARTIN ECCLES, NICK FREEMANTLE,
JAMES MASON

Summary points

- Systematic review is the optimum method of summarising evidence of effectiveness within a clinical practice guideline.
- Within the process of developing a guideline, conducting specific systematic reviews or updating existing ones allows reviews to be focused on the subject area of the guideline and to be tailored to the clinical questions that the group poses.
- There will be occasions when previously available systematic reviews will represent the best available evidence, however, there may be problems in the interpretation and applicability of available systematic reviews.

A systematic review summarising the best available evidence lies at the heart of an evidence-based guideline. However such a review alone is insufficient for guideline development and there are a number of important considerations in using systematic reviews (both 'off the shelf' or conducted *de novo*) within a guideline development process.[1]

There is increasing interest in the development of clinical practice guidelines in the UK[2] and a fast developing clinical effectiveness agenda[3,4] within which guidelines figure prominently. This has been influenced by the increasing body of evidence that guidelines can lead to improvements in both the process and outcome of care.[5,6] Clinical practice guidelines are "systematically developed statements to inform both clinician and patient decisions in specific clinical circumstances".[7] The aim of the guideline development process is to maximise the likelihood that when used, the guidelines will lead to the benefits and costs predicted by them (and thus improve the overall quality of patient care). This is known as guideline validity.[7] Three elements within the guideline development process have been suggested as important in maximising guideline validity: a multidisciplinary guideline development group; systematic review as the method of evidence identification; and evidence linking of the guideline recommendations.[8]

In this chapter we will discuss the issues raised when using systematic reviews within guideline development based on our experiences in the North of England Guideline Development Programme. Systematic reviews and meta-analyses are normally used to summarise the results of randomised controlled trials and we will discuss systematic reviews in this context. However, it is recognised that randomised controlled trials are not the only study design of relevance to guideline development. When a guideline is considering the performance of a diagnostic test then comparison against a gold standard will be appropriate. When describing the natural history of a condition inception cohort studies will be most relevant. As discussed in more detail in Chapter 1, a clear distinction should be made between systematic review and meta-analysis. Whilst the latter may be used as the method for summarising effects within a systematic review, this is not necessarily appropriate. A number of issues specific to meta-analysis will be discussed.

Methods of developing guidelines

The methods of guideline development have been described in North America[7,9] and in the UK[10 16] and are summarised in Box 21.1. Having defined the need for a guideline and its content area, the first step in the process is to convene an appropriately multi-disciplinary guideline development group.[8,16] This group explores, within the clinical area of the guideline, all of the situations for which the guideline might need to offer recommendations. The best available evidence is then identified through systematic review. Papers are summarised quantitatively,[17–20] qualitatively[12,21] or (depending upon the area of the guideline) using a mixture of both.[22] Wherever possible the evidence should encompass not only

---

Box 21.1 Five steps in clinical practice guideline development

1 Identifying and refining the subject area of a guideline
2 Convening and running guideline development groups
3 Assessing the evidence about the clinical question or condition
4 Translating the evidence into a clinical practice guideline
5 External review of the guideline

Box 21.2 Categories of evidence, strength of recommendations and factors contributing to the process of deriving recommendations

Categories of evidence (adapted from AHCPR 1992 [23])
- Ia: evidence from meta-analysis of randomised controlled trials
- Ib: evidence from at least one randomised controlled trial
- IIa: evidence from at least one controlled study without randomisation
- IIb: evidence from at least one other type of quasi-experimental study
- III: evidence from non-experimental descriptive studies, such as comparative studies, correlation studies and case-control studies
- IV: evidence from expert committee reports or opinions and/or clinical experience of respected authorities

Strength of recommendation
- A directly based on category I evidence
- B directly based on category II evidence or extrapolated recommendation from category I evidence
- C directly based on category III evidence or extrapolated recommendation from category I or II evidence
- D directly based on category IV evidence or extrapolated recommendation from category I, II or III evidence

Factors contributing to the process of deriving recommendations
- The nature of the evidence (e.g. its susceptibility to bias)
- The applicability of the evidence to the population of interest (its generalisabilty)
- Resource implications and their cost
- Knowledge of the health care system
- Beliefs and values of the panel

questions of effectiveness but also potential harm, side effects, tolerability and cost. The evidence is categorised according to its susceptibility to bias (Box 21.2) and, finally, guideline recommendations are made in the light of the evidence (or its absence) and implementation issues specific to the clinical setting. Recommendations are explicitly graded to reflect these underlying issues (Box 21.2). The finished guideline is peer reviewed and a future review date is set.

Scale of the review process

The scale of the review process within guideline development is related to the scope of the guideline. Where the focus of the guideline is a relatively narrow clinical area, such as the use of analgesics or NSAIDs in osteo-arthritis,[19] the review is focused and generates relatively small numbers of papers. However, this is not always so. If the subject of the guideline is a broad clinical area, such as the primary care management of asthma in adults, the scale of the review is much larger. Within the North of England Asthma Guideline development process,[21] over 9000 papers were identified as potentially relevant and over 600 had to be retrieved for reading to assess their clinical relevance. Given the scale of this task, if it is possible to use existing systematic reviews to provide off-the-shelf summaries in some of the clinical areas then this may make the task more manageable. However, it is essential to ascertain the quality of methods used in "imported" reviews and confirm the veracity of findings.

Using existing systematic reviews

Systematic reviews used in guideline development can be considered, as with the primary studies, in terms of their internal and external validity. For primary studies the issues of internal and external validity are considered in Chapter 5. Here we suggest that, for a review, internal validity relates to whether or not the review is offering a precise summary measurement of whatever it purports to measure. External validity then relates to the degree to which the findings of the review can be applied, in this case to the health care setting considered within the guideline. In addition, when using existing systematic reviews, there are potential problems with the summary metric used and the possible need to update a review.

Internal validity of reviews

Internal validity relates to the identification of the original studies included in the review and the method of conducting the review. Reviews of selected studies (due to publication bias or failure to find relevant studies, see Chapters 3 and 4) can bias the findings of reviews[24,25] and such reviews cannot be used without further work. Reviews which use inappropriate or flawed methods cannot be taken at face value and are best not used.

Dimensions of evidence

When judging the internal validity of a review a guideline group will also have to decide whether or not it addresses all of the dimensions on which they need evidence in order to derive recommendations. Many systematic reviews are concerned with obtaining summary measures of effectiveness and do not extend to cover other issues of concern to patients such as side-effects, tolerability, or consequences for work-place activities. While this may be a constraint of the studies contributing to the review this is not necessarily the case. Failing to consider significant side effects may offer an inappropriately positive view of an intervention and limit the validity of a review. Similarly, resource implications and costs, not normally the subject of systematic reviews, are likely to be an important consideration in the implementation of a guideline. An intervention with demonstrable cost effectiveness may result in a stronger recommendation within the guideline.

External validity of reviews

The external validity of a review is more likely to be problematic although it is important to recognise that this may again be as much to do with the original studies as with the review.

Characteristics of study participants and study setting

A key aspect of a review is the rationale for including or excluding studies. As with primary studies, the applicability of a review will be limited by the characteristics of the study participants included in it and the settings in which the studies were conducted. Ideally a guideline group wants evidence from studies within which the study participants are typical of those to whom the guideline will be applied. Therefore the minimum requirement is that a review lists the important characteristics of the participants within each study. However, this will not provide information on other aspects such as recruitment rates in studies. The setting in which a study is conducted will also influence its external validity, particularly if it relates to elements of service delivery. Studies of patients with exacerbations of asthma draw patients from emergency room settings; however, the nature of patients and the severity of their asthma may differ between countries where there is a comprehensive primary health care service (such as the UK) and countries where there is not (such as the USA).

Inclusion and exclusion criteria within a review

The exclusion criteria for studies used in a review may be acceptable (for example a trial is not randomised when other available and adequate trials are) or debatable (for example using a different dose of drug from the one used in practice), and should be carefully considered. Often there may not be a clear-cut answer. A guideline group wanting to know about the effectiveness of education delivered in a primary care setting to patients with asthma may question a review including studies from secondary care settings. In such instances the studies have to be reviewed to identify their applicability to primary care health service delivery.

The focus of a review and available endpoints

There are two further ways in which the applicability of a previously published review may be undermined. Firstly, it is unlikely that a review can address the implementation questions posed within a guideline development process. Relevant clinical questions are defined by the guideline development group with the aim of deriving recommendations which can appropriately inform doctor-patient interactions: there may be a substantial contextual component to decision-making. Although well conducted systematic reviews may be available they are unlikely to address all the issues of interest to a guideline group. Indeed it would be surprising if a review conducted outside a guideline development process could second guess all the relevant questions.

Secondly, in a review that uses meta-analysis as a method of summary, the process will require common estimates of effect that can be summarised across studies. Particularly in complex clinical areas where multiple and differing outcome measures have been used within studies, the choice of studies to include in a review may be influenced by factors such as whether or not there are available common endpoints rather than their clinical usefulness.

Summary metric used in reviews

The most commonly used and statistically most robust metric used to summarise effectiveness within systematic reviews is the odds ratio. However, the odds ratio alone is insufficient to summarise the evidence from trials. Used alone it is not readily interpretable and it needs to be considered alongside a summary statistic of absolute risk reduction.[26] Therefore a systematic review that presents the odds ratio alone is difficult, if not impossible, to use. The only option would be to assume that the odds ratio could be applied to the level of baseline risk in the population within which the guideline would subsequently be used.[27] For conditions where this information might be available this strategy involves having to make a number of assumptions. However, for many conditions for which one might want to develop guidelines (depression, non-steroidal anti-inflammatory drug use) levels of baseline risk are not available.

Updating existing reviews

If within a guideline development process a relevant systematic review is identified there may be an issue of its timeliness. A review that was completed two years ago may well have had subsequent relevant papers published but not incorporated into the review. Under such circumstances the ideal is for the review authors to be contacted to update the review. If this is not possible then a guideline process has to either replicate the whole review for itself or consider the new papers alongside but outside the review. Under such circumstances conflicting results may be difficult, if not impossible, to reconcile.

Conducting reviews within the process of guideline development

For any or all of the reasons discussed above, an existing systematic review may be inappropriate for use within a guideline development process. The solution to the issues raised here is to conduct new reviews (or update existing ones) within the process of guideline development. If the reviewers are members of the guideline development group then issues such as the included and excluded studies and the choice of summary metric are more easily addressed. Review decisions are made interactively with the other members of the guideline group. A further advantage of such a process is that the guideline development group can ask questions of the analyst that can be answered either directly or in subsequent meetings. An example of this occurred within the North of England Aspirin Guideline Group,[18] where an existing meta-analysis[28] was replicated and then updated. Having considered the overall effectiveness of aspirin as an anti-thrombotic in various clinical settings, the group asked whether the dose of aspirin used made any difference. Studies were analysed by dose of aspirin used and the results presented to the group at their next meeting. In fact, the benefits appeared if anything to increase with lower dose, a desirable situation as side effects of treatment also decrease with dose (Figure 21.1). Such a degree of interaction allows for questions to be answered much more precisely than would otherwise be possible.

The summary metric used in reviews

From our experiences of working with guideline development groups it is clear that the odds ratio alone is not readily interpretable and that it needs to be considered alongside a summary statistic of absolute risk reduction.[26] However, within a review, included studies will usually have been conducted over differing periods of time and to produce an overall risk reduction within a time period there needs to be a further transformation. This necessitates the use of methods such as incidence rate differences.[29] It is only by using such techniques that the number needed to treat (NNT, see also Chapters 19 and 20) can be calculated meaningfully as a summary

Dose(mg) No. of trials

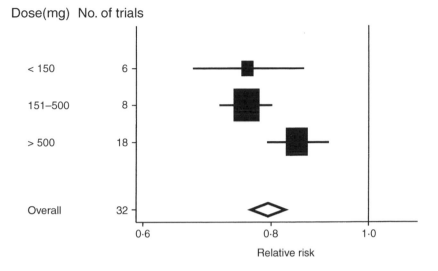

Figure 21.1 – Relative risk of non-fatal myocardial infarction, stroke, or vascular death. Meta-analysis stratified by dose of aspirin used in trials.

measure of a series of trials with different follow-up. Interestingly, this more clinically interpretable result is the least statistically robust. When using such methods it is particularly important to observe the general rules of meta-analysis and only combine studies that it is clinically meaningful to combine.

An example of this method and the advantage that it can bring is provided by the guideline on the primary care use of aspirin as an antiplatelet drug.[18] Meta-analyses of trials of aspirin after acute myocardial infarction or in stable angina show similar odds ratios and similar risk differences for a composite outcome (non-fatal myocardial infarction, stroke or death). However, the incidence risk differences are very different, with 3·3% reduction in outcomes attributable to treatment over 1 month in the acute myocardial infarction trials, and an 0·7% reduction in outcomes attributable to treatment in the stable angina trials over one year (see Table 21.1).

Often use of a range of meta-analytic techniques has proven necessary in the guidelines development process, with routine use of the most interpretable metrics alongside the most robust (e.g. incidence risk differences alongside odds ratios), a mix of continuous and binary outcomes, individual patient data analyses (see Chapter 6) and, on occasions, meta regression analyses (see Chapters 8–11). For the researcher undertaking systematic reviews, work in this context can be rewarding and fascinating.

407

Table 21.1 Aspirin in secondary prevention after myocardial infarction and in stable angina. A comparison of summary metrics.

Trials	Metric	Effect	95% CI
Acute myocardial infarction	OR	0·71	0·65 to 0·77
Stable angina	OR	0·67	0·53 to 0·85
Acute myocardial infarction	RD	−0·038	−0·047 to −0·028
Stable angina	RD	−0·045	−0·071 to −0·018
Acute myocardial infarction	IRD (month)	−0·033	−0·043 to −0·024
Stable angina	IRD (year)	−0·007	−0·017 to 0·004

OR = odds ratio; RD = risk difference; IRD = incidence risk difference.

Concluding remarks

Within the process of guideline development, conducting specific systematic reviews or updating existing ones will usually represent the optimum means of summarising evidence on the effects of interventions. Such reviews will be focused on the subject area of the guideline and the needs of the guideline group, and can be tailored to the clinical questions that they pose. There will be occasions when available systematic reviews will represent the best available evidence, and their use will be necessary when resources are inadequate to conduct a new review. Under these circumstances they may be incorporated into the guideline, but the strength of subsequent recommendations may need to be lowered to reflect any shortcomings of the review.

1 Cook DJ, Greengold NL, Ellrodt G, Weingarten SR. The relation between systematic reviews and practice guidelines. *Ann Intern Med* 1997;**127**:210–16.
2 NHS Executive. *Clinical guidelines: using clinical guidelines to improve patient care within the NHS*. London: HMSO, 1996.
3 Department of Health. *Our healthier nation*. London: HMSO, 1998.
4 Department of Health. *The new NHS: modern, dependable*. London: Department of Health; 1997.
5 Centre for Reviews and Dissemination, Nuffied Institute for Health. Implementing clinical practice guidelines: can guidelines be used to improve clinical practice. *Effect Health Care* 1994;(8):1–12.
6 Centre for Reviews and Dissemination. Getting evidence into practice. *Effect Health Care* 1999;**5**:1–16.
7 Field MJ, Lohr KN, eds. *Guidelines for clinical practice: from development to use*. Washington, DC: National Academy Press, 1992.
8 Grimshaw J, Eccles M, Russell I. Developing clinically valid practice guidelines. *J Eval Clin Pract* 1995;**1**:37–48.
9 Hadorn DC, Baker D. Development of the AHCPR – sponsored heart failure guideline: methodologic and procedural issues. *J Qual Imp* 1994;**20**:539–47.
10 Royal College of General Practitioners. The development and implementation of clinical guidelines: report of the Clinical Guidelines Working Group. Report from Practice 26. London: Royal College of General Practitioners, 1996.

11 Eccles MP, Clapp Z, Grimshaw J, et al. Developing valid guidelines: methodological and procedural issues from the North of England evidence based guideline development project. Quality Health Care 1996;5:44–50.

12 North of England Stable Angina Guideline Development Group. North of England evidence based guidelines development project: summary version of evidence based guideline for the primary care management of stable angina. BMJ 1996;312:827–32.

13 Eccles M, Freemantle N, Mason J. North of England evidence based guideline development project:Methods of developing guidelines for efficient drug use in primary care. BMJ 1998;316:1232–5.

14 Mason J, Eccles M, Freemantle N, Drummond M. A framework for incorporating cost-effectiveness in evidence based clinical practice guidelines. Health Policy 1999;47:37–52.

15 Royal College of Psychiatrists. Clinical practice guidelines and their development. London: Royal College of Psychiatrists. 1994; Council Report CR34.

16 Shekelle PG, Woolf SH, Eccles M, Grimshaw J. Developing guidelines. BMJ 1999;318:593–6.

17 Eccles M, Freemantle N, Mason J, North of England ACE-Inhibitor Guideline Development Group. North of England evidence based development project: guideline for angiotensin converting enzyme inhibitors in the primary care management of adults with symptomatic heart failure. BMJ 1998;316:1369–75.

18 Eccles M, Freemantle N, Mason J, North of England Aspirin Guideline Development Group. North of England evidence based guideline development project: Evidence based guideline for the use of aspirin for the secondary prophylaxis of vascular disease in primary care. BMJ 1998;316:1303–9.

19 Eccles M, Freemantle N, Mason J. North of England evidence based guideline development project: summary guideline for non-steroidal anti-inflammatory drugs versus basic analgesia in treating the pain of degenerative arthritis. BMJ 1998;317:526–30.

20 Eccles M, Freemantle N, Mason JM. The choice of antidepressants for depression in primary care. Fam Pract 1999;16(2):103–11.

21 North of England Asthma Guideline Development Group. North of England evidence based guidelines development project: summary version of evidence based guideline for the primary care management of asthma in adults. BMJ 1996;312:762–6.

22 Eccles M, North of England Evidence Based Guideline Development Project. North of England evidence based guidelines development project: summary version of evidence based guideline for the primary care management of dementia. BMJ 1998;317:802–8.

23 US Department of Health and Human Services; Public Health Service; Agency for Health Care and Policy Research. Acute pain management: operative or medical procedures and trauma. Rockville, MD: Agency for Health Care and Policy Research Publications, 1992.

24 Begg CB, Berlin JA. Publication bias: a problem in interpreting medical data. J Roy Stat Soc 1988;151:419–63.

25 Easterbrook PJ, Berlin JA, Gopalan R, Matthews DR. Publication bias in clinical research. Lancet 1991;337:867–72.

26 Freemantle N, Mason JM, Eccles M. Deriving treatment recommendations from evidence within randomised trials: the role and limitation of meta analysis. Int J Tech Assess Health Care 1999;5:304–15.

27 Smeeth L, Haines A, Ebrahim S. Numbers needed to treat derived from meta-analyses – sometimes informative, usually misleading. BMJ 1999;318:1548–51.

28 Antiplatelet Trialists' Collaboration. Collaborative overview of randomised trials of antiplatelet therapy – I: prevention of death, myocardial infarction, and stroke by prolonged antiplatelet therapy in various categories of patients. BMJ 1994;308:81–106.

29 Ioannidis JPA, Cappelleri JC, Lau J, et al. Early or deferred therapy in HIV infected patients without an AIDS defining illness: a meta analysis. Ann Intern Med 1995;122:856–66.

22 Using systematic reviews for evidence based policy making

J A MUIR GRAY

Summary points

- Policy making, like all other health and healthcare decisions, should be based on best current knowledge.
- Interpretation of evidence by policy makers also takes into account resources and values.
- There is a distinction between decision making and decision taking: scientists can play a part in the former but because the latter always involves values, the final decision has to be taken by representatives of the public affected.
- Scientists and politicians are involved in fundamentally different activities, albeit with the same aim.

There is nothing a politician likes so little as to be well informed; it makes decision making so complex and difficult.

J M Keynes

An aerosol able to dispense confidence that could be inhaled by bankers and investors was how one cynic summarised the economic theories that led to at least one Nobel Prize in economics. There was certainly little evidence to support Keynesian economics and the decision to invest large sums of public money to stimulate the economy was based largely on theory but had an immense effect. Perhaps it was this experience that led to Keynes' dismissive remark, but he would probably have been dismayed when he saw how politicians have reacted to economic problems in the 1990s. They have the evidence of the apparent effectiveness of Keynesian economics but, world wide, they have decided to cut public expenditure and slim the size of the state.

410

Systematic reviews, a high quality source of evidence, should be useful to policy makers. One weakness is, of course, the relative paucity of such reviews but it is perhaps the attitude of the policy makers that is equally important in determining the degree to which the evidence that exists will be used.

There are many different levels in healthcare decision making; excluding the very small proportion of the population for whom cost of care is not a concern, epitomised perhaps by Michael Corleone in *Godfather III* receiving high tech care in penthouse splendour for his ischaemic heart disease. The great majority of most populations receive care from systems which have a finite amount of resources, and the clinical decision comes at the end of a long chain of decisions with the following being recognisable in most countries:

1 How much of our gross national product should we invest in public services?
2 How much of the money allocated for public services should be allocated to health care as opposed to other services which can improve health?
3 How should the money for health care be allocated to different geographical populations?
4 Once allocated to a population, how should the money for health care be distributed between different groups in need, for example, between those who have mental illness and those who have cancer?
5 Once money has been allocated to people with cancer, how can best value be obtained, namely:
   (a) which interventions or services should be funded and which should not?
   (b) how can the population most likely to benefit from intervention or service receive it, and those least likely to benefit be excluded?
   (c) how can we be sure that the service will be delivered to a high quality to those for whom it is actually intended?

There are, of course, variants on this list of questions in different countries. In some countries money is top-sliced nationally for health problems such as cancer or health services such as screening before it is allocated to geographical populations; but these same questions can be identified in most countries and are the stuff of healthcare policy making.

At the end of the chain sit the clinician and the patient, the former little better informed about the range of decisions that have determined the amount of resources they have available to offer the patient, but clearly aware that resources, particularly their own time, are finite and that they must make decisions within this framework. It is for this reason that we

411

distinguish so clearly between evidence based medicine (or evidence based clinical practice to give it its broader term), and evidence based healthcare.

Evidence based medicine and evidence based healthcare

The most widely cited definition of evidence based medicine is reproduced below.

> *Evidence based medicine is the conscientious, explicit and judicious use of current best evidence in making decisions about the care of individual patients. The practice of evidence based medicine means integrating individual clinical expertise with the best available external clinical evidence from systematic research. By individual clinical expertise we mean the proficiency and judgement that individual clinicians acquire through clinical experience and clinical practice.*[1]

Some people argued that it is wrong to absolve the clinician from worrying about the resource consequences of each decision.[2] In our view it is more appropriate to think of evidence based healthcare, namely decision making for groups or populations based on best current evidence, as an activity qualitatively different from evidence based medicine, even though the same evidence is used in both. This distinction leaves the clinician and the patient free to tackle the job that is difficult enough: incorporating current best evidence with the patient's values and baseline condition.

For example, it should be the job of a policy maker or commissioner of health services to decide whether or not tissue plasminogen activator (TPA) should be made available for people with chest pain in a population, basing that decision on the balance of benefit, harm and opportunity cost for the population as a whole. This leaves the clinician to worry about how best to organise the delivery of quick clot-busting to people with chest pain in order to maximise the potential benefit of streptokinase if TPA were not affordable.[3] The clinician is, of course, free to lobby, individually or collectively, for extra resources to be made available for TPA to supplement streptokinase. On a day-to-day, month-by-month, basis clinicians should be freed from the worry of deciding whether or not the particular patient they are seeing justifies the use of resources for TPA, a decision that almost certainly would become more difficult as the financial year progresses.

Evidence based decision making for populations

In making decisions for populations or groups of patients the best available knowledge has to be used and, as with clinical decision making, the systematic review provides the best possible knowledge, although it may

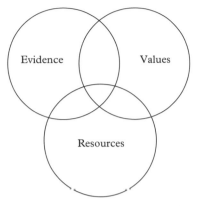

Figure 22.1 Venn diagram of factors which have to be taken into account in evidence based decision making at the population level.

not always be available. However, as in clinical decision making, other factors have to be taken into account, notably values and resources. These are best expressed as a Venn diagram for they overlap and their relative importance in different decisions is usefully represented graphically (Figure 22.1).

Evidence as the dominant driver

In some decisions where resources are not a major issue and the values are relatively straightforward, policy decisions can be based on evidence alone. In the decision not to introduce prostatic cancer screening, the UK government was able to make its recommendations on the basis of two systematic reviews of the evidence, neither of which was able to demonstrate any reduction in mortality from prostatic cancer screening.[4,5] Thus, as screening always does some harm, policy makers were able to conclude that screening would do more harm than good and should not therefore be introduced. On the basis of these systematic reviews, the Secretary of State made a very clear decision and expressed this unequivocally in a circular sent to the National Health Service.

It could be argued that this represented the values of UK decision making which many people, particularly in the USA, see as over-cautious and timid. It is interesting to note, however, that the American Cancer Society, formerly renowned for its aggressive approach to cancer screening, is now itself more cautious and actually suggests a "third way" based on its review of the evidence. In response to an article,[6] the American Cancer Society (ACS) stated that:

413

the casual reader of the article by Stern et al might erroneously construe that ACS supports "mass" screening. Studies have shown that when men are provided with more formal information regarding early detection testing for prostatic cancer, many decline it. The ACS is concerned that men may be undergoing screening without proper pre-test guidance and education and agreed that routine serum prostate specific antigen (PSA) measurement is not appropriate without such education. As was the case with testing for the human immunodeficiency virus, serum PSA measurement should not be bundled in among other routine blood studies that do not require any preamble discussion. The ACS is also concerned that clinicians who do not let men know that early detection testing for prostate cancer is available vitiate a man's right to choose to undergo a relatively simple test that could conceivably save his life.[7]

Resource-driven decisions

Systematic reviews of the cost and effectiveness of screening, for example the Cochrane review on the costs and benefits of colorectal cancer screening,[8] are extremely useful to the policy-maker in reaching a decision. Cost effectiveness studies (see Chapter 23) by themselves do not make policy decisions but they are helpful in decision making. Most policy makers use systematic reviews of cost effectiveness to classify interventions into one of three groups:

1 very inexpensive, a "no brainer" decision which is easy to make and introduce immediately, e.g. physician advice to stop smoking;
2 very expensive in terms of the return obtained and therefore not to be introduced, e.g. TPA in the management of all people with chest pain;
3 the rest (usually the majority of new interventions): the costs per quality-adjusted life year (QALY) are in the same range as standard services such as coronary artery bypass grafting or hip replacement, and more judgement is required based on the values of the decision makers.

In the UK this position will become clarified considerably in the next few years as the work of the National Institute of Clinical Excellence (NICE) evolves. In some countries, notably Canada and Australia, this type of decision making is already more common and more explicit. In decision making within managed care and health maintenance organisations (HMOs) in the USA, particularly those that are for-profit, the decisions are less clear. They are nevertheless the subject of intense scrutiny, speculation, and sometimes spectacle, as in the best-selling novel by John Grisham and the Francis Ford Coppola film *The Rainmaker*, the tale of an idealistic law graduate's quest for justice against a giant insurance company which

414

refuses to pay for a boy's life saving treatment. Resources and values, of course, are interwoven like warp and woof and are difficult to tease apart.

Value-driven decisions

The word "value" is vague and imprecise. Values may usefully be discussed with respect to an abstract system such as utilitarianism but healthcare organisations spend relatively little time, perhaps too little, on this type of abstract thinking. It is often hard to find any record of explicit discussion of theoretical issues in the records of public bodies, but the values are often clear from the decisions that they have made.

The decisions that healthcare organisations responsible for allocation of resources make are generally focused on the needs of their population. For example, the decision to invest in extending a breast screening programme to women aged over 65 will be based in part on the evidence about the effectiveness of breast screening in this age group, and on evidence about the likely rate of uptake, which will influence cost-effectiveness. The decision to stop breast cancer screening at the age of 65 is based on cost effectiveness having a higher value than the value to make services freely available to people irrespective of age, and could be, and has been, interpreted as an ageist decision. Similarly the decision to extend breast cancer screening to women aged over 65 could be a decision driven by values as well as by evidence.

Thus, in health care, the term can also mean more precisely the relative argument of one service in which an investment is made, compared to another in which it is not. It would thus be possible to replace the Venn diagram shown as Figure 22.1 with another diagram in which values and priorities were separated, as shown in Figure 22.2.

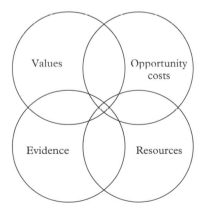

Figure 22.2 Venn diagram separating values and priorities.

415

Where there is no economic reason that makes it obvious either to include or exclude a new screening programme, values come into play and nowhere were values more explicit in recent years than in the debate on mammographic screening for women under the age of 50.

What happened is relatively simple to describe, but was an intense experience for all who were involved. The National Cancer Institute convened its customary panel of experts, who reviewed the evidence. A decision was made that screening for breast cancer in women under the age of 50 should not be recommended. Public and political reaction was sudden, sharp and hostile; at one time the very budget of the National Cancer Institute was threatened by some politicians. Another panel was convened and, as it met only a month after the first, it considered much the same evidence but came (17 to 1) to opposite conclusions, the only dissenting vote being from a woman aged under 50 who had breast cancer. What are the lessons of this episode, called, quite appropriately by a distinguished American analyst, the "Alice in Wonderland world of policy making"?[9]

Who should make value-drive decisions?

Some people felt very indignant about the impact that the media and politicians had had on the decision, but another point of view is that it is right and proper for politicians and the public to make decisions in which values are important. The job of the scientist is to be clear about the evidence and, having reviewed the evidence, it is clear that few people benefit and many people will be harmed and debates about the false positive rate continue to rage. That, perhaps, is the limit beyond which scientists should not go and they have to respect that those who represent the values of society have to clarify those values and make the appropriate decision based on those values.

The main reason why the screening decision about mammography in women under the age of 50 was different in the USA than in Canada (where it was not recommended) may be that Canadian decision making, as is the case with most other countries, starts from a collectivist perspective in which resources are finite. Thus the opportunity costs of every decision have to be borne by people with some other health problem, compared with the individualistic ethos and value system of the USA where it is regarded improper to withhold information from the individual, allowing that individual to seek screening if they can afford it.[9] Neither approach is right or wrong; both reveal that evidence based decision making and policy making is, as the term correctly implies, evidence based.

When thinking about the relationship between the scientist and the politician, it is useful to use a distinction common in management circles about the difference between decision making and decision taking.

416

Decision making is a process in which a number of different elements are brought together. Decision making is the final and definite decision about which of the options identified and appraised during the course of the decision making should be chosen. Some decisions are taken by professionals but where decisions involve the investment of a large amount of resources, the decision to invest these resources in one programme rather than another has to be taken by somebody who can be held to account. Scientists can be held to account only for the quality of the information they have provided, but, as the recent evidence about the framing of management decisions has made clear,[10] scientists can be implicit decision takers by the way they frame the epidemiological evidence, thus increasing their responsibility and accountability.

Box 22.1 Are family preservation services effective? A letter

Dear Dr Tyson,
You will recall that last Thursday when you so kindly joined us at a meeting of the Democratic Policy Committee you and I discussed the President's family preservation proposal. You indicated how much he supports the measure. I assured you I, too, support it, but went on to ask what evidence was there that it would have any effect. You assured me there was such data. Just for fun, I asked for two citations.

The next day we received a fax from Sharon Glied of your staff with a number of citations and a paper, "Evaluating the Results", that appears to have been written by Frank Farrow of the Center for the Study of Social Policy here in Washington and Harold Richman at the Chapin Hall Center at the University of Chicago. The paper is quite direct: "... solid proof that family preservation services can effect a state's overall placement rates is still lacking".

Just yesterday, the same Chapin Hall Center released an "Evaluation of the Illinois Family First Placement Prevention Program: Final Report". This was a large-scale study of the Illinois Family First initiative authorized by the Illinois Family Preservation Act of 1987. It was "designed to test effects of this program on out-of-home placements of children and other outcomes, such as subsequent child maltreatment". Data on case and service characteristics were provided by Family First caseworkers on approximately 4500 cases; approximately 1600 families participated in the randomized experiment. The findings are clear enough. "Overall, the Family First placement prevention program results in a slight increase in placement rates (when data from all experimental sites are combined). This effect disappears once case and site variations are taken into account". In other words, there are either negative effects or no effects.

Keynes was wrong. There is now evidence that allows us to refute Keynes' dismissive proposition quoted at the start of this chapter. Around the world politicians are asking for evidence to help them make decisions. It is true that they may not always like the evidence when they get it, but they are keen for evidence as the letter addressing the effectiveness of family preservation services in the USA eloquently states (see Box 22.1). Perhaps the most exciting development in the world of systematic reviews in 1999 has been the launch of the Campbell Collaboration, a world-wide initiative analogous to the Cochrane Collaboration (see Chapters 25 and 26) to prepare and disseminate systematic reviews of interventions in fields of government policy other than health care.

1 Sackett DL, Rosenberg, WMC, Gray JAM, Haynes RB, Richardson WS. Evidence-based medicine: what it is and what it isn't. *BMJ* 1996;**312**:71–2.
2 Maynard A. Evidence-based medicine: an incomplete method for informing treatment choices. *Lancet* 1997;**349**:126–8.
3 O'Donnell, M. The battle of the clotbusters. *BMJ* 1991;**302**:1259–61.
4 Selley S, Donovan J, Faulkner A, Coast J, Gillatt D. Diagnosis, management and screening of early localised prostate cancer. *Health Technol Assess* 1997;**1**(2):1–96.
5 Chamberlain J, Melia J, Moss S, Brown J. The diagnosis, management, treatment and costs of prostate cancer in England and Wales. *Health Technol Assess* 1997;**1**(3):1–53.
6 Stern S, Altkorn D, Levinson W. Detection of prostate and colon cancer. *JAMA* 1998;**280**:117–18.
7 Rosenthal DS, Feldman G. Talking with patients about screening for prostate cancer. *JAMA* 1999;**281**:133.
8 Towler BP, Irwig L, Glasziou P, Weller D, Kewenter J. Screening for colorectal cancer using the faecal occult blood test, Hemoccult. Cochrane Review. In: *The Cochrane Library*, Issue 1. Oxford: Update Software, 1999.
9 Fletcher S. Whither scientific deliberation in health policy recommendations? Alice in the Wonderland of breast cancer screening. *N Engl J Med* 1997;**336**:1180–3.
10 Tanenbaum SJ. "Medical effectiveness" in Canadian and US Health Policy: the comparative politics of inferential ambiguity. *Health Serv Res* 1996;**31**:517–32.

23 Using systematic reviews for economic evaluation

MIRANDA MUGFORD

Summary points

- Economic evaluation seeks to predict the net change in benefits and costs arising from alternative approaches to providing a particular form of care.
- Methods for economic evaluation and systematic review can inform each other.
- To improve information for optimal decisions in health care:
  - Results of systematic reviews of effectiveness should be used in economic evaluations.
  - Systematic reviews of effects of health care could incorporate more outcomes used in economic analyses.
  - Systematic reviews of economic studies may lead to biased estimates.
  - Reporting of economic studies needs to be transparent about design and methods.

Nearly every health care decision has an impact, not only on health and social welfare, but also on the resources used in the production of health care and health. To make the best decisions, therefore, not only do decision-makers need to know the health benefits, but also the cost, or what is forgone to achieve this benefit. Economics and decision theory offer a framework for weighing up the net value of the costs and outcomes of alternative courses of action.[1-3] Economic evaluation techniques have been developed and applied increasingly in the health field in the last two decades and now appear regularly in clinical and health service research journals.[4] Such studies are sometimes based on primary data collection, but frequently use evidence both about costs and effects from published or other secondary sources. Guidance on the quality of the evidence used in such economic studies is still limited.

419

Systematic review methods are a formal and replicable approach to finding and summarising existing evidence. The approach has evolved in the field of health care in the context of use of selected, sometimes misleading, narrative reviews of evidence in support of advice for decision-makers.[5,6] The methods that have evolved, as this book illustrates, have concentrated on the quality of evidence about the effects of care. This information is necessary, and if it leads either to implementation of new practices or abandoning established ones, will have an effect on resources. Although it is clearly seen that reviews of this type do not provide sufficient evidence for decisions about the allocation of resources, as yet, very little has been written on the methods of systematic review to be used for the synthesis of evidence for an economic decision. The effectiveness of care is usually reported in terms of indicators of health or other clinical indicators, but effects on health service utilization, or on costs, are also considered in many studies, and are potentially important additional information for economic decisions.

In this chapter, I discuss the ways in which both economic evaluation and systematic review techniques can inform each other, and consider what needs to be done to improve the information for optimal decisions about health care.

What is economic evaluation?

Economic evaluation seeks to predict the net change in benefits and costs arising from alternative approaches to providing a particular form of care. There are different forms of analysis which reflect the purpose of the evaluation and the viewpoint from which it is conducted. These include cost-benefit analysis (CBA), cost effectiveness analysis (CEA) and cost-utility analysis (CUA). The approaches have different theoretical origins and are applicable to different types of economic decision (see Box 23.1).

Box 23.1 Economic evaluation terminology

Cost benefit analysis (CBA): Derived from welfare economics, measures net gain or loss to society of a new programme or project and thus considers *allocative efficiency*. The technique incorporates costs to a range of agencies including consumers and producers, as well as narrow health care costs, and usually gives values of benefits in monetary terms.

Cost effectiveness analysis (CEA): Originally derived to assess the *technical efficiency* of alternative projects, with close links to decision theory and operational research, this method compares alternative approaches to care.

Cost-effectiveness ratio: Estimates the value of (additional) resources required (costs) to achieve a particular desired health outcome.

Cost utility analysis (CUA): Overcomes the single dimension of outcome in *CEA*, and compares costs with the *utility* of health gain.

Discounting: A technique for estimating the present value of costs and benefits occurring in different time periods, and therefore having different values because of *time preference*.

Efficiency: Optimising the use of resources. *Technical efficiency* assesses which is the best programme to meet a specific objective. *Allocative efficiency* measures the extent to which programmes improve overall social welfare.

Equity: Fair distribution of access to resources, and/or outcomes.

Marginal analysis: One which considers the costs and benefits of a small change in production or consumption of services.

Opportunity cost: Economists attempt to measure cost as the benefit lost if *resources* are used in a particular way, and are therefore not available for other uses. Agreed money prices for exchange of resources are not always a good measure of opportunity cost, and adjustments must be made.

Resources: The physical means of producing goods and services, including human time and skills, raw materials, equipment, buildings, drugs, supplies etc. All resources have an *opportunity cost*. Sometimes the use of resources is aggregated and expressed in terms of units of service provided such as bed days or general practitioner visits.

Resource use: A measure of the quantity of resources used. Cost is estimated as the quantity of resource use multiplied by the money cost of an item of resource. For example, the cost of hospital inpatient care is sometimes estimated by the number of bed days multiplied by cost per bed day.

Sensitivity analysis: Exploration of uncertainty about assumptions or data included in an economic evaluation. The value of the cost-effectiveness or cost-benefit ratio is recalculated with different values. In one way sensitivity analysis, only one variable is changed at a time, in multiway and extreme scenario analysis, many variables are adjusted at the same time. The method can be used to consider thresholds of patient risk, effectiveness or cost at which a health intervention would be a 'good buy'.

Utility: A term used by economists to sum up the satisfaction gained from a good or service. In health care evaluations, is often expressed in such measures as the quality adjusted life year (QALY) or healthy year equivalent (HYE), thus taking account of quality of life and conflicting outcomes.

Viewpoint: Different agencies commissioning or providing or using health care have different objectives which may or may not conflict with overall societal viewpoint. Economic evaluation studies may consider the impact on these specific objectives, and may therefore not consider some costs and benefits. For example, many evaluations of hospital procedures consider only short term costs to the hospital, and not costs to other agencies.

This abridged glossary is partly distilled from Jefferson *et al.*[7] which provides a more complete introduction to economic evaluation.

421

Whatever form of evaluation is followed, all involve simplification and summing up of information about quantity and value of inputs used and outcomes experienced by those undergoing the alternative forms of health care compared. The information required includes: the predicted change in health, the predicted change in resource use, the utility or value of health gain, and the opportunity cost of resources.

Additional factors will also affect the results, interpretation, and "transferability" of the results of an economic evaluation:

- details of the types of care compared and the context in which they are provided
- characteristics of the patients treated
- how the pathways of care experienced by patients are described in terms of cost-generating events
- the viewpoint of the analysis, which should reflect the stakeholders involved in and affected by the decision
- the time horizon and scale of the decision to be made.

A cost effectiveness ratio is a composite variable, and is subject to the uncertainty about each of its components. Costs and effects can be, and often are, both constructed from synthesised data based on a variety of sources. There is a growing volume of research on statistical properties of costs and cost effectiveness ratios.[8] However, many sources of uncertainty, such as assumptions about discount rates, or about allocation of joint costs, can not usually be treated statistically. Therefore, a key element in economic evaluation is sensitivity analysis, to test thresholds of cost effectiveness, extreme scenarios and the effects of individual assumptions.

Given the range of reasons for differences in the results of economic evaluations, the reliability of the result and of the data used in any evaluation is very hard to judge. For this reason, health economists and those concerned about publishing and making decisions based on valid evidence have been developing guidelines for practising and reviewing economic evaluations of health interventions.[9–13] These guidelines represent a consensus of opinion, and in some cases express a lack of agreement. In some points the recommendations are driven by economic wisdom, such as the recommendation that the value of future costs and benefits should be discounted. In other points, guidelines for economic evaluation have adopted accepted wisdom in health services research. For example, as shown in Box 23.2, guidance from both the USA and the UK recognises the value of avoidance of bias in estimation of effectiveness, preferring evidence based on randomised controlled trials. Economists recognise systematic reviews of effects of care as a possible source for economic evaluation, although in the recommendations published so far, there is still uncertainty about the hierarchy of levels of evidence. For example, the US

Box 23.2 – Recommended sources of effectiveness data for economic evaluation

Outcome probability values should be selected from the best designed (and least biased) sources that are relevant to the question and population under study.

Evidence for effectiveness may be obtained from RCTs, observational data, uncontrolled experiments, descriptive series and expert opinion.

Good quality meta-analysis and other synthesis methods can be used to estimate effectiveness where any one study has insufficient power to detect effects or where results conflict.

Gold et al.[10]

In using the existing published literature for estimates of effectiveness, the economic analyst can either use data from a single trial or, where they exist, data from an overview or meta-analysis of a group of trials.

Drummond et al.[5]

guidelines suggest that systematic review evidence should be seen as second best compared to a single well conducted RCT.[10] Quality criteria for economic evaluations are used by reviewers in the critical abstracts of economic evaluation studies published in the British National Health Service (NHS) Economic Evaluation Database, which is produced by the Centre for Reviews and Dissemination of the NHS.[4]

Very few economic evaluations are entirely based on primary research. Those that are can provide valuable information about the costs and processes of health care in particular settings.[14] However, such studies take as long to complete as the effectiveness research with which they are linked. Decision makers often need an assessment of economic impact at an earlier stage in the diffusion of technology, *before* trials are funded, to assess cost effectiveness in routine practice. Preliminary economic evaluations, or more correctly, appraisals, can be the basis for decisions about the need for further research or indeed about whether to proceed with the new form of health care at all.[15,16] Such studies model the likely costs and consequences based on the *best available data*. Logically, therefore, systematic review techniques should always be used in economic appraisals, for all the categories of data required, and even to derive the structure of the model that is used to predict cost. That this is not yet the case is clear from a look at the studies abstracted in the NHS Economic Evaluation Database. However, methods for economic evaluation are developing.

Using systematic reviews of the effects of health care in economic evaluation

If systematic review of the effects of care is well done, it increases the chance of detecting a true effect of care, and minimises the chance of wrongly finding a form of care effective. Where such evidence is generated, it can provide powerful evidence for a change in health care provision, but does not provide decision-makers with all the evidence they need. Evaluation of the economic implications of the findings of the review is a logical next step. Examples where this has occurred include use of antibiotic prophylaxis at caesarean section to prevent post-operative wound infection,[17] use of antenatal corticosteroids and surfactant for reduction of the risk of neonatal respiratory distress,[18] tamoxifen in treatment of breast cancer,[19] methods for suturing after perineal trauma during childbirth,[20] and many others. In these cases, the typical odds for effects on key outcomes are used to estimate probabilities in decision models, and to infer the use of key services for care. Problems arise in such models when the original systematic review does not generate sufficiently disaggregated data to estimate the probabilities required to construct specific pathways in the decision model.

In each case of economic evaluation based on systematic reviews of effects of care, the model also uses data from other sources about the baseline risks of the key outcomes and the costs of service use. This is often from a single primary study, or health care database. Some economic evaluations use evidence from review of literature for these purposes, but it has been unusual for authors to describe how they found and summed up current evidence, or to set criteria for quality of evidence.

Systematic review protocols have often been developed with a fairly limited clinical viewpoint, which may in turn reflect the emphasis of the trials that are reviewed. Increasingly, however, trials address wider questions and frequently have associated economic evaluations, although these are not always reported in the same journal.[21] Given that such trials are included in systematic reviews, it seems a sad waste of important information where it is not reported in the review. If there is clearly an important economic decision to be made about a form of health care, then systematic review protocols can be developed with a broader objective, and with economic evaluation in mind. For such reviews to come about, however, there is a need for reviewers to understand and judge the methods used for economic evaluation alongside trials, and for their economic advisors to understand the purpose and methods of systematic reviews of evidence. This is being attempted at present in several ongoing reviews, but is still limited by the level of reporting of economic outcomes in most reports of randomised trials.[22]

Systematic review of economic evaluations

Although not often formally used as a source of data in economic evaluation, systematic review techniques are not new in health economics. Efficient methods of electronic and hand searching for economic studies are evolving, and it is clear that methods for identifying economic studies requires very different strategies from those for effectiveness studies.[4,23] Valuable exploratory reviews of studies have been done,[24-26] not primarily to sum up evidence of economic outcomes, but to investigate whether methods used for economic evaluation meet recommendations, and how they affect the results of the reviewed studies.

Taking examples of health care interventions from immunisation and neonatal intensive care, a group of economists investigated whether it might be fruitful to attempt systematic review of economic evaluation studies, with the aim of summing up the economic benefit of a particular health technology. We identified a range of problems. Economic studies of the same form of care often, quite legitimately, have a range of purposes and viewpoints and designs, apply to disparate populations, and refer to different baseline levels of health care. This applied strongly in the cases of immunisation against hepatitis B, and influenza, but less so in the case of giving exogenous surfactant in neonatal intensive care units to prevent neonatal respiratory distress, where the populations, risks and technologies were more homogeneous among studies. Even if the differences among the design of the studies were not a problem, the quality of the reported studies, or the evidence they used, has generally been poor, and many studies would have to be excluded. The conclusion of this investigation was that:

> *economists have not yet developed a formal methodology for reviewing and summing up evidence from individual economic evaluations ... or indeed for assessing whether systematic reviews are possible in this context.*[27]

Since then, further reviews of economic studies have been done and methods are currently being tested for setting quality criteria for inclusion of studies in such reviews.[28,29] There is doubt among some health economists that standardisation of methods is a sensible path to follow, given the wide range of purposes and acceptable formats for economic evaluations. Most agree, however, that there is a need for transparency in reporting economic evaluations.

One problem arising from restricting a review of evidence only to economic evaluations is that much valuable evidence is lost, both about the effectiveness and the costs of alternative forms of care. This occurs because the review will omit high quality trials that did not qualify as economic studies. The review would also omit economic studies, such as cost of

425

Table 23.1 Cost effectiveness estimates for use of exogenous surfactant in neonatal intensive care units to prevent neonatal respiratory distress.

Source of evidence for effects	Number of studies	Countries	Cost per additional survivor (1994 pounds)
Systematic review	2	UK, Netherlands	20 908
Single RCT	3	USA	45 573
Other control	2	USA, Finland	88 350
All	7		50 755

illness or cost comparison studies, which are not classed as economic evaluations. Potentially, therefore, a review based on economic evaluations alone could be quite misleading. This is illustrated in Table 23.1, which shows how the results of economic studies can vary by source of evidence about effects of surfactant. In this example, the country of the study is an additional important source of variation, since health care costs are known to be very much higher in the USA than in Europe. More evidence is needed to judge the degree of bias that is inherent in review of economic evaluation studies.

Conclusions: the role of systematic review in economic evaluation

Economic evaluation is not a single research methodology, but a framework for combining data from different sources about costs and benefits. Methods for economic evaluation are evolving, and health economists increasingly acknowledge the role of systematic review methods, at the same time as the need for economic evaluation is recognised by reviewers of effectiveness. The methodological questions which I have discussed in the previous paragraphs are all the subject of current research by members of Cochrane Economics Methods Group,[30] who are interested in the links between economic evaluation and systematic review of the effects of health care (see Chapters 25 and 26 on the Cochrane Collaboration). Box 23.3 illustrates some of the current tasks faced by the group. On the basis of work underway at the time of writing, it seems likely that in the next few years clearer guidelines for combining evidence from systematic reviews and economic evaluation will emerge.

> **Box 23.3 Work of the Cochrane Health Economics Methods Group**
>
> - Linking reviewers and economic analysts
> - Developing and testing further methods for summing up evidence from economic studies
> - Developing and testing further methods for incorporating the results of systematic review in economic evaluation
>
> **Some research topics on economic evaluation using systematic review**
> - Can valid cost estimates be derived from systematic reviews of effects of health care?
> - Can review protocols be adapted/extended for economic evaluation?
>
> **Examples of current research on economic evaluation studies**
> - Is it possible to define quality standards for economic evaluations?
> - Can economic evaluation guidelines be further developed?
> - Statistical properties of cost and cost effectiveness estimates
> - What do variations in results between studies tell us about methods and contexts?

Acknowledgements

Miranda Mugford is employed by the University of East Anglia. I thank many colleagues for helpful comments, and the Cochrane Economics Methods Group for the discussions and the collaboration which have contributed to this chapter.

1 Mishan EJ. *Cost-benefit analysis*. London: Unwin Hyman, 1988.
2 Sugden R, Williams A. *The principles of practical cost-benefit analysis*. Oxford: Oxford University Press, 1978.
3 Drummond M, O'Brien B, Stoddart G, Torrance G. *Methods for the economic evaluation of health care programmes*, 2nd edn. Oxford: Oxford University Press, 1997.
4 Centre for Reviews and Dissemination. Making cost-effectiveness information accessible: the NHS economic evaluation database. CRD Guidance for reporting critical summaries of economic evaluations. Report No 6. NHS R&D Centre for Reviews and Dissemination, University of York, York, 1996.
5 Mulrow CD. The medical review article: state of the science. *Ann Intern Med* 1987;**104**:485–8.
6 Cochrane AL. *Effectiveness and efficiency: random reflections on health services*. London: BMJ and Nuffield Provincial Hospitals Trust, 1989
7 Jefferson T, Demicheli V, Mugford M. *Elementary economic evaluation in health care*. London: BMJ Publishing Group, 2000.

427

8 Briggs AH, Gray AM. Sample size and power calculations for stochastic cost-effectiveness analysis. *Med Decis Making* 1998;**18**(suppl):S81–S92.

9 Drummond MF, Jefferson TO, on behalf of the BMJ Economic Evaluation Working Party. Guidelines for authors and peer-reviewers of economic submissions to the BMJ. *BMJ* 1996;**313**:275–83.

10 Gold M, Siegel J, Russell L, Weinstein M. *Cost-effectiveness in health and medicine.* New York: Oxford University Press, 1996.

11 Association of British Pharmaceutical Industries (ABPI). Press release 20 May 1994: "Pharmaceutical industry and Department of Health agree guidelines for the economic analysis of medicines". London: ABPI, 1994.

12 Canadian Co-ordinating Office for Health Technology Assessment. *Guidelines for the economic evaluation of pharmaceuticals.* Ottawa: CCHOTA, 1994.

13 Commonwealth of Australia, Department of Health, Housing and Community Services. *Guidelines for the pharmaceutical industry on preparation of submissions to the pharmaceutical benefits advisory committee.* Canberra: Australian Government Publishing Service, 1995.

14 Roberts T, ECMO Economics Working Group on behalf of the ECMO Trial Steering Group. Economic evaluation alongside the UK collaborative ECMO trial. *BMJ* 1998;**317**:911–14.

15 Howard S, Mugford M, Normand C, *et al.* A cost effectiveness analysis of neonatal ECMO using existing evidence. *Int J Technol Assess Health Care* 1996;**12**:80–92.

16 Townsend J, Buxton M. Cost-effectiveness scenario analysis for a proposed trial of hormone replacement therapy. *Health Policy* 1997;**39**:181–94.

17 Mugford M, Kingston J, Chalmers I. Reducing the incidence of infection after caesarean section: cost-effectiveness of prophylactic antibiotics. *BMJ* 1989;**299**:1003–6.

18 Mugford M, Piercy J, Chalmers I. Cost implications of different approaches to the prevention of respiratory distress syndrome. *Arch Dis Childhood* 1991;**66**:757–64.

19 Smith TJ, Hillner BE. The efficacy and cost-effectiveness of adjuvant therapy of early breast cancer in pre-menopausal women. *J Clin Oncol* 1993,**11**:771–6.

20 Howard S, McKell D, Mugford M, Grant A. Cost-effectiveness of different approaches to perineal suturing. *Br J Midwifery* 1995;**3**:587–605.

21 Jefferson T. Commentary: concurrent economic evaluations are rare but should be standard practice. *BMJ* 1998;**317**:915–16.

22 MacLeod A, Grant A, Donaldson C, *et al.* Effectiveness and efficiency of methods of dialysis therapy for end stage renal disease: systematic reviews. *Health Technol Assess* 1998;**2**(5):1–166.

23 Mugford M. How does the method of cost estimation affect the assessment of cost-effectiveness in health care. D Phil thesis, University of Oxford, Oxford, 1996.

24 Gerard K. Cost utility in practice: a policy maker's guide to the state of the art. *Health Policy* 1992;**21**:249–79.

25 Mugford M. The cost of neonatal care: reviewing the evidence. *Soc Prev Med* 1995;**40**:361–8.

26 Jefferson T, Demicheli V. Methodological quality of economic modelling studies: a case study with Hepatitis B vaccines. *Pharmacoeconomics* 1998;**14**:251–7.

27 Jefferson T, Mugford M, Gray A, Demicheli V. An exercise on the feasibility of carrying out secondary economic analyses. *Health Econom* 1996;**5**:155–65.

28 Gift TL, Kassler WJ, Wang G. Assessing the quality of economic studies of health care: searching for an ideal instrument. Poster abstract for *6th Ann Cochrane Colloquium,* Baltimore, October, 1998.

29 Roberts T, Henderson J, Petrou S, Martin M. The quality of economic evidence available to decision makers. Peer reviewed conference presentation abstracts for *2nd Int Conf Priority Setting,* London, October, 1998.

30 Cochrane Collaboration. *The Cochrane Library.* 1999, issue 2. Update Software, Oxford, 1999.

24 Using systematic reviews and registers of ongoing trials for scientific and ethical trial design, monitoring, and reporting

IAIN CHALMERS

Summary points

- Systematic reviews of existing evidence are prerequisites for the scientific and ethical design of new controlled trials.
- Proposals for new trials should take account of information about planned and ongoing trials.
- Ethical and scientific monitoring of ongoing trials should take account of systematic reviews that have incorporated relevant new evidence.
- The results from new trials should be set and interpreted in the context of systematic reviews of all of the relevant evidence available at the time of reporting.
- Up-to-date systematic reviews of existing evidence and registers of planned and ongoing trials are essential for scientific and ethical trial design, monitoring and reporting, and for protecting the interests of patients, and the public more generally.

Authors of previous chapters in this section have discussed the applicability of results of a systematic review to individuals and the issues raised when using systematic reviews for the development of guidelines, economic evaluation and policy making. In this chapter I will suggest that systematic reviews of existing trials and registers of ongoing trials are prerequisites for scientific and ethical trial design, monitoring and reporting, and for protecting the interests of patients, and the public in general.

Questionable use of limited resources

In the first edition of this book, Paul Knipschild[1] noted that researchers who had published reports of controlled trials of pyridoxine for women suffering from premenstrual syndrome had failed to refer to several well-designed earlier studies. As every important trial that they had missed had shown an ambiguous or frankly unpromising result, Knipschild suggested that these researchers might not have embarked on further trials if they had searched for and analysed relevant existing research evidence more systematically.

An expensive controlled trial was sponsored by the US National Eye Institute[2,3] because the results of a non-randomised cohort comparison published in the *New England Journal of Medicine* suggested that neonatal exposure to light increased the risk of retinopathy of prematurity.[4] Critiques of these observational data[5] showed how they might have reflected selection bias, a conclusion that was supported by the results of the controlled trials available at that time.[6] Had the National Eye Institute required a systematic review of the evidence from controlled trials before funding a further study, its investment priorities might have been different.

Ethical concerns

Apart from the inefficient use of limited resources for research, there are worrying ethical concerns raised by failure to prepare systematic reviews of past studies before doing further research, in particular, when this results in failure to recognise that a therapeutic question has already been convincingly addressed. Savulescu and his colleagues[7] suggested that some research ethics committees were behaving unethically by ignoring this issue. As an example, they pointed to the unjustified continued use of placebos in trials of antibiotic prophylaxis for colorectal surgery when there was evidence from earlier trials that antibiotics reduce mortality[8] (Figure 24.1). It is likely that all of the more recent trials were approved by research ethics committees; yet, presented with the evidence shown in Figure 24.1, it seems very unlikely that many patients scheduled for colorectal surgery at any time over the past 20 years would have not wished to have had prophylactic antibiotics, within or outside the context of controlled trials.

In 1997, after considering the influence existing and newly acquired results of research should have on the ethical evaluation of proposals for further controlled trials, the Danish national Research Ethics Committee System concluded that "it is crucial that all relevant literature has been reviewed by the research group before submission". Specifically, they stated that "this will be a precondition when the evaluating committee is

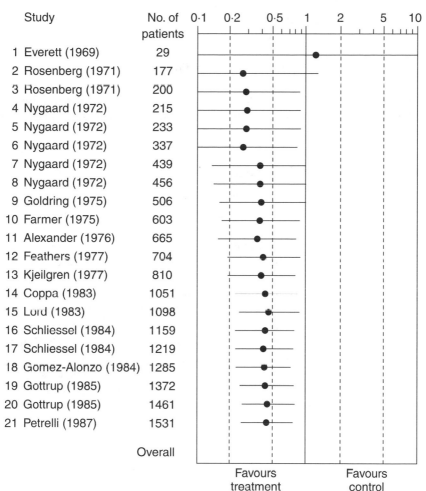

Figure 24.1 Cumulative estimate of the effects on mortality of antibiotic prophylaxis for colorectal surgery. From Lau *et al.*[8]

judging the originality of the project and, for example, the permissibility of using placebo and not an already known treatment in a control group".[9,10]

Over the past half century, researchers, research funders and research ethics committees have presided over an outpouring of controlled trials addressing questions of doubtful or no relevance to patients,[11,12] and they have done so in ways that have been characterised as a scandal.[13] Taking just one area – schizophrenia – as an example, a recent analysis of 2000 controlled trials showed that most were poorly reported, that over 600 different interventions had been studied, and that, in this chronic condition, most trials were of short duration.[14] The 500 reports of trials of nearly 100 different drugs prescribed for the movement disorders caused by medication for schizophrenia, for example, are plagued by methodological problems of small sample sizes, brief interventions, and inappropriate use of the crossover design.[15]

Distorted research agendas

The mismatch that exists between patients' needs and the research actually done often seems to reflect perverse incentives to pursue particular research projects.[11,16,17] There are substantial opportunity costs associated with this situation. For example, investigators are currently being paid substantial amounts of money by drug companies to recruit participants in trials investigating surrogate measures of the effects of new neuroprotective agents. These monetary incentives, together with commercial stipulation that the participants in these trials cannot take part in any other trials, mean that important unanswered questions about many existing elements of treatment are likely to remain unanswered. For example, even though, every year, tens of thousands of patients with severe head injury are hyperventilated and given mannitol, barbiturates and/or corticosteroids, systematic reviews of the available trials have shown that there is uncertainty about whether *any* of these interventions decreases either death or disability.[18–20] Likewise, the effects of treatments for stroke which have limited or no commercial potential, such as phenytoin, magnesium and hypothermia, remain unclear.[21]

Systematic reviews are beginning to make these distortions in the research agenda more visible, and identify which hypotheses are worth pursuing. The trend to prepare systematic reviews to guide decisions about further research in health care began in the 1980s, when it was exemplified by the series of International Studies of Infarct Survival (ISIS) and the programme of trials developed by the Perinatal Trials Service at the UK National Perinatal Epidemiology Unit. A specific example can help to illustrate how the principle can operate in practice.

432

Many (probably most) women find the administration of an enema in early labour distressing and degrading, yet this is still a routine in many maternity hospitals. This practice reflects the fact that some health professionals believe that routine use of enemas shortens labour and reduces the risk of maternal and neonatal infection after birth. A Colombian family physician, Luis Cuervo, was concerned about this mismatch between lay and professional perceptions. At the end of 1994 he consulted the *Cochrane Pregnancy and Childbirth Database* and found a review of the relevant controlled trials. Although the review confirmed his impression that there was good reason to doubt the validity of the professional rationale for administering enemas to women in labour, he was dissatisfied with the quality of the review. The improved review of the available evidence that he prepared[22] revealed that the existing trials were unsatisfactory in a number of respects, and so he designed and completed a further trial addressing many of these deficiencies (Luis Cuervo, personal communication), and the results will be used to update the systematic review in due course.

The principle of building systematically on what is known already is beginning to be reflected in the requirements of research funding organisations. In the UK, for example, the Medical Research Council[23] (Box 24.1) and the National Health Service's Health Technology Assessment

---

Box 24.1 Extract from UK Medical Research Council Proforma for funding applications for new controlled trials (from http://www.mrc.ac.uk/Clinical_trials/ctg.pdf)

2 The need for a trial

2.1 What is the problem to be addressed?

2.2 What are the principal research questions to be addressed?

2.3 Why is a trial needed now?
Evidence from the medical literature – see 2.4 below, professional and consumer consensus and pilot studies should be cited if available.

2.4 Give references to any relevant systematic review(s)* and discuss the need for your trial in the light of the(se) review(s)
If you believe that no relevant previous trials have been done, give details of your search strategy for existing trials.

2.5 How will the results of this trial be used?
E.g. inform clinical decision-making/improve understanding.

* For definition of a systematic review, see Oxman, AD. Checklists for review articles. *BMJ* 1994;**309**:648–51.

Programme have put in place mechanisms for ensuring that information from systematic reviews of past research are available to guide decisions about whether or not to support proposed new research. People proposing new trials to the Medical Research Council are now required to "give references to any systematic reviews and discuss the need for (the proposed) trial in the light of these reviews". If they believe that no relevant previous trials have been done, applicants are required to "give details of (their) search strategy for existing trials" (Box 24.1).

Registration of planned and ongoing trials to inform decisions on new trials

Those planning new research should also take account of planned and ongoing research, to avoid duplication of effort, and to promote collaboration and appropriate replication. Sometimes, information about ongoing trials may lead to a decision not to embark on another trial because it is judged that answers to the questions being considered are likely to emerge soon from work in progress elsewhere. Sometimes information about ongoing trials will prompt researchers to contribute to an existing ongoing trial, both to reduce the infrastructure costs of the research overall, and the time taken to achieve the sample size necessary to obtain statistically robust estimates of effects on important outcomes.

Information about ongoing trials may lead researchers to plan collaborative analyses of similar, but independently organised trials, using an agreed core data set to address questions defined prior to inspecting the data.[24,25] Such prospectively planned meta-analyses seem likely to offer an important way of generating more precise estimates of treatment effects and a way of confronting some of the practical and political problems faced by those organising very large international trials.[26] Better infrastructure is required to support those clinicians and patients who, uncertain about the relative merits of two or more alternative treatments in everyday clinical practice, wish to use randomisation as the preferred option for selecting among treatment alternatives.[27]

Registration of trials to reduce reporting biases

Registration of ongoing trials is also required to contain and reduce the serious problem of reporting biases. There is now substantial evidence that clinical investigators are responsible for biased underreporting of research (see Chapter 3). Compared with studies yielding unremarkable point estimates of effects, studies which have yielded relatively dramatic estimates are more likely to be selected for presentation at scientific meetings; more likely to be reported in print; more likely to be published promptly; more likely to be published as full reports; more likely to be published in journals that are widely read; more likely to be published in English; more likely to be published in more than one report; and more likely to be cited in reports of subsequent, related studies. As emphasised in a report published by the Ethical Issues Working Party of the Faculty of Pharmaceutical Medicine, these reporting biases raise serious ethical questions. "Pharmaceutical physicians", the report states, "have a particular ethical responsibility to ensure that the evidence on which doctors should make their prescribing decisions is freely available . . . the outcome of all clinical trials conducted on a medicine should be reported."[28]

Efforts to tackle reporting biases by trying to identify unpublished studies retrospectively have met with only limited success,[29,30] and Simes' proposal[31] more than a decade ago that the problem should be tackled through prospective registration has become increasingly widely endorsed[29,32–40] (see, in particular, CCT Links Register at www.controlled-trials.com Figure 24.2). In an editorial published in Controlled Clinical Trials in 1998, Meinert wrote "We are a mere dozen years from the dawn of the new century. Let us hope that prospective registration will be the norm for all clinical trials by the time we enter the 21st century. That hope can be realised, but only through a collective resolve and effort to bring it about".[32]

Prospective registration of trials might also have helped to reduce the extent of the disastrous widespread prophylactic use of anti-arrhythmic drugs after myocardial infarction because it would have meant that relevant studies which should have been reported but were not could have been identified. In the light of the evidence of reporting biases summarised above (see also Chapter 3), it is surprising to find that some commentators are still prepared to suggest that "studies that cannot be published in reputable journals are probably flawed and are best disregarded".[41] In 1980, the author of this statement found an increased death rate associated with a class 1 anti-arrhythmic drug, but he and his colleagues dismissed it as likely to be a chance finding and did not report it at the time because the development of the drug "had been abandoned for commercial reasons".[42] They deserve credit for reporting the trial 13 years later as an example of publication bias, noting that had it been reported at the time it was completed, it might have provided warning of trouble ahead.[42–44] Incorporating their data with the data presented in the systematic review of published reports published by Furberg[45] at that time gives 104 deaths (6·5%) among 1609 patients allocated to receive class 1 anti-arrhythmic drugs, and 74 deaths (5·1%) among 1454 control patients, results that suggest that these drugs increase the odds of death by about a third (odds ratio 1·34; 95% confidence interval 0·98 to 1·82).

There will be fewer avoidable tragedies of this kind in future if up-to-date systematic reviews and registers of controlled trials are recognised to be prerequisites for scientific and ethical trial design, monitoring and

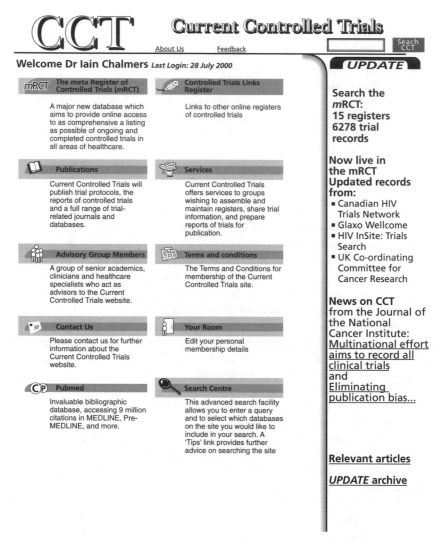

Figure 24.2 Search screen at www.controlled-trials.com, a website established by the publisher Current Science which contains both a meta-register of controlled trials, and electronic links to registers held at other sites on the World Wide Web.

reporting, and if under-reporting of research is seen for what it is – scientific and ethical misconduct.[7,46,47]

For all of the above reasons, summarised in Box 24.2, pressure to establish and maintain registers of ongoing trials has been growing. Until recently such registers have been far from satisfactory because they have

Box 24.2 The need for prospective registration of controlled trials

Prospective registration of information about ongoing controlled trials is needed because:

- Research funding agencies (public, commercial and charitable) want to take their funding decisions in the light of information about relevant ongoing research, both to avoid duplication of effort and to promote collaboration.
- Patients, clinicians and other decision makers wish to be informed about trials in which they can participate or to which they can contribute in other ways.
- People using evidence from controlled trials want to be confident that they are aware of all the trial evidence relevant to a particular question.

relied on voluntary registration.[48] This situation is changing, however, as the importance of prospective registration of trials – on ethical as well as scientific grounds[46] – has become more widely appreciated. Registration of controlled trials is increasingly expected and in many places, it is becoming required. The US Food and Drug Administration Modernization Act of 1997, for example, calls for the establishment of a federally funded database containing information on both government funded and privately funded clinical trials of drugs designed to treat serious or life-threatening conditions.

Prospective registration of controlled trials now also has support at a high level within the UK. For example, the Medical Research Council[49] requires prospective registration of all the trials it supports; the National Research Register assembled within the NHS Research and Development Programme contains information about controlled trials being done within the NHS; and two pharmaceutical companies, Schering Health Care[50] and Glaxo Wellcome,[37] have led the way in making information about commercially sponsored trials publicly available.

These developments, taken together with the potential now offered by the World Wide Web for drawing on information in widely scattered sources, suggest that the time is right to develop a means through which people could obtain information about ongoing trials in many disciplines, pursued in several countries, and supported from a variety of sources.[40] Using records provided by public, charitable and commercial funders of controlled trials, the publisher Current Science has established a website (www.controlled-trials.com) containing both a meta-register of controlled trials, and electronic links to registers held at other sites on the World Wide

Web (Figure 24.2). An international advisory group has been established by Current Science to guide the development of this initiative, and it seems very likely that this will become a crucially important resource for addressing some of the objectives and needs outlined above.

Ethical and scientific monitoring of ongoing trials

The principle of taking into account the results of up-to-date systematic reviews of relevant existing evidence applies not only to decisions about whether to support new research, but also to decisions about whether to continue supporting ongoing research. The dynamic nature of accumulating evidence means that systematic reviews need to be kept up-to-date,[51] and researchers, funding bodies and data monitoring committees need to take account of the changed circumstances which may result.

Proposals for a large trial of thyrotropin releasing hormone for anticipated pre-term delivery, for example, were based on encouraging evidence from a systematic review of the early trials. The new trial was abandoned when the review was updated[52] to take account of evidence which had accumulated from subsequent trials.[53] Similarly, recruitment to Danish and American trials of anti-coagulation in patients with atrial fibrillation was discontinued in the light of the data emerging from other trials (Curt Furberg, personal communication).

There remains inadequate appreciation of the need to use up-to-date systematic reviews in monitoring ongoing trials. The authors of a recently published article in the *Lancet* entitled "The agonising negative trend in monitoring of clinical trials"[54] failed to mention how interpretation of worrying trends in the results of ongoing trials should take account of systematic reviews of relevant external evidence. Two of the specific examples they use in the paper illustrate the potential value of systematic reviews in this situation. Worrying trends in the accumulating results of a large trial of anti-arrhythmic drugs in myocardial infarction[55] could have been informed by the worrying results of systematic reviews of other controlled trials of this class of drugs.[56,57] Conversely, a worrying early trend in a large trial of beta-blockade during myocardial infarction[58] was interpreted conservatively because a systematic review of other trials of these drugs had shown that they were likely to result in a modest but important reduction in mortality.[59]

If systematic reviews are to fulfil this role effectively, they must be up to date. As noted in a contribution to the first edition of this book,[60] one of the few features which currently distinguishes *The Cochrane Database of Systematic Reviews* (see Chapter 25) from other publications is that authors of the reviews it contains are expected to keep their work up to date in the light of new evidence, and as other ways of improving their work are identified. The treadmill into which those who have assumed responsibility for preparing *and maintaining* Cochrane Reviews have stepped is proving a substantial challenge to many of them, and to the Cochrane Collaboration more generally (see Chapter 26). Indeed, efficient maintenance of the reviews published in *The Cochrane Database of Systematic Reviews* is becoming the main challenge facing the Cochrane Collaboration, and seems likely to remain so. As the editor of the *BMJ* has noted, the dynamic nature of Cochrane reviews also creates knock-on challenges for more traditional forms of publication.[61]

Even if the Cochrane Collaboration does not rise to the challenge of maintaining systematic reviews efficiently, others must do so. As long as up-to-date systematic reviews of relevant existing evidence and information about relevant ongoing studies are not readily accessible, those funding, approving, conducting and monitoring research cannot claim that they have taken adequate steps to protect the interests of the patients and others who participate in research.

Interpreting the results from new trials

Finally, systematic reviews are required to implement the recommendation of the CONSORT Group[62] that data from a new trial should be interpreted "in the light of the totality of the available evidence". The public and others will continue to be misled as long as scientists, while attending to the control of biases and imprecision within trials, ignore the need to attend to biases and imprecision in setting the results of a particular trial in context. An analysis of all 25 reports of randomised trials published in the May 1997 issues of the *Annals of Internal Medicine*, the *BMJ*, *JAMA*, the *Lancet* and the *New England Journal of Medicine*[63] revealed that in only two reports (both published in the *Lancet*) had the evidence generated by the new study been presented in the context of updated systematic reviews of other relevant studies. Many of the other articles, including some that claimed (without evidence) to be the first trial addressing a particular question, contained citations to previous trials; but it was not clear whether these citations represented every similar trial, or how they had been identified, or why they had been included. In other words, in terms of the notion of a population of relevant studies,[64] the cited reports were non-random numerators without defined denominators.

Judged by today's *de facto* standards for reporting research, it may seem unreasonable to expect investigators to set the results of new trials in the context of updated systematic reviews of other relevant data. This process will become less onerous, however, if, before embarking on new trials, researchers prepare or refer to relevant systematic reviews of the relevant evidence available at that time. Setting the new data in the context of updated versions of these reviews will then make clear what contribution the new study has made to the totality of the evidence. Electronic publishing now provides the means whereby such detailed reports of research can be handled,[65] and a medium for keeping systematic reviews up to date.[60,66,67]

Returning to the example of the anti-arrhythmic drugs it is worth noting that at least 50 trials of these drugs were conducted over nearly two decades[43] before official warnings about their lethal impact were issued. Had the new data generated by each of these trials been presented within the context of systematic reviews of the results of all previous trials, the lethal potential of this class of drugs would have become clear earlier, and an iatrogenic disaster would have been contained if not avoided.[68]

In summary, up-to-date systematic reviews of existing evidence and registers of planned and ongoing trials are essential for scientific and ethical trial design, monitoring and reporting, and for protecting the interests of patients, and the public more generally.

Acknowledgements

I am grateful to Phil Alderson, Simon Banister, Mike Clarke, Luis Cuervo, Curt Furberg, Richard Horton, Claire Marley, Dale Phelps, Ian Roberts, and Jack Sinclair for providing helpful information and for comments on an earlier draft of this chapter.

1 Knipschild P. Some examples of systematic reviews. In: Chalmers I, Altman DG, eds. *Systematic reviews*. London: BMJ Publishing Group, 1995:9–16.
2 Kupfer C. Differing perspectives: Is meta-analysis a reasonable alternative to large randomized trials? Paper presented at the *6th Ann Int Cochrane Colloquium*. Baltimore, 22–26 October, 1998.
3 Reynolds JD, Hardy RJ, Kennedy KA, Spencer R, van Heuven WA, Fielder AR. Lack of efficacy of light reduction in preventing retinopathy of prematurity. Light Reduction in Retinopathy of Prematurity (LIGHT-ROP) Cooperative Group. *N Engl J Med* 1998;338:1572–6.
4 Glass P, Avery GB, Subramanian KN, Keys MP, Sostek AM, Friendly DS. Effect of bright light in the hospital nursery on the incidence of retinopathy of prematurity. *N Engl J Med* 1985;313:401–4.
5 Commentary and questions session II. In: Flynn JT, Phelps DL, eds. *Retinopathy of prematurity: problems and challenge. Birth defects original article series 24*. White Plains, NY: March of Dimes Birth Defects Foundation, 1988:169–71.
6 Phelps DL, Watts JL. Early light reduction for preventing retinopathy of prematurity in very low birth weight infants (Cochrane Review). In: *The Cochrane Library*, Issue 1. Oxford: Update Software, 2000.
7 Savulescu J, Chalmers I, Blunt J. Are research ethics committees behaving unethically? Some suggestions for improving performance and accountability. *BMJ* 1996;313:1390–3.
8 Lau J, Schmid CH, Chalmers TC. Cumulative meta-analysis of clinical trials builds evidence for exemplary medical care. *J Clin Epidemiol* 1995;48:45–57.
9 Danish Research Ethics Committee System. *Recommendation No. 20: controlled clinical trials – the influence of existing and newly acquired scientific results on the research ethical evaluation.* Copenhagen: Danish Research Ethics Committee System, 1997.

10 Goldbeck-Wood, S. Denmark takes lead on research ethics. *BMJ* 1998;**316**:1189.

11 Chalmers I. The perinatal research agenda: whose priorities? *Birth* 1991;**18**:137–41.

12 Chalmers I. What do I want from health research and researchers when I am a patient? *BMJ* 1995;**310**:1315–18.

13 Altman DG. The scandal of poor medical research. *BMJ* 1994;**308**:283–4.

14 Thornley B, Adams C. Content and quality of 2000 controlled trials in schizophrenia over 50 years. *BMJ* 1998;**317**:1181–4.

15 Soares K, McGrath J, Adams C. Evidence and tardive dyskinesia [letter]. *Lancet* 1996;**347**:1696–7.

16 Dieppe P, Chard J, Tallon D, Egger M. Funding clinical research [letter]. *Lancet* 1999;**353**:1626.

17 Warlow C, Sandercock P, Dennis M, Wardlaw J. Research funding [letter]. *Lancet* 1999;**353**:2250.

18 Schierhout G, Roberts I. Hyperventilation therapy in acute traumatic brain injury (Cochrane Review). In: *The Cochrane Library*, Issue 1. Oxford: Update Software, 2000.

19 Schierhout G, Roberts I. Mannitol in acute traumatic brain injury (Cochrane Review). In: *The Cochrane Library*, Issue 1. Oxford: Update Software, 2000.

20 Alderson P, Roberts I. Corticosteroids in acute traumatic brain injury (Cochrane Review). In: *The Cochrane Library*, Issue 3, 1998. Oxford: Update Software, 1998.

21 Dorman PJ, Sandercock PA. Considerations in the design of clinical trials of neuro-protective therapy in acute stroke. *Stroke* 1996;**27**:1507–15.

22 Cuervo LG, Rodríguez MN, Delgado MB. Enema vs no enema during labor (Cochrane Review). In: *The Cochrane Library*, Issue 1. Oxford: Update Software, 2000.

23 O'Toole, L. Using systematically synthesised evidence to inform the funding of new clinical trials – the UK Medical Research Council approach. Paper presented at the *6th Ann Int Cochrane Colloquium*. Baltimore, 22–26 October, 1998.

24 International Multicentre Pooled Analysis of Colon Cancer Trials (IMPACT). Efficacy of adjuvant fluorouracil and folinic acid in colon cancer. *Lancet* 1995;**345**:939–44.

25 Laupacis A. Research by collaboration. *Lancet* 1995;**345**:938.

26 Berlin JA, Colditz GA. The role of meta analysis in the regulatory process for foods, drugs, and devices. *JAMA* 1999;**281**:830–4.

27 Chalmers I, Lindley R. Double standards on informed consent to treatment. In: Doyal L, Tobias JS, eds. *Informed consent: respecting patients' rights in research, teaching and practice*. London: BMJ Books, 2000.

28 Faculty of Pharmaceutical Medicine, Ethical Issues Working Group. Ethics in pharmaceutical medicine. *Int J Pharmaceut Med* 1998;**12**:193–8.

29 Hetherington J, Dickersin K, Chalmers I, Meinert CL. Retrospective and prospective identification of unpublished controlled trials: lessons from a survey of obstetricians and pediatricians. *Pediatrics* 1989;**84**:374–80.

30 Roberts I. An amnesty for unpublished trials. One year on, many trials are unregistered and the amnesty remains open. *BMJ* 1998;**317**:763–4.

31 Simes RJ. Publication bias: the case for an international registry of clinical trials. *J Clin Oncol* 1986;**4**:1529–41.

32 Meinert CL. Toward prospective registration of clinical trials. *Controlled Clin Trials* 1988;**9**:1–5.

33 Dickersin K. Report from the panel on the Case for Registers of Clinical Trials at the 8th Annual Meeting of the Society for Clinical Trials. *Controlled Clin Trials* 1988;**9**:76–81.

34 International Collaborative Group on Clinical Trial Registries. Position paper and consensus statement on clinical trial registries. *Clin Trials Meta-Analyses* 1993;**28**:199–201.

35 Egger M, Davey Smith G. Meta-analysis: bias in location and selection of studies. *BMJ* 1998;**316**:61–6.

36 Harlan W. Current and future collaboration between the National Institutes of Health and the Cochrane Collaboration. Paper presented at the *6th Ann Int Cochrane Colloquium*. Baltimore, 22–26 October, 1998.

37 Sykes R. Being a modern pharmaceutical company. Involves making information available on clinical trial programmes. *BMJ* 1998;**317**:1172.

38 Horton R, Smith R. Time to register randomised trials. *Lancet* 1999;**354**:1138–9.
39 Horton R, Smith R. Time to register randomised trials. *BMJ* 1999;**319**:865–6.
40 Tonks A. Registering clinical trials. *BMJ* 1999;**319**:1565–8.
41 Hampton JR. Alternatives to mega-trials in cardiovascular disease. *Cardiovasc Drugs Therapy* 1997;**10**:759–65.
42 Cowley AJ, Skene A, Stainer K, Hampton JR. The effect of lorcainide on arrhythmias and survival in patients with acute myocardial infarction: an example of publication bias. *Int J Cardiol* 1993;**40**:161–6.
43 Teo KK, Yusuf S, Furberg CD. Effects of prophylactic antiarrhythmic drug therapy in acute myocardial infarction. An overview of results from randomized controlled trials. *JAMA* 1993;**270**:1589–95.
44 Moore T. *Deadly medicine*. New York: Simon and Schuster, 1995.
45 Furberg CD. Effect of antiarrhythmic drugs on mortality after myocardial infarction. *Am J Cardiol* 1983;**52**:32C–36C.
46 Chalmers I. Underreporting research is scientific misconduct. *JAMA* 1990;**263**:1405–8.
47 Lock S, Wells F. Preface to the second edition. In: Lock S, Wells F, eds. *Fraud and misconduct in medical research*. London: BMJ Publishing Group, 1996:xi–xii.
48 Chalmers I, Soll R. Progress and problems in establishing an international registry of perinatal trials. *Controlled Clin Trials* 1991;**12**:630.
49 Medical Research Council. *MRC guidelines for good clinical practice in clinical trials*. London: Medical Research Council, 1998.
50 Wallace M. Research information and the public interest. Paper presented at the *BMJ Conf 50 Years of Clinical Trials: Past, Present and Future*. 29–30 October, London.
51 Chalmers I. Improving the quality and dissemination of reviews of clinical research. In: Lock S, ed. *The future of medical journals: in commemoration of 150 years of the British Medical Journal*. London: BMJ Books, 1991:127–46.
52 Crowther CA, Alfirevic Z, Haslam RR. Antenatal thyrotropin-releasing hormone prior to preterm delivery (Cochrane Review). In: *The Cochrane Library*, Issue 1. Oxford: Update Software, 2000.
53 Elbourne D. Using external evidence as the basis for stopping a trial: example of the antenatal TRH trial. Paper prepared for the *BMJ Conf 50 Years of Clinical Trials: Past, Present, Future*. 29–30 October, London.
54 DeMets DL, Pocock SJ, Julian DG. The agonising negative trend in monitoring of clinical trials. *Lancet* 1999;**354**:1983–8.
55 Effect of the antiarrhythmic agent moricizine on survival after myocardial infarction. The Cardiac Arrhythmia Suppression Trial II Investigators. *N Engl J Med* 1992; **327**:227–33.
56 MacMahon S, Collins R, Peto R, Koster RW, Yusuf S. Effects of prophylactic lidocaine in suspected acute myocardial infarction. An overview of results from the randomized, controlled trials. *JAMA* 1988;**260**:1910–16.
57 Hine LK, Laird N, Hewitt P, Chalmers TC. Meta-analytic evidence against prophylactic use of lidocaine in acute myocardial infarction. *Arch Int Med* 1989;**149**:2694–8.
58 Randomised trial of intravenous atenolol among 16 027 cases of suspected acute myocardial infarction: ISIS-1. First International Study of Infarct Survival Collaborative Group. *Lancet* 1986;**2**:57–66.
59 Yusuf S, Peto R, Lewis J, Collins R, Sleight P. Beta blockade during and after myocardial infarction: an overview of the randomized trials. *Prog Cardiovasc Dis* 1985;**17**:335–71.
60 Chalmers I, Haynes RB. Reporting, updating and correcting systematic reviews of the effects of health care. In: Chalmers I, Altman DG, eds. *Systematic reviews*. London: BMJ Publishing Group, 1995:86–95.
61 Smith R. What is publication? *BMJ* 1999;**318**:142.
62 Begg C, Cho M, Eastwood S, *et al*. Improving the quality of reporting of randomized controlled trials. The CONSORT statement. *JAMA* 1996;**276**:637–9.
63 Clarke M, Chalmers I. Discussion sections in reports of controlled trials published in general medical journals: islands in search of continents? *JAMA* 1998;**280**:280–2.
64 Jefferson T, Deeks J. The use of systematic reviews for editorial peer-reviewing: a population approach. In: Godlee F, Jefferson T, eds. *Peer review in health sciences*. London: BMJ Books, 1999:224–34.

65 Delamothe T, Müllner M, Smith R. Pleasing both authors and readers. A combination of short print articles and longer electronic ones may help us do this. *BMJ* 1999;**318**:888–9.
66 Chalmers I, Hetherington J, Elbourne D, Keirse MJNC, Enkin M. Materials and methods used in synthesizing evidence to evaluate the effects of care during pregnancy and childbirth. In: Chalmers I, Enkin M, Keirse MJNC, eds. *Effective care in pregnancy and childbirth.* Oxford: Oxford University Press, 1989:39–65.
67 Chalmers I, Altman DG. How can medical journals help prevent poor medical research? Some opportunities presented by electronic publishing. *Lancet* 1999;**353**:490–3.
68 Chalmers I. Foreword. In: Egger M, Davey Smith G, Altman DG, eds. *Systematic reviews in health care: meta-analysis in context.* London: BMJ Books, 2000.

Part VI: The Cochrane Collaboration

25 The Cochrane Collaboration in the 20th century

GERD ANTES, ANDREW D OXMAN
for the Cochrane Collaboration

Summary points

- The Cochrane Collaboration is an international organisation of health care professionals, practising physicians, researchers and consumers.
- The Collaboration aims to help people make well-informed decisions about health care by preparing, maintaining and promoting the accessibility of systematic reviews.
- The main work of the Collaboration is done by about 50 Collaborative Review Groups that take on the task of preparing and maintaining Cochrane reviews.
- The Collaboration fosters the development and improvement of methods used in systematic reviews and the establishment of registers of controlled trials.
- The output of the Collaboration is published in the *The Cochrane Library* which is available on CD-ROM and on the internet. *The Cochrane Library* contains the *Cochrane Database of Systematic Reviews*, the *Cochrane Controlled Trials Register* and other databases.

Health care professionals, researchers, policy makers and people using health services are overwhelmed with unmanageable amounts of information. As discussed in chapter 1 systematic reviews are essential, although not sufficient, to make informed decisions and thus prevent undue delays in the introduction of effective treatments and the continued use of ineffective or even harmful interventions. The Cochrane Collaboration's logo (see Figure 25.1) illustrates a systematic review of seven randomised controlled trials (RCTs) of a short, inexpensive course of a corticosteroid given to women about to give birth too early, comparing the intervention with placebo. A schematic representation of the forest plot (see Chapter 1) is shown. The first of these RCTs was reported in 1972, the last in 1980.

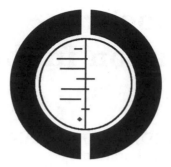

Figure 25.1 The Cochrane logo.

The diagram summarises the evidence that would have been revealed, had the available RCTs been reviewed systematically a decade later: it indicates strongly that corticosteroids reduce the risk of babies dying from the complications of immaturity. Because no systematic review of these trials had been published until 1989, most obstetricians had not realised that the treatment was so effective, reducing the odds of the babies of these women dying from the complications of immaturity by 30–50%. As a result, tens of thousands of premature babies have probably suffered and died unnecessarily, and needed more expensive treatment than was necessary. By 1991, seven more trials had been reported, and the picture had become stronger still.

The ambitious aim of the Cochrane Collaboration is to prepare, maintain and promote the accessibility of systematic reviews in all areas of health care. The Cochrane Collaboration is intrinsically linked to the development of the science of systematic review and much of the progress described in this book was to some extent influenced, if not driven, by the Collaboration. In this chapter we will describe the historical developments that led to this unique enterprise, which has been compared to the Human Genome Project in its potential implications for modern health care.[1] We will discuss the Collaboration's remit and structure and describe its output at the end of the 20th century. The second chapter in this section will address the considerable challenges that the Cochrane Collaboration faces going into the next millennium.

Background and history

In 1972 the British epidemiologist Archie Cochrane drew attention to our great collective ignorance about the effects of health care in his influential book "Effectiveness and efficiency. Random reflections on health services"[2] Cochrane recognised that people who want to make informed decisions about health care do not have ready access to reliable reviews of the available evidence.[3] His book and the discussion stimulated by it inspired what in retrospect can be seen as a pilot project for the Cochrane Collaboration.[4] Beginning in 1974 all controlled trials in perinatal medicine were systematically identified and assembled in a trials register. By 1985 the register contained more than 3500 reports of controlled trials, leading to the preparation of around 600 systematic reviews in the late 1980s. In 1987, the year before his death, Cochrane referred to a collection of systematic reviews of randomised controlled trials (RCTs) of care during pregnancy and childbirth, based on this work, as "a real milestone in the history of randomised trials and in the evaluation of care". He suggested that other specialities should follow this example.[5] In the same year, the scientific quality of reviews published in major medical journals was shown to leave much to be desired.[6] Subsequently, the need for systematically prepared reviews became increasingly recognised.

In response to Cochrane's call for systematic, up-to-date reviews of all relevant RCTs of health care, the Research and Development Programme, initiated to support the British National Health Service (NHS), provided funding to establish a "Cochrane Centre", to "facilitate the preparation of systematic reviews of randomised trials of health care". This centre was opened in Oxford in October 1992.[7,8] Facilitated by a meeting organised by the New York Academy of Sciences six months later,[9] the idea spread around the world and led to the formal launch of the Cochrane Collaboration at the first Cochrane Colloquium, which was held in Oxford in October 1993. By the end of 1994 six further Cochrane Centres had been founded in Europe, North America and Australia. Ten groups were established to prepare reviews within different areas of healthcare and groups were formed to address methodological issues. The Collaboration was registered as a charity in May 1995. A steep increase in activities followed. New groups were established, attendance at the annual colloquia grew rapidly and the number of contributors to the Collaboration grew exponentially. At the end of the 20th century, more than 4000 health professionals, scientists and consumers participate in the Collaboration, in a structured and transparent framework of over 80 registered entities. These are open to anyone who wants to contribute to the enormous task that the Collaboration has undertaken.

Mission, principles and organisation

The Cochrane Collaboration is an international organisation that aims to help people make well-informed decisions about healthcare by preparing, maintaining and promoting the accessibility of systematic reviews of the effects of healthcare interventions.

Box 25.1 Principles of the Cochrane Collaboration

- Collaboration, by internally and externally fostering good communications, open decision-making and teamwork.
- Building on the enthusiasm of individuals, by involving and supporting people of different skills and backgrounds.
- Avoiding duplication, by good management and co-ordination to maximise economy of effort.
- Minimising bias, through a variety of approaches such as scientific rigour, ensuring broad participation, and avoiding conflicts of interest.
- Keeping up to date, by a commitment to ensure that Cochrane reviews are maintained through identification and incorporation of new evidence.
- Striving for relevance, by promoting the assessment of healthcare interventions using outcomes that matter to people making choices in health care.
- Promoting access, by wide dissemination of the outputs of the Collaboration, taking advantage of strategic alliances, and by promoting appropriate prices, content and media to meet the needs of users worldwide.
- Ensuring quality, by being open and responsive to criticism, applying advances in methodology, and developing systems for quality improvement.
- Continuity, by ensuring that responsibility for reviews, editorial processes and key functions is maintained and renewed.
- Enabling wide participation in the work of the collaboration by reducing barriers to contributing and by encouraging diversity.

The work and the organisation of the Collaboration in its efforts to achieve these aims are guided by ten principles (Box 25.1). These principles and a transparent structure are crucial in light of the enormous diversity in disciplinary and cultural backgrounds of the people who are working together in the Collaboration. The Collaboration consists of five types of entities, in addition to a Steering Group. Each of these is described below and a detailed description of each registered entity is maintained in *The Cochrane Library*, which is described below.[10] To register as an entity within the Collaboration a group must formally apply to the Steering Group. This process and the criteria that are used to assess applications for each type of entity are described in the Cochrane Manual (Box 25.2). The Collaboration is a decentralised organisation in which each entity is responsible for its own management and securing its own funding. The Steering Group together with the Cochrane Centres are responsible for monitoring the progress of entities as well as registering, or should the need arise, de-registering entities.

Box 25.2 Information about the Cochrane Collaboration

Web sites
Adelaide, Australia: *www.cochrane.org.au/*
Hamilton, Canada: *http://hiru.mcmaster.ca/cochrane/*
Freiburg, Germany: *www.cochrane.de*

Additional sites can be found at any of the above addresses, including mirror sites, sites in other languages, and sites maintained by Cochrane entities: www.cochrane.org/cochrane/ccweb.htm

Documents

Cochrane brochure	*www.cochrane.org/cochrane/cc-broch.htm*
Cochrane leaflet	*www.cochrane.org/cochrane/leaflet.htm*
Cochrane Manual	*www.cochrane.org/cochrane/cc-man.htm*
Cochrane Reviewers' Handbook	*www.cochrane.org/cochrane/hbook.htm*
Steering Group minutes	*www.cochrane.org/cochrane/document.htm*
Cochrane Consumers Network	*www.cochrane.org/cochrane/consumer.htm*
About the Cochrane Library	*www.update-software.com/cochrane.htm*

Email discussion lists
A list of the Collaboration's email discussion lists can be found at: *www.cochrane.org/cochrane/maillist.htm*
   Information about how to subscribe to CCinfo, the Collaboration's primary discussion list, can also be found there.

Newsletters and contact details
A selection of current newsletters, including Cochrane News, the Collaboration's newsletter, are posted on the Collaboration's Web sites: *www.cochrane.org/cochrane/newslet.htm*

   Information about additional newsletters can be found in *The Cochrane Library*, in the description of each entity (under "About the Cochrane Collaboration") or by contacting relevant entities.
   Contact details for all entities in the Collaboration can be found at: *www.cochrane.org/cochrane/crgs.htm*

NHS Centre for Reviews and Dissemination (CRD)
Additional information about the CRD, DARE and other databases prepared and maintained by CRD can be found at: *www.york.ac.uk/inst/crd/*

Collaborative Review Groups

The main work of the Collaboration is done by about 50 Collaborative Review Groups that take on the central task of preparing and maintaining Cochrane reviews. The members of these groups, including researchers, health care professionals, people using the health services (consumers), and others, have come together because they share an interest in ensuring the availability of reliable, up-to-date summaries of evidence relevant to the prevention, treatment and rehabilitation of particular health problems or groups of problems. Each Collaborative Review Group has an editorial base that includes a co-ordinating editor, a review group co-ordinator, a secretary and in many cases a trials search co-ordinator. Others, such as statistical and health economics advisors, and research fellows may also be located at the editorial base. The editorial base is responsible for maintaining a register of all relevant studies within the scope of the Review Group, co-ordinating and supporting the preparation and updating of reviews, and managing the Group's editorial processes.

Each Collaborative Review Group is responsible for preparing a module of reviews within the Group's scope that, together with the modules prepared by other Review Groups, form the Cochrane Database of Systematic Reviews, described below. Other members of the editorial team include additional editors, who must come from more than one country and discipline, a criticism editor, and a consumer representative. Reviewers who prepare and update the reviews included in each Review Group's module come from a variety of countries, disciplines and backgrounds. Other contributors to Collaborative Review Groups include people who help by handsearching journals to identify studies, peer referees and translators.

Cochrane Centres

The work of Collaborative Review Groups and other entities is co-ordinated and supported by 15 Cochrane Centres around the world. Each centre is responsible for providing guidance, training and support for all of the entities and individual contributors within the geographical area for which it is responsible. The Centres are also responsible for providing information to people and organisations wishing to learn more about the Collaboration or wanting to become involved, and for promoting the aims of the Collaboration within the areas for which they are responsible.

Method Groups

Methods Groups advise the Collaboration on the methods it uses to prepare, maintain and promote the accessibility of systematic reviews, promote and support relevant empirical methodological research and help

452

to prepare and maintain systematic reviews of relevant methodological research. For example, the Statistical Methods Group is, among other things, assessing ways of handling different kinds of data for statistical synthesis, and the Applicability and Recommendations Methods Group is exploring important issues surrounding the application of the results of reviews in making decisions and formulating recommendations. The results from ongoing methodological research are presented and discussed at the annual Cochrane Colloquia. Publications, other reports, workshops and meetings of each Methods Group are included together with a description of the Group's background, scope and contributors in *The Cochrane Library*.

Fields

Fields (or Networks) are groups of people with a broad interest that cuts across a number of Collaborative Review Groups. The focus can be on the setting of care (e.g. primary care), the type of consumer (e.g. older people), the type of intervention (e.g. vaccines), or a broad category of problems (e.g. cancer). Fields contribute to achieving the aims of the Collaboration by searching for trials within their area of interest and contributing these to the *Cochrane Controlled Trials Register*, described below. They help to ensure that priorities and perspectives in their sphere of interest are reflected in the work of Collaborative Review Groups by commenting on systematic reviews relating to their area of interest. They link reviewers from their area of interest to appropriate Collaborative Review Groups and help to train and support them. They liaise with relevant organisations within their area and over time they may elect to develop specialised databases of reviews plus other information to support decision making by people within their area of interest.

The Consumer Network

Consumers participate throughout the Cochrane Collaboration. Collaborative Review Groups, Fields, and Cochrane Centres all seek input and feedback from consumers, which is considered essential in order to fulfil the Collaboration's aims. The Consumer Network has been established to reflect consumer interests within the Cochrane Collaboration. The basis for the Network is a belief that involvement by consumers in the work of the Collaboration is important, and that this involvement will be enhanced by collaboration among consumers and others. The Consumer Network aims to provide information for consumers and encourage and support the involvement of consumers throughout the Cochrane Collaboration's activities.

Additional information about the Consumer Network can be found on the Collaboration's World Wide Web sites (Box 25.2).

453

The Steering Group

The official membership of the Collaboration consists of all registered entities. Each entity, in turn, determines its own membership, who is eligible to vote for candidates to represent that type of entity on the Collaboration's Steering Group. The Steering Group has fourteen elected members, who meet twice a year, once during the annual Cochrane Colloquia and on one other occasion. The minutes of its meetings are on the Collaboration's web sites (Box 25.2). The Steering Group has overall responsibility for overseeing the development and implementation of policy affecting the Collaboration, and legal responsibility as the Board of Directors for the Collaboration as a registered charity. Subgroups and advisory groups accountable to the Steering Group are described in the Cochrane Manual (Box 25.2).

Communication

The creation and maintenance of electronic internet-based communication structures are an essential part of the Collaboration's work, which enables it to function as an efficient global network, at relatively low costs. Several electronic mailing lists exist for exchange of information (Box 25.2). The "CCinfo" list is the primary email list for the Cochrane Collaboration. It aims to keep members of the Collaboration well informed about the activities and policies of the Collaboration. It is moderated (all items are checked for suitability before being distributed to subscribers) and compiled several times each month. It is open to anybody with an interest in the Collaboration.

A wealth of material is found on the Collaboration's web pages, which are mirrored at several places to allow quick access from all parts of the world (Box 25.2). The pages contain general information about the Collaboration, including contact details, information about workshops and meetings and the abstracts of all Cochrane reviews. Cochrane web pages can also be found in languages other than English and several entities have their own web pages. Documents, such as the Cochrane Reviewers' Handbook, and the Collaboration's Review Manager software (see Chapter 15) are available on the web sites and file transfer protocol (FTP) servers.

In addition to this wide array of electronic communication, many entities publish newsletters and a number of publications describing the Collaboration are available. Cochrane News, published by the Collaboration, and a number of other Newsletters published by Cochrane entities, are also available on the Collaboration web sites.

Output of the Cochrane Collaboration

The efforts of the Cochrane Collaboration are focussed on producing and maintaining up-to-date systematic reviews, which are available, together with other databases, in *The Cochrane Library*. *The Cochrane Library* may be purchased on CD-ROM or subscribed to on the internet directly from its publisher[10] or from several other providers. Both the CD-ROM and online versions of *The Cochrane Library* are currently updated quarterly. Increasingly the Library is being made available to individuals through group subscriptions and it is the aim of the Collaboration to minimise cost as a barrier to access to its products.

The Cochrane Library contains the following databases that can be searched simultaneously with the search engine provided:

- The Cochrane Database of Systematic Reviews (CDSR). CDSR is a rapidly growing collection of regularly updated, systematic reviews of the effects of health care, maintained by the Cochrane Collaboration. This is the primary product of the Cochrane Collaboration.

  A unique feature of The Cochrane Database of Systematic Reviews is that Cochrane reviews, unlike other published reviews, can be updated when new data become available or in the light of comments, criticisms and suggestions. The Comments and Criticisms System that is an integral component of The Cochrane Database of Systematic Reviews is not yet being used as extensively as we would wish, but it holds the promise of a "democratisation" of "post-publication peer review", and the potential to reduce the time required to identify and correct errors.

- Database of Abstracts of Reviews of Effectiveness (DARE). DARE aims to include structured abstracts of all recent non-Cochrane systematic reviews of the effects of health care and diagnostic test accuracy published in journals and elsewhere. The NHS Centre for Reviews and Dissemination (CRD) at the University of York critically appraises the reviews, prepares the structured abstracts and maintains DARE (see Box 25.2).

- The Cochrane Controlled Trials Register (CCTR). CCTR is a bibliography of controlled trials, downloaded from databases like MEDLINE and EMBASE or identified as part of an international effort to hand-search the world's journals and create an unbiased source of data for systematic reviews (see Chapter 4 for a detailed description of CCTR).

- The Cochrane Review Methodology Database (CRMD). CRMD is a bibliography of articles and books on the science of research synthesis and evaluations of the effects of health care.

- About the Cochrane Collaboration. This is a compilation of descriptions of each entity within the Collaboration maintained by the respective entities.

- Other sources of information. This currently includes the list of internet sites relevant to evidence based practice which is produced by the School of Health and Related Research (ScHARR) at the University of Sheffield. A collection of titles and abstracts of reports from various health technology assessment agencies is also included in this section.

The Library also includes the Cochrane Reviewers' Handbook,[11] which describes policies and provides guidelines for preparing and maintaining Cochrane reviews, and a glossary of terminology used in the Cochrane Collaboration and relevant methodological terms. Future plans for *The Cochrane Library* include improving the interface and adding additional databases, including databases of economic analyses (maintained by CRD), systematic reviews of diagnostic test accuracy (under development), and systematic reviews of methodological research (prepared by the Cochrane Empirical Methodological Studies Methods Group).

Box 25.3 Articles that provide useful descriptions of the Cochrane Collaboration and its development.

Chalmers I, Enkin M, Keirse MJNC. Preparing and updating systematic reviews of randomized controlled trials of health care. *Milbank Q* 1993;**71**:411–37.

Chalmers I. The Cochrane Collaboration: preparing, maintaining, and disseminating systematic reviews of the effects of health care. *Ann NY Acad Sci* 1993;**703**:156–65.

Chalmers I, Haynes RB. Reporting, updating and correcting systematic reviews of the effects of health care. *BMJ* 1994;**309**:862–5.

Bero L, Rennie D. The Cochrane Collaboration: preparing, maintaining and disseminating systematic reviews of the effects of health care. *JAMA* 1995;**274**:1935–8.

Chalmers I, Sackett D, Silagy C. The Cochrane Collaboration. In: Maynard A, Chalmers I, eds. *Non-random reflections on health services research*. London: BMJ Publishing Group, 1997:231–49.

Dickersin K, Manheimer E. The Cochrane Collaboration: evaluation of health care and services using systematic reviews of the results of randomized controlled trials. *Clin Obstet Gynecol* 1998;**41**:315–31.

Conclusion

Six years after its foundation and after a period of dynamic evolution, the Cochrane Collaboration has established guiding principles, a set of policies, an organisational structure and mechanisms for communication that offer a rich environment for reviewers and other contributors to achieving its aim of preparing, maintaining and promoting the accessibility of systematic reviews of the effects of healthcare. The rapidly growing number of reviews published in the Cochrane Database of Systematic Reviews demonstrates that this support is appreciated by an increasing number of individuals in all areas of healthcare. The Collaboration's growth is driven by the improved acceptance of systematic reviews in many countries around the globe. However, the continuing international expansion leads to new challenges by introducing a new level of diversity, with respect to differences in cultural and social background, available resources and language. As discussed in the following chapter the transformation of a group of enthusiastic individuals into an efficient international organisation is at the heart of this process. Looking back on the work of the last six years there is ample reason to believe that the forthcoming challenges will be met successfully.

Acknowledgements

We would like to acknowledge the generous efforts of the thousands of contributors to the Cochrane Collaboration who together have helped turn a bright idea into a reality and collectively continue to define the Collaboration and determine its development. This chapter is based in part on the Cochrane Collaboration brochure and other source documents listed in Box 25.2.

1 Naylor CD. Grey zones of clinical practice: some limitations to evidence-based medicine. *Lancet* 1995;**345**:840–3.
2 Cochrane A. *Effectiveness and efficiency. Random reflections on health services.* London: Nuffield Provincial Hospital Trust, 1972. See http://www.cochrane.org/cochrane/cchronol.htm for a chronology of the development of the Cochrane Collaboration.
3 Cochrane AL. 1931–71: a critical review, with particular reference to the medical profession. In: *Medicines for the Year 2000.* London: Office of Health Economics, 1979:1–11.
4 Chalmers I. The work of the national perinatal epidemiology unit. *Int J Technol Assess Health Care* 1991;**7**:430–59.
5 Cochrane AL. Foreword. In: Chalmers I, Enkin M, Keirse MJNC, eds. *Effective care in pregnancy and childbirth.* Oxford: Oxford University Press, 1989.
6 Mulrow CD. The medical review article: state of the science. *Ann Intern Med* 1987;**106**:485–8.
7 Chalmers I, Dickersin K, Chalmers TC. Getting to grips with Archie Cochrane's agenda. *BMJ* 1992;**305**:786–8.
8 Anon. Cochrane's legacy. *Lancet* 1992;**340**:1131–2.

9 Chalmers I. The Cochrane Collaboration: preparing, maintaining and disseminating systematic reviews of the effects of health care. In: Warren KS, Mosteller F, eds. *Doing more good than harm: the evaluation of health care interventions. Ann NY Acad Sci* 1993;**703**:156–63.
10 *The Cochrane Library*. Oxford: Update Software, 1999.
11 Clarke M, Oxman AD, eds. *Cochrane Reviewers' Handbook 4.0* (updated July 1999). In: *The Cochrane Library* Issue 1. Oxford: Update Software, 2000.

26 The Cochrane Collaboration in the 21st century: ten challenges and one reason why they must be met

ANDREW D OXMAN

Summary points

- While the Cochrane Collaboration has a simple aim, there are formidable challenges that must be met to achieve this aim.
- Ethical and social challenges include finding ways to continue to build on enthusiasm while avoiding duplication and minimising bias, to promote access while ensuring continuity, to ensure sustainability and to accommodate diversity.
- Logistical challenges include finding ways to efficiently identify trials and manage criticisms and updates of reviews.
- Methodological challenges include developing sound guidelines for deciding what types of studies to include in reviews, effective ways of communicating the results of reviews and summarising the strength of evidence for specific effects, and effective ways of involving consumers.
- These challenges must be met because there is no acceptable alternative.

As described in the previous chapter, the Cochrane Collaboration is an international organisation that aims to help people make well informed decisions about healthcare by preparing, maintaining and promoting the accessibility of systematic reviews of the effects of healthcare interventions. In this chapter I will discuss major challenges to achieving these aims, six years after the Collaboration began in 1993. These include ethical, social, logistical and methodological challenges (Box 26.1). While these challenges are most relevant to contributors to the Cochrane Collaboration and users of its products, anyone who shares the desire to have available

Box 26.1 The ten challenges and one reason why they must be met

Ethical challenges
  1   Building on enthusiasm while avoiding duplication
  2   Building on enthusiasm while minimising bias
  3   Promoting access while ensuring continuity

Social challenges
  4   Ensuring sustainability
  5   Accomodating diversity

Logistical challenges
  6   Identifying trials
  7   Managing criticisms and updating reviews

Methodological challenges
  8   Deciding what types of studies to include in reviews
  9   Summarising the strength of evidence
  10   Effectively involving consumers

Why these challenges must be met
There are no acceptable alternatives

systematic summaries of current best evidence for people making decisions, both within and outside of healthcare, must address similar issues.

Ethical challenges

Ethical challenges arise when there is a conflict between principles.[1] For example, the principle of doing good (beneficence) is frequently in conflict with the principle of allowing people to make their own decisions (autonomy). When the balance shifts too far towards beneficence this might be considered paternalistic, whereas it might be considered irresponsible if the balance shifts too far towards autonomy. Different people, of course, may have different views of what the appropriate balance is with respect to specific decisions or actions. The Cochrane Collaboration's work is based on ten key principles (see Chapter 25). Not surprisingly, conflicts arise between these principles and finding the right balance is a challenge. Three such challenges are considered here.

Building on enthusiasm while avoiding duplication

Preparing and maintaining systematic reviews is demanding work. Getting it done and doing it right depend on the enthusiasm of the people who undertake this work, particularly reviewers. Because there are so few people with the enthusiasm, skills and resources to prepare and then keep up-to-date systematic reviews, it is important to avoid duplication of effort. In addition to being a poor use of scarce resources, undesired duplication can result in confusion and conflict. Finding an appropriate balance between building on the enthusiasm of individuals and avoiding duplication of effort has been a challenge for the Collaboration from its beginning.

Individuals who have organised themselves around common interests such as stroke, schizophrenia and sexually transmitted diseases undertake the work of the Collaboration. It was agreed when the Collaboration first started that the best way to organise these groups, called Collaborative Review Groups (CRGs), would be around problems. However, peoples' enthusiasms do not fall naturally into non-overlapping sets of problems. In forming CRGs we have, for the most part, tended to rely on the principle of building on enthusiasm. After six years there are approximately 50 review groups that cover most of healthcare with relatively few holes. Thus far, there has been almost no conflict between review groups as to which group should be responsible for reviews that are of interest to more than one group; e.g. hypertension in diabetes or malaria prophylaxis in pregnancy. This is largely a tribute to the extent to which people adhere to our first principle: collaboration. However, deciding how to form questions that fit together in a coherent framework (with minimal undesired duplication), while responding to and supporting the enthusiasm of individual reviewers who may have questions that do not fit neatly into that framework, is still a challenge.

As with any research the first and most important step is asking the right question. There is no simple answer to how big or small a question should be for a review or to what makes a good question. It is desirable to avoid reviews that ask questions that are "too large" or "too small". Reviews that are too large and complex may be difficult for people to use and difficult to maintain. On the other hand, because of the risks of subgroup analysis,[2-4] a review should not arbitrarily focus on a subgroup of studies based on patient characteristics, the setting, or characteristics of the intervention; unless there is a solid rationale for doing so. Focusing on a subgroup of studies can result in spurious conclusions, as illustrated by the miracle of DICE therapy for acute stroke,[5] or miss an important effect, such as mortality associated with general anaesthesia compared with local or regional anaesthesia across different surgical procedures.

Cochrane reviews should almost never be split-up based on outcomes, both because of the duplication of effort that this is likely to involve and because it is unlikely to make sense from the perspective of someone using a review to make a practical decision. For example, someone deciding about hormone replacement therapy is likely to be interested in all its important effects, including possible benefits, such as reducing the risk of fractures and cardiovascular disease, and possible adverse effects, such as increasing the risk of breast cancer. From this perspective, it would be unhelpful, as well as inefficient, for each of the many review groups with an interest in this intervention to focus only on the outcomes that they consider within their scope.

There remains a large middle ground between reviews that are too large or small where, hopefully, through both experience and methodology we will find the right balance. The human challenge is more difficult; i.e. how to accommodate the interests of enthusiastic individuals with overlapping interests and avoid any pretence of monopolising areas. It is unlikely that a permanent fix will be found for this challenge. Ongoing vigilance is required from both within and outside the Collaboration. We must remain open to criticism and responsive to people with new ideas. If we do not, the Collaboration will stagnate.

In addition, we must ensure that there is enthusiasm for addressing important questions, whether there is evidence to answer those questions or not. Unfortunately, academic and other incentives are likely to generate the most enthusiasm for questions where there is evidence, even though those questions may sometimes be of trivial importance. Often it is more important to address questions where little or nothing is known, to make this clear to people making decisions now, and to support decisions to undertake new research to answer important questions for which there is no evidence.

Building on enthusiasm while minimising bias

A fundamental argument for the Cochrane Collaboration, and systematic reviews in general, is to provide summaries of what we know, and do not know, that are as free from bias as possible. However, there are at least three important ways in which balancing our need to build on the enthusiasm of contributors with our aim to minimise bias represents a major challenge. Firstly, people who have an enthusiasm for summarising the evidence on a particular topic often have strong opinions, which can sometimes result in biased judgements about how a review is done or how the results are presented, discussed and interpreted. Since our experience and our surroundings influence us all in various ways, this problem will never be completely eliminated. By continually striving to develop ways of making both the methods and assumptions underlying a review as explicit and clear as possible, we can reduce this problem. Because the methods and assumptions underlying Cochrane reviews are published first in protocols that describe the process that will be used in preparing a review, and subsequently in completed reviews, these are open to criticism and revision both before and after completion of a review. To succeed this must be coupled, again, with remaining open and responsive to criticisms. Although explicit declarations of potential conflicts of interest might also help, relatively little is known about how to ensure that important conflicts of interest are identified and reported. How often important potential conflicts of interest are hidden behind the standard "none known" statement under this heading is unknown, although there is some evidence that financial conflicts of interest are underreported.[6] Underreporting is likely to be at least as common for other types of conflicts of interest. Studying this problem and developing an empirical basis for reducing the risks of conflicts of interest is a challenge that is likely to remain so at least until the next edition of this book.

Secondly, enthusiasms that are related to competing interests, that is interests that are secondary to achieving the aims of the Cochrane Collaboration, can be a problem in other ways, particularly interests that are related to funding. For example, review groups may be tempted to lower their standards for reviews or to split reviews inappropriately, if their funding is contingent on the quantity of reviews they produce. Reviewers may be slow to respond to criticisms and update reviews, if their initial enthusiasm was related to the availability of external funding for preparing a review and there is no funding for maintaining it. A lack of academic recognition for maintaining a review after it is first published might have a similar effect. Maintaining enthusiasm and avoiding bias and other problems arising from competing or conflicting interests depends firstly on recognising these problems. Beyond this, it is necessary to foster a culture and conditions within the Cochrane Collaboration in which quality and the importance of keeping reviews up-to-date are highly valued, and to promote these values outside of the Collaboration.

Thirdly, enthusiasm alone is not sufficient to enable people to contribute effectively to Cochrane reviews. This is especially true for people from low and middle-income countries who do not have the resources to participate in the Collaboration. If we do not actively promote and seek resources to support their participation, we risk having a biased perspective in reviews, if reviewers make assumptions based on circumstances in wealthier countries. We also risk having a biased selection in the topics that are reviewed, with inadequate coverage of problems that are most important to the majority of the world's people. While this may simply reflect the distribution of resources for both healthcare research and health services in the world, we must strive to do better than this.

463

Promoting access while ensuring continuity

The third ethical conflict that I would identify as being amongst the most important challenges that must be addressed by the Cochrane Collaboration is between promoting access to Cochrane Reviews and ensuring the continuity of our work. A great deal of work goes into preparing a systematic review. Cochrane reviews require an ongoing commitment after they are first published: to update searches for new relevant studies, to respond to valid criticisms, and to update reviews in the light of new developments. The main responsibility for maintaining a review lies with the reviewers, almost all of whom do this because of a personal interest in the topic of the review. This is often done in connection with a professional responsibility to keep up-to-date on a topic. However, preparing, maintaining and promoting the accessibility of the *Cochrane Database of Systematic Reviews* requires the collaboration of thousands of people to search for studies, translate, provide methodological training and support, referee and edit material, provide administrative and technological support, and to co-ordinate this work. Although the Cochrane Collaboration is built on shared aims and the principles summarised in chapter 25, achieving our aims requires resources. Balancing the need to secure these resources, while at the same time trying to ensure that the results of all this effort are available, and affordable, to everyone is indeed challenging. I believe this is primarily a challenge in the short term and that we will meet this challenge. It reflects the transitional phase in which we are: transforming from a relatively small group of idealistic individuals to a large, efficient international organisation. The challenge is to make this transition without sacrificing our principles.

Social challenges

Ensuring sustainability

Cochrane review groups have between zero and 150 completed reviews and up to 65 protocols each. The number of completed reviews is growing by over 200 new reviews per year and the number of new protocols is growing more rapidly, indicating an increase in the production of new reviews as CRGs become established. This alone requires a tremendous effort. On top of this, CRGs must continue to develop and maintain specialised registers of trials within their scope, update an increasing number of reviews each year, respond to criticisms and keep up with methodological, technological and organisational developments. Although this work is shared by thousands of people around the world, this represents more of a workload for some than for others and there are signs of exhaustion from many people with heavy workloads within the Collaboration.

There is a great deal of pressure on the Collaboration to constantly improve both the quantity and the quality of its work. This comes from those that fund the work, users and, perhaps most, from those who are doing the work, our selves. The *Cochrane Database of Systematic Reviews* contains hundreds of reviews and protocols, but these represent only a fraction of the questions that are important to people making decisions about healthcare. We need to and want to act quickly and well to fill the large void that exists for people who want to make better-informed decisions about healthcare interventions. However, this pressure is taking its toll. For the Collaboration to survive, and achieve its aims, we must have reasonable expectations of how quickly we can progress. These expectations must be constantly adjusted and conveyed both internally and externally. Above all, we must value and nurture the most precious resource we have, the many hard working people who are needed to achieve the aims of the Collaboration.

Accommodating diversity

The Collaboration requires a wide range of people from different backgrounds and cultures who bring with them different types of expertise. This diversity is a strength of the Cochrane Collaboration. It is also a challenge to find ways of accommodating this diversity. This requires good communication across different languages and varying degrees of background knowledge and familiarity with the Collaboration. It also requires avoiding ways of communicating that are understood by those that are inside the Collaboration but exclude those who are not. One sign that the Cochrane Collaboration is succeeding is the fuzzy boundaries that exist between contributors and users. At the same time, there is a risk inherent in this: neglecting the needs of active contributors within the Collaboration and not adequately supporting their continuing education and development. Finding the right balance between these sometimes-competing needs is not easy. It is most clearly manifest at the annual meetings of the Cochrane Collaboration (Cochrane Colloquia, see Chapter 25). Over the past several years we have striven to ensure that newcomers are welcome at the Colloquia. However, in avoiding exclusivity we have to some extent sacrificed opportunities to meet the needs of active contributors to the Collaboration.

Many difficulties arise in communication arising from language differences, cultural norms relating to interpersonal interactions, and power relations between north and south (partly arising from vestiges of colonialism and partly from imbalances in resources). Much has been done to address these difficulties already, particularly by some CRGs, Cochrane Centres and individuals. However, we still have a long way to go. We must continually struggle to improve and to address imbalances due to language or resource differences, and we must avoid assumptions based on any particular set of cultural norms.

Logistical challenges

Identifying trials

Over 1100 journals are being hand-searched by the Cochrane Collaboration, and MEDLINE, EMBASE and other bibliographic databases are being systematically and thoroughly searched for trials. This is a huge effort, which has resulted in the identification of over a quarter of a million reports of trials (see Chapter 4). There are still thousands of journals that are not being hand searched and many other electronic search strategies that might be used to identify trials. However, the backlog of completed healthcare trials is likely to be less than half the one million estimated by Chalmers and Haynes in 1994.[7] Because of overlap among different sources and because sources with the highest yield are being searched first, there are steeply diminishing returns on additional efforts to identify trials. Moreover, as long as the focus of these search strategies is on published reports, the results are likely to be biased (see Chapter 3).[8-11] The only way to avoid this bias is through prospective registration of trials.[10-12] In the same way that reviews are limited by the quality of the evidence that is available, the work of the Cochrane Collaboration in identifying trials is limited by the availability of complete registers of trials. Although the Cochrane Collaboration can support the development of registers of trials, ultimately this will depend on a commitment from governments, research funders, ethics committees and others. The need for prospective registration has been identified for well over a decade.[13] Although responses to this recognised need have been frustratingly slow, there are reasons for increased optimism now (see Chapter 4).[14-17] As prospective registration becomes more widely implemented, the role of the Cochrane Collaboration in identifying trials should change dramatically. Meanwhile, for at least the next five years, we will need to continue to struggle at the margin. To a large extent, this reflects the need to clean up after over five decades of healthcare trials with inadequate systems for organising the results of this extensive investment of resources.

Managing criticisms and updating reviews

Cochrane reviews, like other systematic reviews and research reports, must be read critically (see also Chapters 5 and 7). Publication in the

Cochrane Database of Systematic Reviews does not guarantee that a review is free of bias or errors. Empirical research indicates that Cochrane reviews are, on average, more methodologically rigorous, more frequently updated and less likely to show evidence of bias than meta-analyses published in journals.[18,19] This does not mean that Cochrane reviews do not have shortcomings or that there are not ways in which Cochrane reviews in general can be improved. While critics of the Collaboration are quick to point out general shortcomings, the majority of feedback received through our criticism management system, from systematic assessments of various aspects of Cochrane reviews and provided informally, comes from people working within the Collaboration. Nonetheless, the amount of criticism is already a burden on review groups, which are expected to respond promptly to criticisms and comments. Ingenuity will be needed to develop mechanisms that encourage submission of valid criticisms that will lead to improvements in reviews, while not overwhelming review groups.

Similarly, ingenuity is needed to find ways of supporting reviewers and CRGs in their efforts to update reviews in the light of new evidence. A unique feature of Cochrane reviews is that they are updated. Although the Collaboration has a policy that reviews should be updated at least yearly, this has proven difficult to implement. Some reviews published in the *Cochrane Database of Systematic Reviews* are already seriously out of date. Addressing this problem is at least as important as producing new reviews that address other important questions.

One way in which this problem must be addressed is by ensuring that people who first express an interest in preparing a Cochrane review understand that this carries with it an obligation to update the review on an ongoing basis. It is mutually beneficial for CRGs and organisations that commission systematic reviews to use those resources to prepare Cochrane reviews. However, in doing so it is essential that we adhere to the principle of building on the enthusiasm of individuals, who have an interest in updating a review beyond the period for which they are funded to first prepare the review. Ignoring this principle may help produce new Cochrane reviews, but it will create serious problems with maintaining those reviews.

Methodological challenges

Although meta-analyses have been published for almost a century (see also Chapter 1),[20-23] the science of systematically reviewing research is young.[24-25] It is only during the past two decades that attention has been paid to the scientific quality of reviews in the social sciences and healthcare. Nonetheless, there has been a heartening growth of both interest and empirical research regarding the methods that are used to summarise

467

evidence. The Cochrane Review Methodology Database contains over 1000 references relevant to systematic reviews of the effects of healthcare, many of which are reports of empirical methodological research.[27] This includes studies and papers that address a wide range of methodological issues regarding the formulation of questions, identification of studies, data collection, assessment of study quality, meta-analysis, and interpreting and reporting the results of reviews. There are many unanswered questions concerning decisions about what methods to use when preparing a review. Among these there are three questions that I will highlight here as being particularly important challenges for the Cochrane Collaboration.

Deciding what types of studies to include in reviews

There are both logical arguments and an empirical basis for using randomised controlled trials (RCTs) to evaluate the effects of healthcare interventions and to restrict systematic reviews to RCTs.[4,28] However, it may sometimes be appropriate to conduct a systematic review of non-randomised studies of the effects of healthcare. For example, occasionally the course of a disease is so uniform or the effects of an intervention are so dramatic that it is unnecessary and unethical to conduct RCTs. Under such circumstances it would not be sensible to restrict a review to RCTs. RCTs might also be difficult, impossible or inappropriate for evaluating the effects of some interventions or some effects, such as rare adverse effects. While attention to the risk of bias should guide decisions about what types of study designs to include in a review, currently individual reviewers and review groups must decide what types of studies are best suited to specific questions. This is a pragmatic solution to deciding where to set the cut-off for what types of studies to include in Cochrane reviews, but *ad hoc* decisions about what types of studies to include may be even more arbitrary than only including RCTs, and they can introduce bias.

The inclusion of non-randomised studies puts additional demands on reviewers to locate studies, assess their quality and analyse the results.[4] Moreover, inconsistency from review to review regarding what types of studies are included is likely to cause confusion and mistrust, if decisions about this appear arbitrary. While the Cochrane Collaboration should continue to focus on systematic reviews of RCTs and non-randomised controlled trials, coherent and transparent decision rules are needed for deciding when only to include RCTs, when to include non-randomised controlled trials and when to include other types of evidence. So far as possible, there should be an empirical basis for these decision rules, as well as logical arguments. Developing that empirical basis is a major challenge (see also Chapters 12–14).

Summarising the strength of evidence

Cochrane reviews should aim to provide the best possible summary of current evidence of the effects of healthcare. Deciding what evidence to include is a first step in doing so. One of the last steps is to summarise the overall level of evidence for each important effect, together with the best estimate of the magnitude of each effect. Developing effective and efficient ways of communicating the evidence is an important challenge for the Cochrane Collaboration, particularly ways of communicating the overall level of evidence for specific effects.

Over the past two decades approaches to characterise explicitly the level of evidence underlying recommendations and the strength of the recommendations have been developed for clinical practice guidelines (see also Chapter 21).[29-33] These have been motivated, in part, by recognition that, although the strength of recommendation should reflect the level of evidence, it also involves other types of information and judgements. Occasionally, the results of a review will be such that no additional information or judgements are needed to make a recommendation. For example, if the effects of an intervention are unequivocally harmful, without any benefit, it may be reasonable to conclude that the intervention should not be used without the need for additional information. More often, healthcare interventions are likely to have some beneficial effects, some harmful effects and costs. There is always some degree of uncertainty about all of these, and other information and judgement are needed to make a decision or recommendation about what should be done. Those making decisions or recommendations must, either implicitly or explicitly, make an assessment about the level of evidence for each effect that is or should be considered. Advantages of doing this systematically and explicitly are that this may reduce the chance of bias, result in more reliable assessments, and make it easier for others to appraise the judgements that were made.

One of the first such approaches was that used by the Canadian Task Force on the Periodic Health Examination.[29] Since then a variety of other approaches have been proposed. To some extent all of these approaches have suffered from lack of clear definitions of what is meant by level of evidence and strength of recommendation, and from difficulties in simplifying a complex assessment into a simple model. For example, the Canadian Task Force and a number of other approaches rely on study design alone to determine the level of evidence. While this is admirable for its simplicity, it ignores many other factors that are relevant to assessing the level of evidence.

If level of evidence is defined as the extent to which one can be confident that an estimate of effect or association is correct, the following considerations are relevant, which are similar to considerations for assessing causal inferences:[4]

469

- How good is the quality of the included studies?
- How large and significant are the observed effects?
- How consistent are the effects across studies?
- Is there a clear dose-response relationship?
- Is there indirect evidence that supports the inference?
- Have other plausible competing explanations of the observed effects been ruled out?

In addition to using an approach that is systematic and explicit, a standard approach across reviews and review groups is desirable to help ensure that the approach is understood by and useful to users of Cochrane reviews. Development of a sensible, empirically based approach to summarising levels of evidence in Cochrane reviews would be an important contribution to ensuring good communication of the results of reviews and achieving the aims of the Collaboration.

Effectively involving consumers

As noted above, preparing, maintaining and promoting the accessibility of systematic reviews of the effects of healthcare interventions requires contributions from a large number of people with different types of expertise and backgrounds. From the beginning of the Cochrane Collaboration it has been recognised that healthcare consumers should be involved in developing Cochrane reviews because they are the ultimate beneficiaries of the work and the reason why we bother, and to help ensure that reviews are:

- targeted at problems that are important to people
- take account of outcomes that are important to those affected
- accessible to people making decisions
- adequately reflect variability in the values and conditions of people, and the circumstances of healthcare in different countries.

Consumers can be involved in reviews in a number of ways, including: helping to determine topics and issues for reviews, as co-reviewers and as referees. While there are strong arguments for involving consumers, relatively little is known about the effectiveness of various means of involving consumers in the review process or, in healthcare research more generally. Involving consumers involves ethical, logistical and social challenges. To address these challenges, it is essential that we learn how to effectively involve consumers in preparing, maintaining and promoting the accessibility of Cochrane reviews. We must develop and evaluate methods to ensure that consumer involvement is not simply a mantra, but an integral – and effective – mechanism for helping to ensure that the aims of the Cochrane Collaboration are achieved.

470

Why these challenges must be met

If the Cochrane Collaboration is to succeed, it will require ongoing efforts to address formidable methodological and logistical challenges. The ethical and social challenges that the Collaboration faces are likely to be even more difficult to address and more important. The boundaries between what I have called ethical, social, logistical and methodological challenges are fuzzy. Others might choose to label them differently, or not use these labels at all. In any case, it is important that we do not neglect any of these challenges, or the ethical, social, logistical and methodological aspects of the challenges that must be addressed.

While I have raised these challenges specifically in the context of the Cochrane Collaboration, they are challenges for anyone who recognises the importance of having summaries of current best evidence readily accessible to decision makers. Similar issues are likely to be important for other types of evidence, such as evidence about diagnostic test accuracy (see Chapter 14), environmental health risks or cost effectiveness (Chapter 23), as well as for evidence about the effects of healthcare. They are also likely to be relevant for evidence of the effects of other types of interventions, such as educational and social interventions.

As formidable as these challenges are, the alternatives to attempting to address them are unacceptable. One such alternative is to rely on non-systematic, out-of-date summaries of evidence, using the occasional systematic, up-to-date summary when one can be found, or delaying a decision until an up-to-date systematic review can be prepared. Another is simply to make decisions without concern for evidence of what the likely consequences are. While these alternatives are common practice today, thanks to the generous, collaborative and often exhausting efforts of thousands of people around the world, they will hopefully not be common practice in the future.

Acknowledgements

I would like to thank Mike Clarke, Monica Fischer, Jini Hetherington, Patrice Matchaba, Chris Silagy and Jimmy Volmink for their helpful comments on a draft of this paper. Untold credit should be given to the many hard working people who are already addressing the challenges discussed here through their contributions to the Cochrane Collaboration. Archie Cochrane, after whom the Cochrane Collaboration is named, issued the challenge that led to the Cochrane Collaboration. Iain Chalmers is responsible for conceiving the Cochrane Collaboration in response to Cochrane's challenge and, as a consequence, creating all of the challenges discussed here for himself and the rest of us.

1 Beauchamp TL, Cildress JF. *Principles of biomedical ethics*, 3rd edn. Oxford: Oxford University Press, 1989:5.
2 Yusuf S, Wittes J, Probstfield J, Tyroler HA. Analysis and interpretation of treatment effects in subgroups of patients in randomized clinical trials. *JAMA* 1991;**266**:93–8.
3 Oxman AD, Guyatt GH. A consumer's guide to subgroup analyses. *Ann Intern Med* 1992;**116**:78–84.
4 Clarke M, Oxman AD, eds. *Cochrane Reviewers' Handbook* (updated July 1999). In: *The Cochrane Library*, Issue 1. Oxford: Update Software, 2000.
5 Counsell CE, Clarke MJ, Slattery J, Sandercock PAG.The miracle of DICE therapy for acute stroke: fact or fictional product of subgroup analysis? *BMJ* 1994;**309**:1677–81.
6 Krimsky S, Rothenberg LS, Stott P, Kyle G. Scientific journals and their authors' financial interests: a pilot study. *Psychother Psychosom* 1998;**67**:194–201.
7 Chalmers I, Haynes RB. Reporting, updating and correcting systematic reviews of the effects of health care. *BMJ* 1994;**309**:862–5.
8 Egger M, Smith GD. Bias in location and selection of studies. *BMJ* 1998;**316**:61–6.
9 Ioannidis JP. Effect of the statistical significance of results on the time to completion and publication of randomized efficacy trials. *JAMA* 1998;**279**:281–6.
10 Dickersin K. How important is publication bias? a synthesis of available data. *AIDS Educat Prev* 1997;**9**:15–21.
11 Stern JM, Simes RJ. Publication bias: evidence of delayed publication in a cohort study of clinical research projects. *BMJ* 1997;**315**:640–5.
12 Chalmers I. Underreporting research is scientific misconduct. *JAMA* 1990;**263**:1405–8.
13 Simes RJ. Publication bias: the case for an international registry of clinical trials. *J Clin Oncol* 1986;**4**:1529–41.
14 Sykes R. Being a modern pharmaceutical company involves making information available on clinical trial programmes. *BMJ* 1998;**317**:1172–80.
15 The metaRegister of Controlled Trials (mRCT). Current Controlled Trials. http://www.controlled-trials.com/frame.cfm?nextframe=mrct. Accessed 21 November 2000.
16 Funded Research. Community of Science. http://fundedresearch.cos.com. Accessed 21 November 2000.
17 The National Research Register. Update Software. http://www.doh.gov.uk/research/nrr.htm. Accessed 21 November 2000.
18 Jadad AR, Cook DJ, Jones A, *et al*. Methodology and reports of systematic reviews and meta-analyses: a comparison of Cochrane reviews with articles published in paper-based journals. *JAMA* 1997;**280**:278–80.
19 Egger M, Smith GD, Schneider M, Minder C. Bias in meta-analysis detected by a simple, graphical test. *BMJ* 1997;**315**:629–34.
20 Pearson K. Report on certain enteric fever inoculation statistics. *BMJ* 1904;**3**:1243–6.
21 Cochran WG. Problems arising in the analysis of a series of similar experiments. *J Roy Stat Soc* 1937;**4**(suppl):102–18.
22 Yates F, Cochran WG. The analysis of groups of experiments. *J Agric Sci* 1938;**28**:556–80.
23 Cochran WG. The combination of estimates from different experiments. *Biometrics* 1954;**3**:101–29.
24 Glass GV. Primary, secondary, and meta-analysis of research. *Educat Res* 1976;**5**:3–8.
25 Jackson GB. Methods for integrative reviews. *Rev Educat Res* 1980;**50**:438–60.
26 Light RJ, Pillemer DB. *Summing up: the science of reviewing research*. Cambridge: Harvard University Press, 1984.
27 Clarke M, Olsen KL, Oxman AD, eds. Cochrane Review Methodology Database. In: *The Cochrane Library*, Issue 3. Oxford: Update Software, 1999.
28 Kunz R, Oxman AD. The unpredictability paradox: review of empirical comparisons of randomised and non-randomised clinical trials. *BMJ*. 1998;**317**:1185–90.
29 Canadian Task Force on the Periodic Health Examination. *Can Med Assoc J* 1979;**121**:1193–254.
30 US Preventive Services Task Force. *Guide to clinical preventive services*, 2nd edn. Baltimore: Williams & Wilkins, 1996:xxxix–lv.

31 Guyatt GH, Sackett DL, Sinclair JC, Hayward RC, Cook DJ, Cook RJ, for the Evidence-Based Medicine Working Group. Users guides to the medical literature. IX. A method for grading health care recommendations. *JAMA* 1995;**274**:1800–4.

32 Eccles M, Clapp Z, Grimshaw J, *et al*. North of England evidence based guidelines development project: methods of guideline development. *BMJ*. 1996;**312**: 760–2.

33 Levels of Evidence and Grades of Recommendations. Centre for Evidence-Based Medicine. http://cebm.jr2.ox.ac.uk/docs/levels.html. Accessed 21 November 2000.

Index

Page numbers in **bold** type refer to figures; those in *italic* refer to tables or boxed material.